FUNDAMENTALS OF WOUND MANAGEMENT

FUNDAMENTALS OF WOUND MANAGEMENT

edited by

Thomas K. Hunt
M.D., F.A.C.S.

Professor of Surgery
University of California
San Francisco
School of Medicine

J. Englebert Dunphy
M.D., F.A.C.S.

Professor and Chairman,
Emeritus, Department of Surgery
University of California
San Francisco
School of Medicine

Appleton-Century-Crofts/New York

This book is dedicated to our many friends, colleagues, and forebearers who made it possible through their research and wisdom. We cannot recognize them enough.

79 80 81 82 83 / 10 9 8 7 6 5 4 3 2 1

Prentice-Hall International, Inc., London
Prentice-Hall of Australia, Pty. Ltd., Sydney
Prentice-Hall of India Private Limited, New Delhi
Prentice-Hall of Japan, Inc., Tokyo
Prentice-Hall of Southeast Asia (Pte.) Ltd., Singapore
Whitehall Books Ltd., Wellington, New Zealand

Library of Congress Cataloging in Publication Data
Main entry under title:

Fundamentals of wound management.

  Bibliography: p.
  Includes index.
  1. Wounds.   I. Hunt, Thomas K.   II. Dunphy,
John Englebert, 1908–
RD93.F86   617'.1   79–1266
ISBN 0-8385-2837-6

Text design: James M. Wall
Cover design: Susan F. Rich

PRINTED IN THE UNITED STATES OF AMERICA

CONTRIBUTORS

John F. Burke, M.D.
Helen Andrus Benedict, Professor of Surgery, Harvard Medical School, Boston, Massachusetts

Clifford W. Deveney, M.D.
Assistant Professor of Surgery, University of California, San Francisco, School of Medicine

J. Englebert Dunphy, M.D., F.A.C.S.
Professor and Chairman, Emeritus, Department of Surgery, University of California, San Francisco, School of Medicine

Milton Edgerton, M.D.
Professor and Chairman, Department of Plastic Surgery, University of Virginia School of Medicine, Charlottesville

Richard F. Edlich, M.D., Ph.D.
Professor of Plastic Surgery, University of Virginia School of Medicine, Charlottesville

R. Bruce Heppenstall, M.D., F.A.C.S.
Associate Professor of Orthopedic Surgery, The University of Pennsylvania School of Medicine, Philadelphia

Thomas K. Hunt, M.D., F.A.C.S.
Professor of Surgery, University of California, San Francisco, School of Medicine

Lynn D. Ketchum, M.D., F.A.C.S.
Director, Hand Rehabilitation Center, University of Kansas Medical Center, Kansas City

Stanley M. Levenson, M.D.
Professor of Surgery, Albert Einstein College of Medicine of Yeshiva University, New York, New York

James M. Malone, M.D.
Assistant Professor of Surgery, University of Arizona Center for the Health Sciences, Tucson

Jonathan L. Meakins, M.D., D.Sc.
Assistant Professor of Surgery and Microbiology, McGill University Faculty of Medicine, Montreal, Quebec, Canada

Wesley S. Moore, M.D.
Professor and Chairman, Section of Vascular Surgery, University of Arizona Center for the Health Sciences, Tucson

George T. Rodeheaver, Ph.D.
Assistant Professor, Department of Plastic Surgery, University of Virginia School of Medicine, Charlottesville

Eli Seifter, Ph.D.
Associate Professor of Biochemistry and Surgery, Albert Einstein College of Medicine of Yeshiva University, New York, New York

John G. Thacker, Ph.D.
Assistant Professor, Department of Mechanical Engineering, University of Virginia, Charlottesville

Walton Van Winkle, Jr., M.D.
Professor of Surgical Biology, Emeritus, University of Arizona College of Medicine, Tucson

Donald E. Willard, M.D.
Associate Professor, Department of Ophthalmology, Temple University School of Medicine, Philadelphia, Pennsylvania

Richard E. Wilson, M.D.
Professor of Surgery, Harvard Medical School, Boston, Massachusetts

Contents

7

Preface

This book is an outgrowth of a series of monographs on the fundamentals of wound management, produced by Chirurgecom, Inc., and distributed to residents and physicians by Smith, Kline, and French Laboratories. The enthusiastic reception given to the original papers has prompted the publication of this updated and consolidated volume.

The editors acknowledge the enthusiastic cooperation and participation of Mr. Walter Herz, President of Chirurgecom, in all aspects of the original monographs as well as this volume.

We deeply appreciate the authoritative, up-to-date contributions of each of the distinguished contributors, all of whom are outstanding authorities in the broad field of wound healing and regret that in a publication of this type it has not been possible to give adequate and specific credit to the many surgeons and basic scientists who have made important and original contributions to this field.

This publication is intended to be a broadly informative and useful reference for practicing surgeons in all of the surgical specialties as well as a vademecum for investigators, new and old, in the fascinating realm of injury, repair, and regeneration.

Finally, we are indebted to our publishers, Appleton-Century-Crofts, for their advice and help.

FUNDAMENTALS OF WOUND MANAGEMENT

1

NORMAL REPAIR
Thomas K. Hunt
Walton Van Winkle, Jr.

CONCEPTS OF REPAIR AND REGENERATION

Regeneration and repair are fundamental facts of life and occur in literally all organisms. Unicellular organisms repair themselves essentially by regenerating portions of lost or damaged cellular structure. The process of regeneration becomes more complex as the organism becomes more complex, and regeneration of whole limbs is common in some species. However, as complexity increases, tissue injury is more and more frequently healed through the reconstruction of connective tissue, its vasculature, and covering epithelium, the process known as "wound healing" or "repair." While amphibia are the most advanced animals in which regeneration of a lost extremity, for instance, can occur, limited regeneration of epithelium and endothelium and partial regeneration of liver are still seen in the human.

Regeneration of connective tissue, i.e., repair, has its own value, however, and is not just a remnant of regeneration. Some form of "glue" to connect cells has been found in literally all multicellular animal organisms studied and remarkably few substances act as this intercellular cement. Vertebrate connective substance is always collagen and proteoglycans (i.e., mucopolysaccharide), and in invertebrates it is chitin and proteoglycans. Reformation of connective substances is a prime concern to multicellular organisms which depend on differentiation, specialization, and interconnection of function among cells. Renewed synthesis and deposition of connective substances is the natural reaction to forceful separation of cells whose functions depend on close interconnections. Thus, the basic mechanisms for connective tissue regeneration are found in the cells of the most primitive animals.

Repair is a normal reaction to injury and is often essential to prolonged life in a hostile environment. It is the keystone on which surgery is founded. Despite the lessons of surgical history, it seems that most surgeons still, as they always have, regard repair as an inevitability, a process that will or will not occur, and, having occurred, will be "normal," i.e., a single immutable sequence. However, a glance at history reveals that the most fundamental advances in surgery have coincided with sudden new insights into the reparative mechanism. Witness the struggles of such surgeons as de Chauliac, Paré, and Lister to separate the fact of sepsis from surgeons' concepts of normal repair. Though it had been recognized periodically for centuries that reunion of two cut edges of tissue could occur without evidence of infection or excessive inflammation, such an event was so unpredictable that surgeons adopted the idea that local infection and extreme scarring were a part of normal healing. In that concept of repair "laudable pus" was a sign that eventual repair might be expected. We now know that pus was merely an expression that a potentially invasive infection had probably been contained.

When cleanliness had become an ideal, and the microbial theory had become a fact, the stage was set for prophets such as Semmelweis, Lister, and others to advance a concept so important that it literally made modern surgery possible. They realized that sepsis and repair were separate phenomena. They learned to expect repair without sepsis. Yet, ironically, only 100 years ago, Lister was ostracized for exhorting his fellow surgeons to accept this unorthodox concept which so expanded the profession. One wonders how much "inertia" remains in the practice of surgery, since there can be no doubt that the surgeon's concept of repair and its capacities still often governs his judgment, technique, and expectations.

Refinements in aseptic technique, the introduction of antibiotics, and improvements in surgical technique now make primary repair the rule rather than the exception. Today, Lister's argument would seem to have been won—but has it? In fact, we differ only in degree with the disapproving surgeons of Lister's early days. Sepsis and delayed union are no longer considered inevitable; they are only considered inevitable some of the time.

Furthermore, as a profession, surgeons have not yet grappled fully with the concept of scarring. Just as early surgeons "expected" infection, surgeons today "expect" scar. Some scar seems to be a biologic necessity, but can excessive scarring be divorced from the concept of repair? May it become possible to control keloid, hypertrophic scar, arthritic scarring, and other related manifestations? History and science suggest that it may be possible. Plastic surgeons, of course, accept the argument as a technical challenge. Is it not possible to accept it biologically and pharmacologically?

It probably is not possible today, as it was 100 years ago, for one discovery such as aseptic technique to initiate such a magnificent change in medical practice. The times are too sophisticated for that. It is in anticipation of important "smaller" advances, as well as in recognition of very real advances that are already made, but unused, that this book is written. Repair is not simply the surgeon's ally; repair is his lifeline. Unless the surgeon arranges his priorities to aid the forces of repair, to mobilize resistance to infection, and to control excessive scarring, he will be little more than a surgeon of the last century who, somehow, found a modern operating room. The knowledge to use, foster, and perhaps even control, many of the forces of repair is now within the grasp of every surgeon; it is his to use, if he is willing.

The setting for optimal repair is a healthy organism with a healthy vascular system. Maintaining or establishing that setting will be covered in later phases of this book. In this first chapter, it is assumed that the basic health of the patient is assured. Therefore, the surgeon's concern with repair begins at the moment of injury.

THE INJURY AND THE RESPONSE

At the instant of injury, a complex series of events occurs that, in the healthy individual, inevitably proceed to repair and ultimately to scar formation. At that instant, the wound begins its short life as an organ dedicated to obviating the need for its own existence. The major mysteries of repair have always been, and continue to be: *what* in the injury stimulates repair, and *how* does the wound recognize that it is no longer needed, that is, *why* does healing stop?

When tissue is disrupted, vessels are injured, cells are broken, and platelets and collagen intermingle and interact. The complement cascade is initiated, and the local microvasculature soon shows that the injury has been sensed. Injured vessels thrombose. Nearby vessels, especially the venules, soon dilate. Platelets and white cells begin to stick to the endothelial lining, and the leukocytes migrate between the endothelial cells and into the area of injury. Within a few hours, the edge of the injured area is infiltrated with granulocytes and macrophages. In the case of connective tissue and bone injury, the tissue is now overladen with highly metabolic white cells that will soon be replaced by rapidly metabolizing fibroblasts—all this in an area of damaged vasculature. Thus, at the very time that connective tissue and bone have their greatest metabolic need, their local circulation is least able to supply it. A local "energy crisis" is inevitable.

Within a few days, fibroblasts become visible. In most injuries, fibroblasts seem to stream from the perivascular connective tissue cells. In the cornea of the eye, they seem to spring from keratocytes or fibrocytes. In the wall of the artery or vein, they seem to spring from smooth muscle cells. These fibroblasts gradually replace the majority of white cells, and, as they do, the momentum of collagen synthesis increases. If a wound is primarily closed, it begins to gain strength through collagenous links by about the third postinjury day.

Neovascularization is a constant feature of repair, at least partly because the needs of inflammation and repair overwhelm the injured nutritional supply. By the third or fourth day, beginnings of a new circulation can be seen bridging the wound space of a primarily closed wound; and in open wounds, a roseate hue can be seen where the first new vessels are appearing.

This morphologic sequence can be translated into more chemical terms. At the moment of injury, vessels and cells are injured. Within a few moments, blood coagulation is activated and platelets have bound to the exposed collagen and have released their phospholipids stimulating the intrinsic coagulation mechanism. Injured cells have released thromboplastin that activates the extrinsic coagulation mechanism. The end result is a blood clot. At the same time, the aggregating platelets, and perhaps white cells, release proteolytic enzymes that initiate the cascade of proteolytic enzymes in the complement system. As this enzymatic cascade rapidly amplifies the distress signals of injured tissue, chemotactic substances accumulate and call forth the inflammatory cells that are first seen sticking to the sensitized endothelial membranes of local vessels. The cells follow the chemical signals to the area of injury and bind their membranes to injured tissue (i.e., spent platelets, inactivated blood cells, and blood and tissue macromolecules). The phagocytic cells ingest these altered substances as if to "lick the wound."

The chemical signals that call forth the sudden burst of fibroblast replication near the area of injury are only just becoming known. The evidence suggests that platelets and phagocytic macrophages release a substance or substances that can stimulate replication of fibroblasts. Both seem to do so with the aid of the coagulation system since thrombin activates the platelet factor and plasminogen activator seems to potentiate macrophage factor(s). No matter what the signal, the evidence is clear that the vast majority of the total fibroblast population originates in the wound itself, probably stemming mainly from cells located in or around local small vessels.

Fibroblasts in cell culture do not necessarily make collagen. It seems necessary to stimulate them to do so. The most prominent stimulators of collagen synthesis in cultured fibroblasts are ascorbic acid and lactate ion, which "activate" enzymes necessary for collagen synthesis. Ascorbic acid remains in its reduced (active) form only in hypoxic conditions and lactate obviously accumulates most rapidly in the same environment. The hypoxia and the concentrations of ascorbate and lactate necessary to stimulate collagen synthesis in cultured cells are actually present in wounded tissue. As the numerous cells that are called into the wound reach the environment of damaged vasculature and limited oxygen supply, anaerobic metabolism inevitably results. The extracellular P_{O_2} in this area falls well below 10 torr, a point probably below the *critical* or lowest optimum P_{O_2} for aerobic metabolism in both fibroblasts and leukocytes. Possibly for this reason, fibroblasts and new epithelial cells start their lives with a prominent capacity for anaerobic metabolism. Furthermore, leukocytes and macrophages, when "activated" by the ingestion of altered substances or a foreign body, have a prodigious capacity for lactate production no matter what their environment. Within a few days, lactate in the extracellular fluid of the central dead space of wounds is in the region of 10 to 15 mM, which is quite sufficient, in the test tube, to stimulate fibroblasts to produce collagen.

THE WOUND MODULE

By about the third day after injury, the wound cells form a rather vague "module of repair." In the van of the advancing wound edge is the macrophage. Wound macrophages seem to be chronically "activated" and are usually found with ingested substances in their digestive vacuoles. Granulocytes on the surface seem to combine with macrophages in the defense against bacteria. Just behind these cells are some maturing but still youthful fibroblasts, apparently the product of nearby cells that are actively dividing. Fibroblasts in mitosis are found most frequently between the most distal functioning capillary and the first maturing fibroblast of the wound edge. The most distal functioning blood vessel is about 50 to 75 μ from the wound edge, and it is sprouting new capillary buds which are destined to complete an arcuate path through the injured or healing tissue, either 1) to unite with a vessel from the other side in primary repair,* 2) to unite with a cut vessel end in a skin graft, or 3) to join another similar bud from a lower or higher pressure point in the granulation tissue of an open or dead space wound.† The new and tender microcirculatory loops find external support in a collagen gel secreted by the immature fibroblasts and in a fine network of collagen that the endothelial cell probably secretes itself. Without such support they would inevitably rupture as soon as they were exposed to the pressure of the arterial system. As each new capillary loop becomes functional, more oxygen becomes available to nearby cells. The fibroblasts can then synthesize more collagen and can migrate further until they again run out of oxygen. The macrophage can advance on the support given by the fibroblast. The process continues in a cyclic fashion. As the "module" proceeds, the collagen-synthesizing fibroblasts are left behind to continue their work of constructing and reconstructing the new connective tissue.

The "wound module" then can be defined as a loose knit but exquisite ecologic cooperative made up of new blood vessels, macrophages, granulocytes, and fibroblasts.

The concept of the advancing "module" implies that there are metabolic gradients in the wound that probably govern its

---

*"Primary" repair is the term used to describe a sharply made wound that is accurately reapproximated within hours of the incision and heals with minimal space between its edges. It is sometimes called "repair by primary intention."

†Healing of a dead space or open wound is said to occur by secondary intention. It involves filling of a tissue defect through formation of large amounts of new connective tissue, new vessels, and epithelium in many cases. The term usually implies an external, open wound, but the repair involved is much the same as in healing a closed space such as a pneumonectomy space, or a serum collection as often occurs after mastectomy. The new tissue which fills the space is frequently called "granulation tissue" (Fig. 1.1).

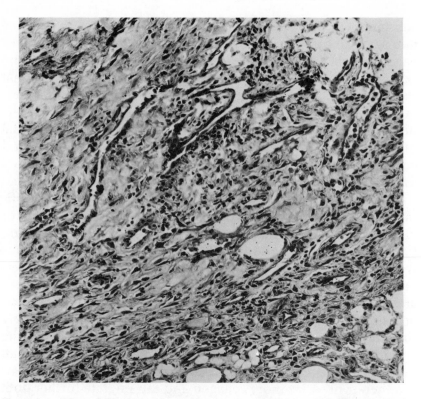

Figure 1.1 "Granulation tissue" from a dead space wound in a rabbit. The wound edge is in the upper right corner. All this tissue has grown into a wire mesh cylinder. Therefore, it is all new. Small vessels can be seen emptying into the dead space. Macrophages can be seen on the surface, with fibroblasts on the surface and just below. A little remodeling can be seen with fat cells and looser collagen weave in the lower right corner.

form and motion. One would expect that if the above description is accurate, there would be a very low oxygen tension at the surface of the macrophage in the wound module. In fact, this is true. Measurements of oxygen gradients show that the P_{O_2}, which is in the region of 50 torr over the arteriolar portion of the capillary, falls to near zero torr at the surface of the macrophages and in the dead space. The lactate, the pH, and P_{CO_2} gradients are in the other direction; that is, high in the dead space and lower near the functioning vessels (see Fig. 1.18).

Thus the elements that are mobilized to form the module of repair are many. It is probably impossible to achieve anything but simple collagenous gluing of cells in fibroblast culture, where there is little to perform the functions of the blood-vascular circulation, liver, heart, lungs, and many aspects of the metabolic response to injury. The cells that are prominent in the local area of the injury are macrophages, lymphocytes, polymorphonuclear granulocytes, fibroblasts, and vascular endothelial cells. The milieu of these cells is a composite of the effects of their own metabolism and the delivery and removal of various substances by the vascular system. The physical support for all these cells is provided by the local synthesis and deposition of collagen and its accompanying proteoglycans.

Leukocytes—The Macrophage

In the first few days after injury, the polymorphonuclear leukocyte predominates. However, by about the fifth day, macrophages predominate and they remain until the reparative sequence is done. Thus, the macrophage seems to retain one or more roles throughout the life of the wound.

Primary repair occurs uninhibited even by major reductions in the numbers of circulating and tissue polymorphs and lymphocytes in the system. Their role is to inhibit and kill contaminating bacteria. However, when the macrophage is eliminated from the healing wound, even primary repair suffers.

Fibroblasts are rarely far from macrophages. Macrophages are wandering mononuclear cells found in tissues and tissue spaces. The tissue monocyte, the pulmonary macrophage, the peritoneal macrophage, the Kupffer cell, and other members of the reticuloendothelial system all fit the single classification of "macrophages." They are large, mobile, and well fitted for metabolism in any environment. They can live in the most or least nourished of tissues. They are actively phagocytic and can kill organisms in a manner apparently similar to polymorphs. They can ingest macromolecules and excrete the products of digestion into the surrounding environment. Recent laboratory research suggests that local macrophages can play a nutritional role by acting as "the digestive tract of the wound."

Probably most important, however, is that macrophages seem to act as director cells, to release chemotactic substances in order to bring in other macrophages, to release stimulatory substances in order to cause multiplication of fibroblasts, and to release substances which ultimately stimulate neovascularization. For instance, when wound macrophages are placed in the cornea of the eye, nearby keratocytes are stimulated to form fibroblasts that are stimulated, in turn, to make collagen. New blood vessels sprout from the limbus to tunnel through the peripheral cornea as if to supply a healing wound. The mere injection of an equal amount of fluid used to suspend the macrophages produces only a transient edema without fibroblast replication, collagen synthesis, and neovascularization. If these macrophages are mixed with an activator such as latex granules, even more vessels form and more fibroblasts appear. These experiments are confirmed by cell culture studies in which products of macrophages stimulate multiplication of fibroblasts, smooth muscle cells, and vascular endothelial cells. This action is potentiated by thrombin and plasminogen activator, both found in high concentration in serum. If activated macrophages are mixed with activator and then disintegrated by exposure to ultrasound, "wound healing" occurs. However, on microscopic sectioning, one finds not only debris of broken macrophages, but viable macrophages and polymorphs as well, both obviously attracted by the macrophagic debris. If polymorphs or lymphocytes are injected instead of macrophages, almost no reaction occurs.

If macrophages are eliminated from a newly made incised wound in tissue by the use of antimacrophage serum, repair is clearly inhibited. Injured cells and tissue are not debrided. Development of wound strength (i.e., collagen synthesis) is poor. Thus, the case is strong that the macrophage is the key cell of the inflammatory response to injury. It (1) debrides injured tissue, (2) processes macromolecules to useful amino acids and sugars, (3) attracts more macrophages, (4) probably signals for fibroblast formation and activation, (5) may signal for neovascularization, and (6) secretes lactate that in turn stimulates collagen synthesis by fibroblasts.

In some unknown manner, vitamin A aids the entrance of macrophages into the wound. This important vitamin is vital to the initiation of repair. If macrophage entry is prevented by antiinflammatory steroids, repair can usually be stimulated by giving vitamin A. In this case, the vitamin A administration is followed by increased leukocyte and macrophage entry into the wound. This is an important effect that will be explained further in the next chapter.

Vascular Endothelium

One of the most important and least appreciated aspects of repair is the regeneration of new blood vessels. Neovascularization is seen in injuries, infarcts, areas of inflammation (especially those attended by certain types of macrophagic inflammation), and is prominent in tumor growth. The function of neovascularization, or angiogenesis, in wounds is to nourish tissue that obviously cannot be well nourished unless new vessels can replace and supplement the old, injured system. Present concepts rest on two major facts: 1) new vessels always originate from existing vessels, and 2) whatever their ultimate size or function becomes, all new vessels begin as capillary buds (Fig. 1.2; see also Figs. 1.1, 1.19–1.22).

In general, angiogenesis takes three forms. The first is the generation of a whole new vascular network where a large tissue defect has to be filled. The second is the joining with an unused circulation as when the host bed provides circulation to a skin graft. The third is the joining or rejoining of vessels across a primarily healing wound.

It seems most instructive to consider the generation of a whole new vascular network first. The clinical circumstance in which it is found is healing of a dead space in tissue, e.g., a severe fracture. First, the injured vessels thrombose. The wound module is assembled, and from the functioning vessels nearest the wound, sprouts of vascular cells appear from the bases of the existing endothelial cells. (Capillary sprouts are pictured in Figure 1.2.) These new vessels somehow join with similar sprouts from other venular or arteriolar branches to form a functioning capillary loop. Later on, this loop will either participate in formation of a larger vessel or will stop functioning and disappear. Blood clot, contrary to popular belief, does not aid neovascularization.

The basement membrane is incomplete in the newest vessels. Therefore, for a while after cannulation has occurred, the new endothelial cells fit loosely and the vessels are fragile and "leaky." Large particles in blood leak between the cell junctions and are engulfed by local phagocytic cells, perhaps "activating"

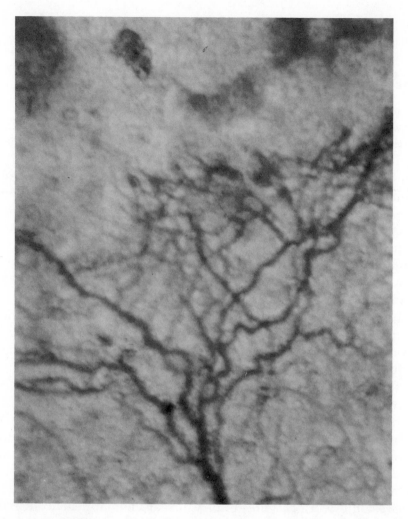

Figure 1.2 Photomicrograph of the advancing arterial circulation in a healing dead space wound. All of these vessels are new. The whole pictured field is from the center of what was once a dead space in tissue. In the upper portion, one can see a number of small vessels that are buds growing out from the established circulation. Below this one can see how the buds have joined to form capillary loops. Magnification × 325. *(Slide courtesy of Ian Silver, Professor of Comparative Pathology, Department of Pathology, University of Bristol, England.)*

them. For instance, colloidal carbon penetrates between cells and is found in macrophages. Some vascular sprouts appear to have no lumen. Others appear to be open-ended tubes through which red cells may escape. This last type would seem to predominate in primary repair or revascularization of a skin graft (see Fig. 1.1, upper right).

An explanation for the stimulation of new vessel formation has not been completely formulated. The molecular signals emanate from macrophages and platelets. One can only speculate that, somehow, hypoxia also plays a role. When platelets and thrombin are injected into the rabbit cornea, new vessels appear. Exactly how the stem vessels become larger and larger as more tissue is supplied is a totally unsolved mystery.

The surgeon has a unique chance to observe one form of neovascularization in skin graft repair. The skin graft is applied essentially bloodless and cadaveric, in the white-skinned patient. Within two days, the graft appears purple. One might simply attribute this to blood between the graft and the recipient bed were it not that microscopic sections show blood cells in the vessels of the graft. Within a few days, small areas of the "purple" graft become pink and blanch somewhat on direct pressure. These areas of reestablished circulation enlarge and coalesce. Experimental studies leave no doubt that the "old" vessels first passively fill with red cells and then establish a functioning circulation.

In primary repair, reestablished circulation bridging the wound can be noted by the second or third day. The manner in which reconstruction of somewhat larger vessels occurs is not understood. It seems likely, however, that thrombosed vessels may be reopened by the thrombolytic mechanism. Most vessel endothelia contain fibrinolysin. This may open "holes" in the fibrin that initially "glues" the wound edges together. Pathways for blood cells may thereafter form, just as oft-walked paths in a field become worn by constant use. Such a path would be an ideal guide for regenerating endothelial cells. One can now understand why immobilization is so helpful to skin graft "takes."

Vascular regeneration is, as one might expect, a delicate process. Histamine depletion and numerous cytoplasmic poisons used in chemotherapy can stop it. It is poor in tissue showing chronic changes of radiation exposure. Clinically, however, we find that the placement of an autograft or heterograft on viable but wounded and radiation-damaged tissue, followed by administration of oxygen to maintain the arterial Po_2 in the region of 200, is followed by obvious evidence of neovascularization hitherto unseen in these chronically scarred and wounded tissues.

Vascular regeneration is also poor in steroid-treated patients. Once again, vitamin A seems to restimulate the process, further indication that monocytes have a role in neovascularization. The process is also inhibited in ischemic tissue. Needless to say, as neovascularization goes, so goes the wound.

Lymphatics also regenerate—smaller ones by new vessel formation, as with blood vessels in granulation tissue; while it appears that some larger channels, as in skin grafts, may reconnect. If lymphatic recanalization or regeneration does not occur, an edematous, easily infected wound results. Very little is known about the details of lymphatic growth and regeneration in wounds.

The Fibroblast

The fibroblast synthesizes and deposits collagen and proteoglycans. There has been controversy in determining the origin of fibroblasts. The basic reason for the controversy has been that the fibroblast, as seen in the actively healing wound, is not seen in normal tissue although one can find spindly cells with nuclei rather like fibroblasts in the cornea (the keratocyte) and in the adventitia of local arteries and veins. Since fibroblasts are rare in uninjured tissue, they were once thought to be derived from blood spilled into the injury. However, extremely sophisticated experiments with symbiotic animals and with radiation inhibition of cells in wounded tissue give the answer that all, or almost all, fibroblasts found in the wound originate in the injured tissue. Most fibroblasts appear to arise from perivascular cells. Whatever the signal, the response is extraordinary, especially in connective tissue where a relatively acellular tissue converts to one which is almost all cells within a few days. This response has caused a number of observers to remark on the similarity to malignancy. In fact, a favorite pathologist's trick is to fool the neophyte into diagnosing a fracture callus as an osteogenic sarcoma. Some have even postulated that if we could find the reason why wounds stop healing, we might find a means of changing malignancies into more orderly and cooperative tissues. This seems unduly optimistic, but the wound seems an ideal place to study the effects of the environment (as modified by the cell's own metabolism) on the form and function of the metabolizing cell. The local feedback loop of a cell releasing a metabolite that leads to a change in the cell probably is an important biologic mechanism.

The mature fibroblast is pictured in Figures 1.3 to 1.5 and diagramed in Figures 1.6 and 1.7. It is richly endowed with endoplasmic reticulum, Golgi apparatus, and mitochondria, as are other protein-synthesizing cells. It is mobile, and migrates in tissue culture. Its mobility is subject to contact inhibition, leading some to say that the contact of fibroblasts on one side of a wound with the fibroblasts on the other side is the signal that turns off repair. Unfortunately, this concept does not withstand even the initial examination since the object of repair is not edge-to-edge fibroblasts. It is edge-to-edge connective tissue. Density inhibition may serve as a means of limiting the wound population during the most intense phases of fibroplasia, but any role it has in limiting the totality of repair must be small.

The fibroblast is a hardy cell. It can survive the most hostile environments. Unfortunately, however, it cannot function outside a rather specific environment. It favors a solid surface on which to attach and migrate. It will stick to glass or many types of plastic. In wounds it seems to adhere to fibrin and collagen. It makes collagen best in a slightly acidic environment with an oxygen tension more than about 10 to 20 torr, but below that of room air. It needs a reducing environment, usually rich in ascorbate, to produce collagen, and as outlined above, it makes more collagen if there is a high concentration of lactate.

The immature fibroblast is rounded, while the mature one is elongated with long cell processes that aid its mobility. These processes can even guide a fibroblast over or under a nearby fibroblast. Some fibroblasts have a rich supply of myofibrils and appear to be a hybrid "myofibroblast," (Fig. 1.5). This cell will contract and relax in response to the usual stimuli. Such cells are found in contracting wounds where they seem to supply at least part of the contractile force. They are also seen in large arteries where they participate in the process of arteriosclerosis. The tiresome argument about whether cells in atheromata are fibroblasts or smooth muscle cells is over: they are both.

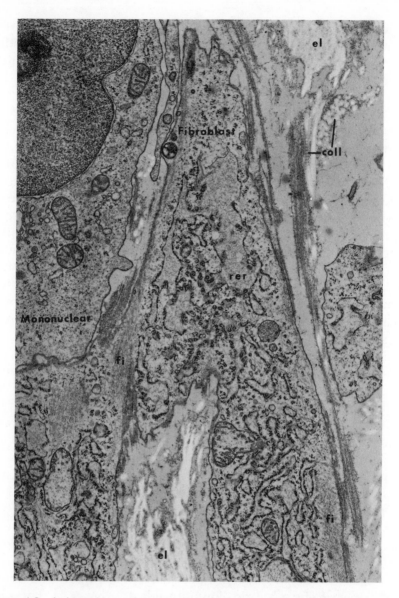

Figure 1.3   A photomicrograph showing the often intimate relationship of fibroblasts and mononuclear cells. The mononuclear cell has less endoplasmic reticulum, has free cytoplasmic ribosomes and regular cristae in the mitochondria. Note the fine myofilaments in the periphery of the fibroblast. Magnification × 17,000. *(Courtesy of Russell Ross, Ph.D., University of Washington Medical School, Seattle, Washington.)*

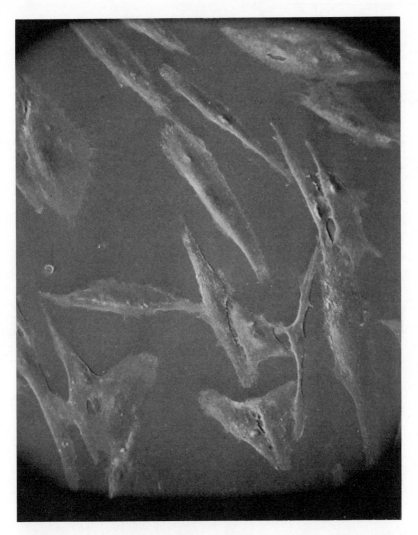

Figure 1.4 Scanning electron micrograph of fibroblasts in culture. Note the long foot processes and the flat cell shape.

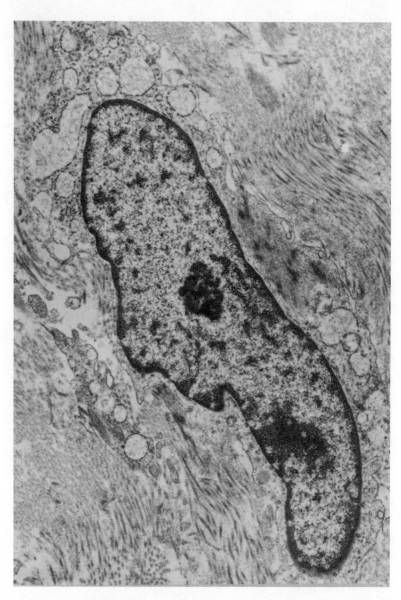

Figure 1.5 Transmission electron microscopy of a myofibroblast. Note the prominent microfilaments in the periphery of the cell just above the nucleolus.

In view of modern genetic theory, it seems possible that almost any mesenchymal cell could become a fibroblast. Almost every animal organism ever analyzed has contained collagen-proteoglycans or chitin-proteoglycans. The genetic code for collagen synthesis would seem to be present in all vertebrate cells. In fact, even some epithelial and endothelial cells have been induced to produce collagen.

The fibroblast has a full complement of metabolic pathways. It synthesizes collagen, of course, but also synthesizes proteoglycans and elastin. It can also synthesize cholesterol and has a full range of enzymes for the Krebs cycle, as well as the glycolytic pathways, and so on. Thus, its requirements probably include most of the B vitamins as well as ascorbate, oxygen, amino acids, and trace metals such as zinc, iron, and copper. Metabolic needs are met by circulating sugars, fats, amino acids, oxygen, ascorbate, and other nutrients. One function of the macrophage is to break down local large molecules into reusable amino acids for fibroblast use. Last, the fibroblast itself is pinocytic and may supply some of its glucose and amino acid requirements through hydrolysis of more complex molecules.

COLLAGEN

Collagen is the principal structural protein of the body and is the major constituent of skin, tendons, ligaments, bones, cartilage, fascia, and the septa of various organs. Of more importance at the moment, it is the principal component of scar tissue. It has many chemical and structural properties to distinguish it clearly from other proteins.

When we use the word *collagen* we now mean not a single substance, but a group of glycoproteins that have the following attributes in common:

1. They are composed of three separate linear peptide chains of approximately equal length, each containing about 1000 amino acids. These are alpha chains. Each chain is made up of one-third glycine, one-third proline and hydroxyproline, and one-third other amino acids. Glycine occurs in every third position making a repeating structure of glycine-X-Y. X and Y may be any amino acid, but hydroxyproline or hydroxylysine is usually found in the Y position.

2. Each alpha chain is twisted into a right-handed helix, three of which lie parallel to each other and the entire structure is then twisted into a left-handed "superhelix." This compound helical formation is unique to collagen and accounts for its rigidity despite its enormous length of 3000 A and width of only 15 A—a length-to-width ratio of 200 to 1.

Hydroxyproline and hydroxylysine are almost unique to collagen. (They occur to a small extent in complement.) The analysis of hydroxyproline has been a precise means of measurement of collagen content.

Table 1.1 Structurally and Genetically Distinct Collagens

Type	Tissue Distribution	Molecular Form	Characteristics
I	Bone, tendon, skin, dentin, ligament, fascia, arteries, and uterus	$[\alpha1(I)]_2\alpha2$	Most prevalent form of collagen in the mature vertebrate organism; composed of two chain types; low content of hydroxylysine and glycosylated hydroxylysine
II	Hyaline cartilages	$[\alpha1(II)]_3$	Relatively high content of hydroxylysine and glycosylated hydroxylysine
III	Skin, arteries, and uterus	$[\alpha1(III)]_3$	High content of hydroxyproline; contains interchain disulfide bonds
IV	Basement membranes	$[\alpha1(IV)]_3$	High content of hydroxylysine and glycosylated hydroxylysine; contains interchain disulfide bonds and may contain large globular regions

Four distinct types of collagen with the above attributes are now recognized (Table 1.1). Type I collagen, found in adult dermis, fascia, bone, and so on, is the most common. Two of its three α chains, termed α-1 chains, are identical. The third, termed α-2, is similar but not identical to the α-1 chains. Type II collagen is found only in cartilage and has three identical α-1 chains that differ slightly in amino acid sequence from the α-1 chains of Type I collagen. Type III collagen is found principally in embryonic connective tissue, but is present in small amounts in some adult tissue such as wounds, dermis, and aorta. It also contains three identical chains that differ somewhat from the chains of types I and II collagen. A type IV collagen has been identified in certain basement membranes.

Some type III collagen is laid down initially in dermal wounds but as the wound matures it is replaced by type I collagen. This is the first hint of an important concept in which we see that collagen composition in wounds changes as time passes. In other words, the collagen that is initially deposited may be removed and replaced during maturation of the wound. This may be particularly important in bone where fracture callus changes from fibrous to cartilagenous to bony tissue. This suggests that types I and III collagen may give way to type II collagen that is then replaced by type I collagen. Several turnovers of collagen occur before bone can be fully healed. Since type III collagen is the "embryonic" form, there seems to be a reversion to more primitive mechanisms in early repair.

Collagen Synthesis (Figs. 1.6–1.9). Collagen is synthesized much the same as any other protein. However, there are a few unique steps that make a knowledge of collagen synthesis of great interest to the surgeon and of great potential value in the treatment of healing tissue (see Figs. 1.6, 1.7).

When collagen synthesis is stimulated, the nuclear DNA forms the messenger RNA (transcription). The messenger RNA travels into the cytoplasm to control the makeup of the ribosomal network. Transfer RNA brings specific amino acids to the growing polypeptide chains while they are still attached to the ribosomes (see Figs. 1.6, 1.7). No transfer RNA for hydroxyproline or hydroxylysine exists, and these two amino acids cannot be directly incorporated into collagen. Instead, proline and lysine are included in the growing chain, and while the chain is still on the ribosome, significant numbers of each of these amino acids are hydroxylated through the action of specific enzymes, prolyl hydroxylase or lysyl hydroxylase, with the other substrate being molecular or dissolved oxygen. The cofactors are ferrous iron, alpha ketoglutarate (a constituent of the Krebs cycle), and a reducing agent such as ascorbic acid or light-activated riboflavin, but the rapid collagen synthesis of repair seems to proceed at best speed only with vitamin C. In the absence of vitamin C, prolyl and lysyl hydroxylase, which

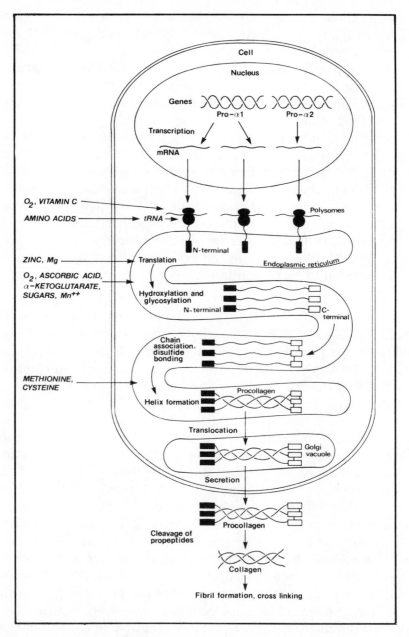

Figure 1.6 Diagrammatic representation of steps in collagen synthesis from translation to secretion. Note the cleavage of the registration peptide (the rectangles at the ends of the molecule) that occurs in the extracellular space before final polymerization. Important nutrients at certain steps are noted on the left.

24

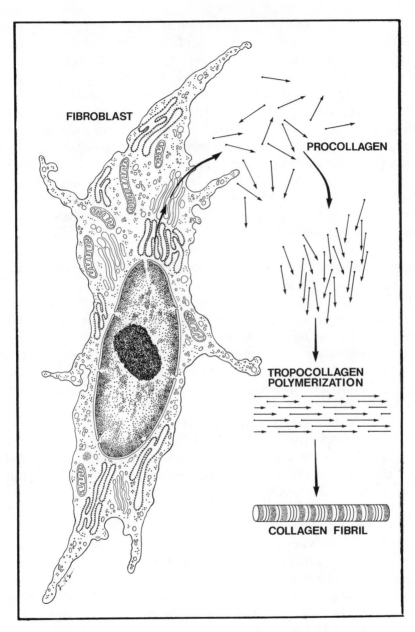

FIBROBLAST

PROCOLLAGEN

TROPOCOLLAGEN POLYMERIZATION

COLLAGEN FIBRIL

Figure 1.7 Representation of collagen synthesis from the ribosome to the Golgi and to the extracellular space. After collagen is excreted, the registration peptides (see Fig. 1.6) are cleaved and polymerization is begun.

exist in an inactive monomeric state, will not aggregate into the active enzyme, and oxygen will not be transferred to proline or lysine. Somehow, through an unknown mechanism, lactate participates in the activation (but not de novo synthesis) of these enzymes; and as noted above, the synthesis of collagen and the activity of prolyl hydroxylase are very much increased in the presence of lactate. Without ascorbate, underhydroxylated collagen is produced and little of this substance escapes from the cell. That which does escape fails to form characteristic collagen fibers. The condition we recognize as scurvy develops, wounds fail to heal, capillaries become fragile because of failure of basement membrane formation, fractures will not unite, and many other consequences of failure of connective tissue repair occur.

The basic chain of collagen can be made with energy derived from anaerobic glycolysis. Without oxygen to hydroxylate proline and lysine (Fig. 1.8), however, finished collagen production is halted and wound healing cannot occur. As one might expect, a local condition resembling scurvy tends to occur. The mechanism by which ascorbate aids in hydroxylation other than hydroxylase activation is still unclear. It appears now that when ascorbate is oxidized in the presence of Fe^{++}, a high energy form of oxygen called superoxide ion (O_2^-) results. When more O_2^- is made available, as when more O_2 is present, collagen synthesis is enhanced. When O_2^- is produced by photochemical stimulation of riboflavin, collagen synthesis is enhanced as with ascorbate. This may seem rather technical, but the same mechanism becomes important later in the oxidative microbicidal mechanism in leukocytes.

The molecule resulting from assembly of the alpha chains is transported to the Golgi apparatus where galactose is attached, a step of controversial significance. After glycosylation occurs, this molecule, procollagen, is excreted from the cell. Somehow, the microtubule is also important to collagen transport, perhaps for excretion from the cell. Colchicine, which interferes with microtubular function, inhibits microtubular transport, and slows collagen secretion.

The collagen molecule, the monomer, when excreted from the cell, contains a terminal peptide at each end (Fig. 1.6). These extensions contain several residues of cystine found otherwise only in the alpha chains of type III collagen. This

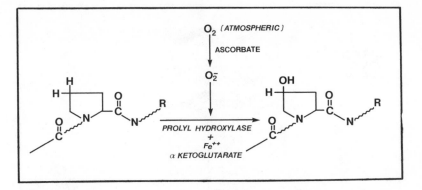

Figure 1.8 Schematic representation of proline hydroxylation as it occurs in the assembling chain. The hydroxylation of lysine is similar.

molecule is called procollagen. The terminal peptides are called "registration peptides" and enable the alpha chains to assemble in proper parallel array and proper distance so that they may assume the superhelical configuration. Before the molecules can aggregate into fibers, however, the terminal peptides must be removed. This is done by one or more enzymes termed procollagen peptidase. The resultant molecule is termed tropocollagen. Deficiency of the enzymes that cleave the registration peptides results in a disease called dermatosparaxis, which is now grouped as one form of Ehlers-Danlos syndrome. This syndrome is caused by genetic defects, resulting in fragility and weakness of collagen structure (see Chap. 2).

Tropocollagen aggregates with other tropocollagen molecules to form fibrils. The initial attracting forces are probably ionic interaction between oppositely charged polar groups in adjacent molecules. These ionically charged groups occur in clusters along the alpha chains. Partly for this reason and partly because of the registration of peptides, each tropocollagen unit is displaced by one-quarter of its length from the adjacent tropocollagen molecules. This "quarter-stagger" arrangement with groupings of the ionically charged polar residues accounts for the characteristic band pattern of collagen seen in transmission electron microscopy.

Before and during the assembly of tropocollagen molecules, certain of the lysine residues are acted upon by a specific

27

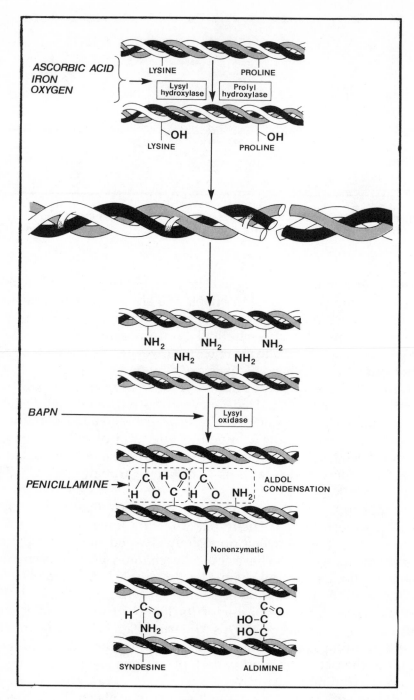

Figure 1.9

monamine oxidase, lysyl oxidase. This copper-containing enzyme removes the ϵ amino group and converts the terminal carbon into an aldehyde which then reacts with another aldehyde from another lysine forming an intermolecular crosslink. When this link occurs within each molecule, it may not have much significance, but when other lysines from adjacent molecules condense, forming an aldimine bond, strong organic, intermolecular connections are formed. These intermolecular cross-links, which "mature" gradually, are responsible for a major portion of the strength of the collagen fibril. Lysine-lysine links are the major source of cross-linking in elastin as well, although the chemistry is somewhat different.

A disease in cattle and other animals, called lathyrism, is characterized by fragility and weakness of all connective tissues. Bone deformities, skin fragility, and arterial aneurysms are characteristic. This condition is caused by ingestion of sweet peas from the genus *Lathyrus odoratus*. The active principle is a compound called β-aminoproprionitrile (BAPN), which is a specific inhibitor of lysyl oxidase thus repressing the formation of intermolecular cross-links in both collagen and elastin. (see Fig. 1.9). Fibril formation proceeds normally, but the fibers have no strength and are soluble in dilute neutral salt solution. Removal of the BAPN allows cross-links to form normally.

COLLAGEN SYNTHESIS IN WOUND HEALING

New collagen can be found in healing wounds as early as the second day. The peak rate of synthesis in a primarily healing wound appears to occur about the fifth to seventh day. The early collagen is highly disorganized, and views obtained by scanning electron microscopy suggest that collagen exists almost as a gel. The collagen synthesized on the very surface of a wound that is "granulating in" by second intention also exists basically as a gel and can be identified as collagen only through sophisticated immunochemical techniques. The slightly deeper, slightly older collagen appears much more mature and strong.

Figure 1.9 Schematic diagram of the extracellular assembly of collagen fibrils. Remember that the molecules align in the "quarter stagger" as shown in Figure 1.7. The various manipulable steps in collagen secretion and cross-linking are shown.

29

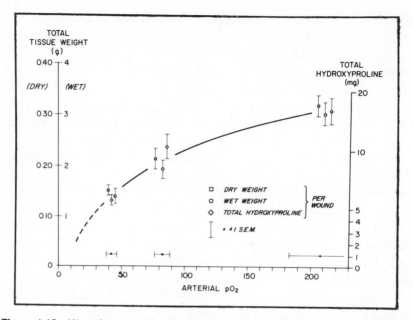

Figure 1.10 Wound tissue and collagen content as a function of blood oxygen tension.

Collagen synthesis in a wound depends to a critical degree on its vascularity and on the degree to which the circulatory system perfuses it. In the normal clinical situation, collagen synthesis is dependent on oxygen supply. Figure 1.10 shows how increased arterial P_{O_2} changes the rate of accumulation in dead space wounds. Disorders of collagen synthesis in wounds will be discussed in the next chapter.

Collagen synthesis remains rapid for many months after injury, often up to six months or a year. Why, then, does the wound not become hypertrophic and slowly amass collagen until it protrudes from the surrounding tissue? Some scars will continue to amass collagen and become keloids or hypertrophic scars. *However, in the fact that the vast majority do not lies the simple but powerful concept that even as collagen is being synthesized, it is being lysed and removed in a constant process of collagen turnover.*

COLLAGEN LYSIS

It may be possible to make an ideal wound if one should use an infinitely sharp knife, protect the wound edge from water loss,

30

and close the wound primarily without sutures within a few seconds of its making. In such a case, little surrounding tissue would have to be debrided before the conditions for repair would be suitable. In practice, however, wounds are not made with infinitely sharp instruments, wounds are exposed and contaminated, and surgeons tend to leave islands of strangulated or coagulated tissue behind them. Before repair can occur, then, the "damaged face of the wound" must be removed. This process involves collagen lysis as well as removal of noncollagenous protein. This job is generally left to the macrophage. Polymorphonuclear cells also contribute collagenase. The macrophage secretes lysosomal enzymes into the extracellular fluid which can digest protein, including denatured collagen. These enzymes probably can digest some native collagen as well, although this point is controversial. Besides mounting an enzymatic attack on damaged tissues, the macrophage can ingest fragments of tissue and can hydrolyze them to amino acids within the digestive vacuole through the action of lysosomal enzymes.

Collagen lysis continues to play a constructive role as normal repair proceeds. At first, newly deposited collagen is essentially a gel, and wound strength is poor. Thus, much of the early collagen deposited must be broken down, probably ingested, and reduced to amino acids, and these amino acids resynthesized into collagen, all in the wound site. This process is essential to maturation of the wound. In order to continue resynthesis, however, amino acids must be brought in from elsewhere because, inevitably, some of the original amino acids will be lost to diffusion or deamination and carbohydrate metabolism. Furthermore, some of the byproducts of collagen metabolism will inevitably be hydroxyproline and hydrosylysine, neither of which can be resynthesized into collagen. Therefore, the proline and lysine must be replaced from external sources.

The principal extracellular enzyme involved in collagen lysis is collagenase. This enzyme cleaves native collagen monomer about one-third of the distance between its end at neutral pH. The fragments are susceptible to other proteases and to ingestion by cells. The intimate details of collagenase action are still controversial. It is produced by inflammatory cells including polymorphonuclear leukocytes and macrophages. It is also produced by regenerating epidermis. Its presence or its activity seems to be enhanced by steroids and inflammatory reactions. Because collagen lysis is a destructive process, energy demands are less than the constructive process of collagen synthesis. Therefore, lysis continues despite (and may even be accelerated by) starvation, or specific protein deficiency. If collagen synthesis proceeds normally and is not depressed by malnutrition or oxygen deficiency, it balances collagen lysis. When the balance is tipped, however, collagen lysis may predominate, and the wound may literally melt away. The reparative process is so delicate that malnutrition or sepsis may turn a normal balance into self-destruction.

THE BALANCE OF SYNTHESIS AND LYSIS

The most commonly known example of collagen lysis exceeding collagen synthesis in wounds is the well-known proclivity of even apparently healed wounds to break down in a patient who contracts scurvy (see Fig. 1.11). Here, collagen synthesis and collagen lysis are probably proceeding at a relatively low rate, but in the absence of ascorbic acid, collagen lysis inevitably predominates, and the wound breaks down and falls apart.

The burn surgeon sees a similar event. A patient who has developed a red, lush granulation tissue and is ready for grafting sometimes contracts sepsis or shock from a distant source. When this is not corrected within a few hours, the lytic mechanism plus the death of the acutely malnourished cells result in a complete loss of the red granulation tissue, leaving only a thin translucent film over apparently unchanged fat. Needless to say, this can be a disheartening experience.

The solubility of collagen as well as its susceptibility to enzymatic destruction is partly dependent on the extent of cross-linking and stability of the cross-links. Native collagen, in the triple helical configuration, is resistant to the action of such naturally occurring proteolytic enzymes as pepsin, trypsin, or acid proteases. If native collagen is denatured by heat or four molar urea or similar denaturing agents, the triple helix is destroyed, and the individual alpha chains separate as random coils that are susceptible to digestion by most proteolytic enzymes. Some collagen can be denatured at temperatures as low

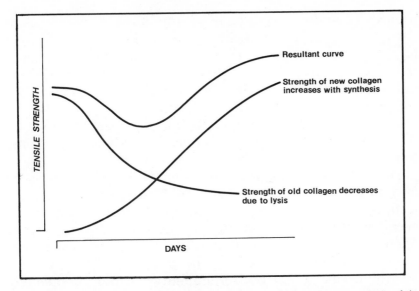

Figure 1.11 Concept of wound strength expressed as a balance between lysis of the old collagen holding the sutures and of the new collagen welding the wound edges. Any deficit of synthesis or exaggeration of lysis makes the wound weak point even weaker for a longer time.

as 39 C and it is even theoretically possible that high fevers can result in collagen loss through denaturation.

Tissue collagenases have been found in the upper portions of dermis and the epithelial cells of the gastrointestinal tract, in regenerating squamous epithelium, macrophages, in granulocytes, and in the term and postpartum uterus as well as other organs. Collagen digestion in the normal organism is limited partly by an inhibitory factor in the globulins of serum. Some individuals lack the full degree of collagenase inhibitor factor and may be susceptible to wound consequences as a result.

Neutral mammalian collagenase is a large molecule, and there is some evidence that its activity in wounds is particularly directed toward the already established, highly insoluble collagen. Several studies involving radioactive labeling of old collagen before wounding, or of new collagen after wounding, in rat colon have shown that the old collagen is preferentially destroyed. The end result is that tissue strength suffers until the new collagen can be adequately cross-linked. Every anastomosis passes through a nadir of strength on its way to maturity (normally about the third to fifth day). Normally, collagenolytic activity is found up to approximately 7 mm away from the wound. Within this region, tissue strength diminishes; and sutures, when placed within this distance from the wound may well cut through. For this reason, it has become customary to close wounds that represent a dehiscence danger with internal retention sutures placed more than 5 mm from the wound edge.

The infliction of major trauma stimulates collagen lysis not only in the area of injury, but a generalized collagen lysis as well. As lean body mass is lost, collagen is lost. As the wound becomes larger and the degree of injury is increased, the reparative ability of each portion of the wound diminishes. Furthermore, other structures may be weakened. For instance, a disproportional number of aortic aneurysms found at operation for some other indication will rupture in the postoperative period. Presumably, they are weakened by the collagenolytic mechanism. Many vascular surgeons realize this problem and consider it urgent to repair aneurysms detected in this manner.

Although the technical details of collagen lysis in wounds are not available, it is obvious that collagen lysis is an important biologic fact. The balance of collagen synthesis and collagen lysis represents the well-being of the wound. Inasmuch as the surgeon holds this balance in his hands, he holds the well-being of his patient.

As stated above, the peak rate of collagen synthesis in a primarily healing wound is reached at about five to seven days. This corresponds with the most rapid rate of increase of tensile strength (Fig. 1.12). By about the third week, the primarily healing wound has about the greatest mass it will have. This mass is often described as the healing ridge whose absence by the seventh to ninth day may signify the possibility of dehiscence of the wound.* This mass, perhaps a simplified counterpart of fracture callus, then recedes; and the tissue softens while its collagen content diminishes. Paradoxically, the strength of the wound increases during this time. The obvious conclusion is

---

*The converse is also true. A wound that has a healing ridge throughout its length will not dehisce. Sutures, even retention sutures, can safely be removed.

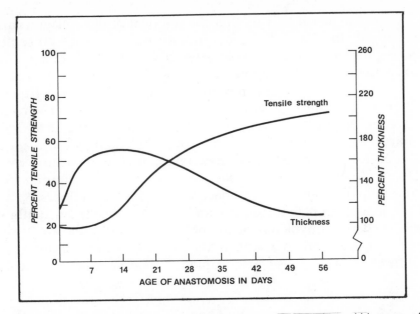

Figure 1.12 Tensile strength development in the wound. Note the rapid increase of strength after the initial "lag phase." The initial peak in thickness is clinically defined as the healing ridge. The late, slow increase in strength despite loss of thickness reflects collagen turnover and remodeling. *(Courtesy Lange Medical Publications. In Dunphy JE, Way LW (eds): Current Surgical Diagnosis and Treatment, 3rd ed., 1977, p. 113. Adapted from Douglas DM.)*

that there is remodeling of the structure of the wound and a more effective structure is being made with less collagen. The best analogy, perhaps, is in the development of materials for aircraft. "Honeycombed" or corrugated structures sandwiched between thin layers of aluminum can be designed to be stronger than an equal weight of solid metal. The major point is that the new structure is not achieved by intelligent *subtraction* of collagen molecules. Instead, it is achieved by intelligent *replacement* of the total collagenous structure. The closely packed, even gel-like, collagen structure in the early wound gives way to an open "basket-weave" tissue structure. Scanning electron microscopic views of normal, early and well remodeled collagen structure from primary wounds in animals are shown in Figures 1.13–1.15. In this manner, the wound is remodeled repeatedly for six months to a year.

Common sense tells us that the removal of old collagen can occur only to a limited distance into the normal tissue. At some point, the new collagen must interact with the old collagen to form a bond. New collagen may physically unite with the ends or sides of old collagen in a sort of "weld"; or new collagen fibers might interlace with the old, providing a sort of woven junction or "darn." Probably, both occur. It is difficult to find sharply cut collagen ends even in an early healing wound and, therefore, we presume that they have united with wound collagen. However, it is also easy to see, as shown in Figure 1.15, that new collagen fibers interlace with old collagen fibers.

If, in a given patient, significant inhibitors of collagen synthesis, such as hypovolemia or chemotherapeutic agents, are present, the surgeon may anticipate possible wound trouble. If inhibitors of synthesis are coupled with significant enhancers

Figure 1.13   Normal skin collagen magnified about × 10,000. Note the definition of the collagen fibrils and the large fibers.

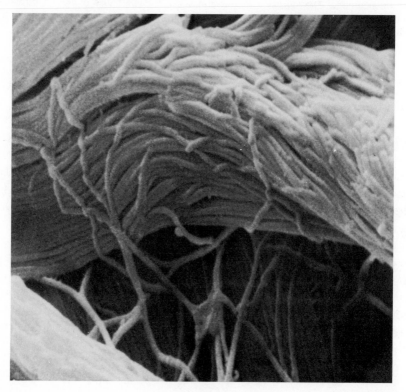

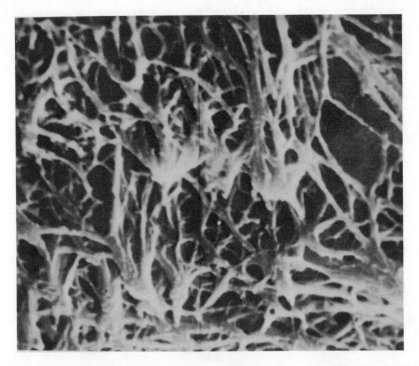

Figure 1.14 Wound collagen at 10 days by scanning electron microscopy. Note the lack of definition of collagen fibrils and the small fibers. Magnification × 10,000.

of collagen lysis, such as starvation, steroid hormones, or inflammation, impaired wound healing is probable. When infection is also present, a technically precarious suture line is almost certainly doomed.

Normal Collagen Turnover and the Effect of Mechanical Stress on Repair As collagen in the maturing wound is turned over, its synthesis and deposition probably follow a somewhat different set of rules than on the first synthesis and deposition. The vascular system, which was relatively inadequate the first time around, is now complete. The wound, now having united, is subjected to a continuity of stresses and strains as if the tissue were once again normal. The electrical charges produced by these stresses probably result in an alignment of the proteoglycans and collagen fibers. When slight force is applied to the wound periodically during its maturation phase, the wound is

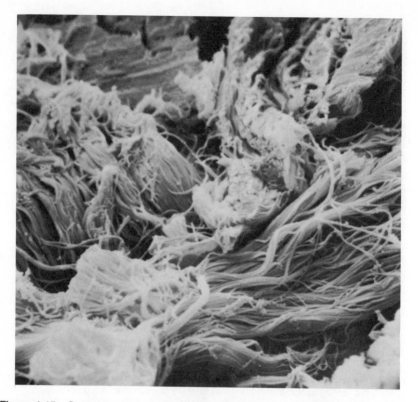

Figure 1.15 Scanning electron microscopy of collagen near a rat colon anastomosis. Note the relatively disorderly new collagen fibrils (side view) interlacing with the more densely packed and orderly older fibers (end view in most cases). Magnification × 2800.

stronger than if it is protected from those forces. Perhaps this relates to the observation that animals, allowed freedom to move about after wounding, heal their wounds more securely by an earlier date. Fibroblasts and collagen tend to line up along lines of tension. For instance, in tissue healing around grafts to the abdominal aorta, there is a fibroblastic and collagenous pattern reminiscent of the normal architecture of the muscularis and adventitia of the original vessel. While there is no doubt that mechanical factors affect repair, the mechanism is entirely unknown and can only be surmised. Nevertheless, it seems reasonable to allow patients freedom of movement after the initial fragility of the wound is gone. Theoretically, too much protection of the hernia repair from mechanical stress, for instance, is harmful.

PROTEOGLYCANS—GLYCOSAMINOGLYCANS (MUCOPOLYSACCHARIDES)

Among the noncellular components of connective tissue, comprising a substantial portion of what is known as "ground substance," are the glycosaminoglycans. These substances are largely polysaccharides composed of chains of repeating disaccharide units that are in turn composed of glucuronic acid or iduronic acid and a hexosamine. The hexosamine is sulfated in varying degrees, usually at the four or six position. Glycosaminoglycans rarely exist free in the body but instead couple to proteins. The combinations are called proteoglycans. The glycosaminoglycans are linked with the carrier protein through an O-glycosidic linkage to a serine, or occasionally a threonine, residue. There may be several such chains linked to a single protein and the chain line may vary from about 2000 disaccharides in the case of hyaluronic acid to as few as 10 in the case of keratan sulfate or heparitan sulfate.

Much less is known of the protein core of the proteoglycans. Probably several proteins are involved, all quite large, linear, randomly coiled chains about 4000 A in length. Thus, proteoglycans are very large molecules and, because of the presence of numerous sulfates and glucuronic groups, are highly charged. The charges tend to repel one another, and the complex molecule occupies considerable space. This space, because of the charge and steric influences, limits the type and size of molecule that can penetrate it. Large, negatively charged molecules generally cannot pass through the proteoglycans' domain. Smaller positively charged molecules may pass through or can even be trapped within the space and bind to the proteoglycans. Thus the ground substance that contains large amounts of proteoglycans can act as a molecular filter, exactly as does a chromatographic column.

Collagen has groups of charged residues along the alpha chains. These can interact with the charge groups on proteoglycans. The nature, extent, and significance of these interactions are still under investigation. Fiber orientation or size may be influenced or directed by proteoglycans but this is questionable. We know that different connective tissues with different architectures each contain a predominance of one or the other type of proteoglycan and that collagen fiber diameter and orientation are each characteristic for these types of connective tissue. For instance, dermis is composed of large collagen fibers that are coiled about one another in an apparently random fashion. However, when skin is stretched, the majority of fibers orient themselves along the lines of stress. The principal glycosaminoglycan of skin is dermatan sulfate. On the other hand, the collagen fibers of cornea are small, and are highly oriented in planes with unidirectional fibers in each plane at approximately right angles to the underlying or overlying fiber bundles. The principal glycosaminoglycan in cornea is keratan sulfate. In corneal scars, however, collagen fibers are randomly arranged and vary greatly in size. The major glycosaminoglycans found in corneal scars are chondroitin sulfate and dermatan sulfate (as in other scars).

Hyaline cartilage presents a special and interesting case of collagen-proteoglycans interaction. The collagen in hyaline cartilage is type II and contains a large number of glycosylated hydroxylysine residues. The collagen fibers are small and rarely show a typical banding pattern with the electron microscope. Nearly 50 percent of the mass of cartilage is proteoglycans. This mixture binds water and releases it slowly under pressure thus accounting for the elastic and compressive qualities of cartilage. Injury to cartilage is not repaired by the formation of new hyaline cartilage. If repair occurs at all it occurs by deposition of fibrocartilage that contains type I collagen and a small quantity of proteoglycans. The product of repair obviously is inferior to the real cartilage. One can imagine the gradual loss of the function of intervertebral disc with wear and the scars of time. Thus scarring in cartilage is very much like scarring in the cornea. There is a loss of normal function accompanying the replacement of the normal collagen proteoglycans matrix with scar tissue.

The precise role played by proteoglycans in healing is not understood. Shortly after injury, hyaluronic acid content of wounds rises rapidly. Some of it comes from the local circulation, arriving as a result of microvascular permeability. As healing progresses, the hyaluronic acid decreases and chondroitin sulphates increase. As maturation occurs, the concentration of proteoglycans falls, eventually, to a low level. At some point, a small amount of proteoglycans is incorporated into the collagen fiber. As proteoglycans are lost, water is also lost; and the wound assumes its dense, white appearance due to its high content of tightly packaged collagen fibers.

EPITHELIZATION

Since epithelia cover all external surfaces of the body, they are probably the most frequently injured tissues. They have their own style of repair which usually entails multiplication of the cells at the wound edge, migration across the wound of the resulting new cells, and then maturation of the one or two cell layers into an almost (but not quite) normal structure.

Squamous Epithelium

Squamous epithelium consists of stratified layers of epithelial cells. The lowermost cells, basal cells, rest on the connective tissue of the dermis. Above the basal layer are several layers of cells undergoing mitosis or differentiation known as "prickle cells" because of the prominent desmosomes, or plate-like intracellular connections. Above these are well-differentiated cells producing keratin, and the outermost layers are dead cells and keratin. Epidermis can be visualized as a structure made of modular columns of cells starting at the basal cells and differentiating outward through the prickle cell stage and eventually becoming a dead keratinized residue that constitutes the horny layer of the skin. The outer layers are constantly being desquamated and replaced from below.

When a defect is made in squamous epithelium, the basal cells at the margin of the wound flatten and begin to move toward the area of cell deficit. Mitoses appear at the wound edge and the cells thus produced migrate. Migration is usually started within hours of the injury. There seems to be some tumbling or "leapfrogging" of cells, and, as they move, basement membrane forms beneath. As the wound becomes covered with flat migrating epithelial cells, those farthest from the margin begin to assume a more cuboidal or rectangular shape and begin to divide. Daughter cells, products of these divisions, move outward, forming once again the characteristic columnar module of the epithelial barrier (Fig. 1.16).

Epithelial cells will migrate only over viable tissue. Thus, the cells often move into the underlying tissue below the wound debris, blood clot, or eschar. The cells, as one would expect, seek a blood and nutritional supply adequate to meet their needs. As the "tongue" of epithelium burrows between the eschar and the living tissue, it must release collagen lytic enzymes that must literally cleave through the collagen connecting the viable and nonviable tissues. Any eschar therefore, impedes epithelization. If the wound is kept moist and is pro-

Figure 1.16 A. A tongue of epithelial cells is shown migrating under an eschar. Note that the basal layer lies on essentially healthy tissue and the advancing tongue is penetrating the collagenous tissue at the point which divides viable from nonviable. The epithelial cells seem to be seeking their environment. **B.** A lower power view of C, showing the epithelium advancing over damaged but still viable abraded tissue. A nest of epithelial cells is seen to the left where it is expanding from a skin appendage. **C.** Epithelization at the edge of a superficial abrasion which was protected from drying by the use of a plastic film dressing. One can see the mitoses and cellular activity in the tongue of epithelium which is pointing downward. However, since eschar formation was inhibited, the actual epithelization proceeded across the top of the wound. *(Photomicrographs courtesy of Howard Maibach, M. D., Department of Dermatology, University of California, San Francisco, School of Medicine.)*

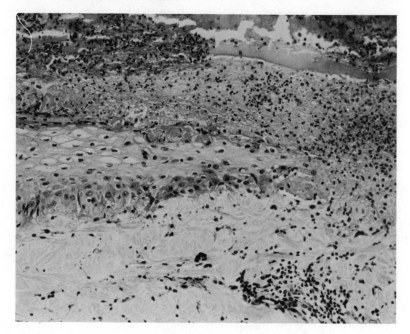

A

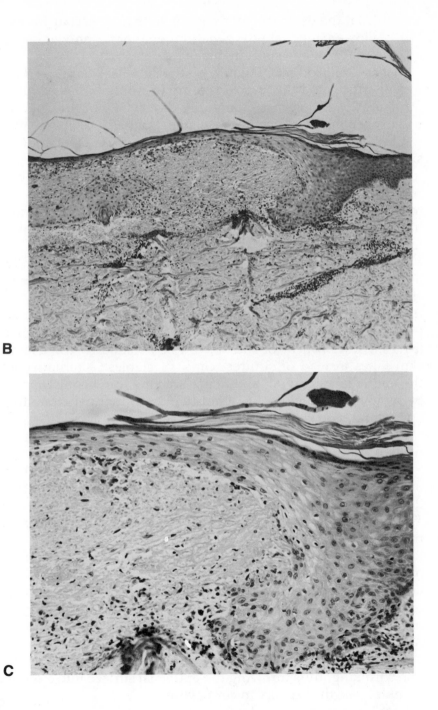

B

C

tected from the external environment so that no eschar forms, but is allowed adequate oxygenation, epithelization will occur on its surface, at a maximum rate.

Just as for fibroblasts, the new epithelial cell is "born" as if its parent anticipated the hypoxic nature of wounds. Its enzymes for energy metabolism are primarily glycolytic, but the cell can use oxygen when it becomes available. Epithelial cells can subsist but cannot divide or migrate in anoxia. Their rates of division and migration are P_{O_2}-dependent.

There is dispute over what stimulates epithelial repair. Currently, the most accepted theory is that a "chalone" responsive to catecholamines constantly holds the cells in check. Wounding is said to interrupt the local supply of catecholamines and mitosis results.

Skin sutures create a microwound. Epithelial cells migrate into these wounds just as they do in the major wound. Occasionally, a plug of keratinized epithelium will be trapped in the tract when final healing occurs, and small cysts may appear at the side of the mature wound. The epithelized suture tract leaves a scar, which, of course, can be avoided by the use of skin tapes instead of sutures, clips, or staples. Alternatively, the epithelial migration, and hence scarring, can be minimized by removing fastenings (in about two days) that penetrate the epithelium, and replacing them with tapes.

Epithelization over linear defects, however, is only a minor portion of the wound healing that epithelial cells perform. Superficial injuries, e.g., second degree burns epithelize not only from the wound edge but from hair follicles and other deep dermal appendages that supply live squamous cells. Third degree burns, however, can heal only from the edge of the injury.

The intense cellular activity at the edge of an open wound produces a thickened, active looking hyperplastic zone that disappears after epithelization is complete. Nevertheless, the completed epithelial scar is thin, flat, and devoid of dermal papillae. The surface of the scar is often ridged, however, because epithelization is so often accompanied by contraction. That is, while the covering is becoming complete, the wound is also shrinking, thus throwing the epithelial surface into a set of wrinkles (see the section on contraction).

Local environment is obviously important to the regenerat-

44

ing squamous cell. Epidermis regenerates faster in hyperbaric oxygen. The underlying blood vessels also regenerate better or are better preserved. Epithelization of second degree burns is faster under homograft or under microporous tape. The mechanism is not entirely clear. The acceleration due to these coverings seems to result from the conservation of energy that might otherwise have been dissipated through heat radiation or evaporative water loss, but that now can be used for more creative metabolic activity. This has a number of useful clinical correlates. For instance, second degree burns heal more rapidly under intact, uninfected blisters, a fact proved by many investigators. If possible, uninfected blisters should be left intact. However, infection slows epithelization. Infected blisters should be debrided. Epithelium heals poorly under so-called wet-to-dry dressings. In such conditions, the clean, moist environment encourages epithelium to grow so it can then be torn off with the dried-on dressing. With this technique one may debride dead tissue, but one also debrides new epithelium which, being only a few cells thick, is easily overlooked.

Squamous repair is dependent on the underlying wound. The two influence each other by signals yet unknown. Deep repair of inflammation due to a superficial second degree injury will not occur until epithelization is complete. As epithelium covers granulation tissue, the red, soft tissue loses vessels, shrinks, and its collagen matures. There are many other examples of "mesenchymal-epithelial interactions."

Respiratory Epithelium

Respiratory epithelium repairs in a somewhat different manner. Tracheal and bronchial epithelium differs from other epithelia in that it is columnar and ciliated on the surface. Among these surface cells are goblet cells that secrete mucous. Injury involving removal of tracheal epithelium leads to a repair process similar to that seen in epidermis, with some important exceptions. Flattening and migration of cells at the edges of the wound occur. However, it is not only the basal cells that migrate, but those that overlie the basal layer. Furthermore, two cell layers usually migrate together. The replacement of cells by mitosis begins to occur after about 48 hours, but at first the new cells are neither columnar nor ciliated and the area over the wound appears to be covered by transitional cells. After about 96 hours, differentiation of the new cells begins by arrangement into a layer of low cuboidal cells overlying one or more layers of flattened basal cells. Eventually, the upper layer becomes columnar and cilia appear.

If the injury destroys tissue underlying the epithelial layer, scarring results. In this case, the elastic lamina is lost, and the epithelium that eventually covers the defect does not differentiate into ciliated columnar epithelium. Remodeling of this scar can produce stricture or closure of the airway. Attempts to prevent stricture with prosthetic implants or "stents" may be successful in maintaining an airway. However, the epithelial covering which develops under a "stent" will not contain normal ciliated columnar cells. Secretions, dust, etc., cannot be transported upwards and pulmonary infection, atelectasis and other complications may occur. The history of reconstructive surgery of the airways is marred by this problem. An obvious solution, therefore, is to work towards a narrow "hairline" scar. Microsurgical technique might well improve clinical results in this type of reconstruction.

Differentiation of respiratory epithelium depends upon some sort of specific inductive effect of the underlying mesenchymal structures. Thus, repair of tracheal wounds seems to be aimed at preventing scars and restoring the integrity of the natural supporting structures so that normal migration and differentiation of ciliated epithelium can occur.

Esophageal and Intestinal Epithelium

Esophageal epithelium is stratified squamous epithelium. Regeneration of esophageal epithelium is essentially the same as that of epidermis except that it is slower.

Intestinal epithelium is columnar, formed into finger-like folds that project into the lumen. As in the stomach, these cells are constantly being shed and replaced as a result of the continuous mitotic activity of the cells in the crypts of Lieberkühn. The mitotic cycle is about one and one-quarter hours and the upper intestinal epithelium is completely replaced in two and one-quarter to two and three-quarter days. It is not surprising, therefore, that defects in the epithelial lining of the intestine can be repaired with great rapidity. The cells that migrate are formed by mitoses in crypt cells. The cells flatten as they migrate and after a few days they commence mitosis again and form new crypts by downgrowth into the underlying connective tissue. If the submucosa and muscularis are destroyed, crypts are not reformed and fibrous scar, superficially resembling a thick submucosal layer, results.

The stomach mucosa is perhaps the most interesting of all. At first, it seems amazing that any wound of the stomach would ever heal since the delicate new cells are exposed to hydrochloric acid and powerful digestive enzymes. However, the stomach has a remarkable capacity to heal and does so very quickly.

Epithelial cells of the stomach are highly specialized and they are constantly being replaced as a result of continuous mitotic activity of cells in the neck of gastric glands at the base of gastric pits. The life of a surface cell is about 24 hours. Disorders such as stress ulcers are encountered much less frequently than might be expected in the presence of such a dynamic process. At the base of the gastric pits in the fundus are mucus-secreting cells. In the body and pylorus, many of the pit cells are either parietal cells that produce hydrochloric acid or chief cells that produce pepsin. Most of the surface epithelium consists of mucus-producing cells.

When a wound is made in the stomach, the gastric mucosa at the wound edge shows considerable disorganization. The glands in this region show no differentiation into chief or parietal cells. Instead, all are the mucus-secreting variety, and these are the cells that migrate over the wound bed. Mitosis is not confined to cells at the neck of glands, but involves the depths of the glands as well as the surface epithelium. Once coverage is obtained, maturation again occurs, but once more the result is not quite normal unless the injury was extremely superficial. After toxic doses of total body radiation, gastric epithelial repair is "paralyzed," and usually within 24 hours a hemorrhagic gastritis or enteritis begins.

Colon Epithelium

Colon epithelium heals the same as the small intestine except at a considerably slower rate. Instead of a few days to resurface an epithelial defect, it may take as long as three months for epithelium to resurface a moderately large defect in the colon. Infection, so much more likely in the colon, is undoubtedly one deterrent to epithelization, but it is not the only factor. The lesser colon blood supply also probably is important. However, the full cause of this slow healing is still not fully understood.

Rectal lesions heal poorly. Epithelization is slow and is modified by extensive growth of granulation tissue in denuded areas. Usually, wound contraction begins before epithelization is complete and the scarring and contraction may lead to stricture. Diseases such as lymphogranuloma venereum characteristically cause colon stricture. Pain due to inflammation and infection leads to spasm of the rectal sphincter which encourages contracture and inhibits epithelization.

Regeneration of bladder mucosa is rapid. All layers of epithelium participate in cell migration and multiplication when the bladder wall has lost its mucosa. It has even been reported that the bladder will regenerate. However, the evidence for true regeneration of the bladder wall is equivocal. Other reports indicate that fibrous tissue lined with urothelium is all that is produced. While this may serve as a passive reservoir for urine, it cannot be equated with a functioning urinary bladder.

The confusion regarding regeneration of the urinary bladder probably stems from failure to identify the cell types in the newly formed tissue. When the original reports of bladder regeneration were published, fibroblasts were probably identified as smooth muscle. Later work has shown that the cells in newly formed granulation tissue are contractile, collagen-secreting "myofibroblasts." While these cells resemble smooth muscle cells in certain morphologic aspects and in their response to pharmacologic agents, they cannot fully substitute for them in functioning smooth muscle organisms (see section on contraction).

CONTRACTION

Wound contraction is the movement of full thickness skin toward the center of the skin defect. It is an active process by which a wound shrinks by "drawing in" surrounding normal skin. The term contraction should not be confused with "con-

48

tracture," which is the end result of shortening of scar tissue, usually limiting the motion of a joint. (See Chapter 2.)

For the most part, contraction is a friendly process by which large wounds become small without the necessity for secondary closure or skin graft. In occasional instances, when the tissue available for movement across the defect is limited, contraction may shorten or narrow a structure, such as the esophagus. Normal tissue does not "grow" into the wound by contraction; it is pulled or pushed there with stretching of the normal tissue, usually skin. If that skin cannot be stretched, either contraction will stop, or a stricture may result.

If a rectangular piece of full thickness skin is excised where the skin is freely moveable, the edges of the wound will immediately retract so that the wound area becomes larger. The retraction is due to the normal skin tension often noted as Langer's lines. After three or four days, the area of the wound begins to decrease. Careful examination will show that although epithelization may have begun, the decrease in area of the wound is due more to the movement of the original wound edges toward the center. The center point of each side of the rectangle will have moved more rapidly than the corners. Eventually, the wound edges will meet, leaving a linear scar in the shape of two Y's, tail-to-tail. Wounds that can heal by contraction often heal to the best cosmetic and functional result in this manner. However, whereas almost any wound in an animal can heal by contraction, many wounds in the human cannot. For instance, wounds on the anterior aspect of the lower leg that are fixed closely to the tibia will not close by contraction at all. Wounds of the face will contract, but because the skin is fixed to so many structures nearby, there is a purse-string effect and distortion of the features may result. For instance, the lower eyelid may be pulled down if a malar wound contracts shut. The lips may be pulled into the distorted position if a cheek wound is allowed to contract. On the other hand, on the back of the neck, even the largest wounds may eventually close with small scars. On the abdomen or the breasts, almost any wound will contract to a size smaller than it began.

Over the years, various theories to explain wound contraction have been advanced. Even today, the last word on this subject has probably not been written. Nevertheless, certain basic facts have been determined:

1. Collagen is not essential for wound contraction. Contraction proceeds normally in the scorbutic animal.
2. The motive force for contraction comes from a cell. Any event that interferes with the viability of cells in the wound edge will inhibit wound contraction.
3. The cells that supply the motive force appear to be a special type of contractile cell having attributes of both the fibroblast and the smooth muscle cell. These cells have been termed "myofibroblasts" (see the section on the Fibroblast and Figs. 1.3 and 1.5).

Under light microscopy, the myofibroblasts appear similar to any fibroblast, for that matter, to any smooth muscle cell. Under electron microscopy, however, these cells appear to be basically fibroblasts with rough endoplasmic reticulum. But in the periphery of the cytosol, there are contractile myofibrils essentially identical to those found in smooth muscle cells. These cells have been cultured and have been shown to synthesize and deposit collagen. They have desmosomes and tight intercellular junctions. They become attached to the underlying substrate and respond appropriately to smooth muscle stimulants and relaxants. Therefore, wound contraction can be inhibited by local application of smooth muscle relaxants. However, it can also be inhibited by antimicrotubular drugs such as colchicine and vinblastine. As one might expect, myofibroblasts also contain microtubules. It appears, therefore, that wound contraction is due to contraction of myofibroblasts utilizing the motile force of microfilaments and somehow involving the function of microtubules. Certain fibrotic contractures, such as Dupuytren's contracture, also contain myofibroblasts. Strangely, or perhaps fittingly, myofibroblasts are not found in ordinary incised and closed wounds, even in areas of skin in which contraction of an open wound would inevitably occur. No one knows what determines whether a mesenchymal cell will differentiate into a myofibroblast or into an ordinary fibroblast. In granulating tissue, cell types vary from pure fibroblasts to fully developed contractile myofibroblasts. Myofibroblasts are also found in high concentrations in wounds of arteries.

Epithelization and wound contraction proceed simultaneously and independently. Neither process seems to affect the other. If a thin split thickness skin graft is placed on an excised and contracting wound, contraction may be slowed, but the wound will continue to contract sometimes to the same extent as if the graft were not present at all. Clinically, one sees this phenomenon in split thickness skin grafts which at first lie smooth on a burn wound but later become wrinkled by the contraction of the wound bed. If, however, the wound edges are mechanically splinted so that contraction cannot occur, and if a skin graft is applied immediately, and the graft and splints remain for at least seven days, contraction will not occur after the splint is removed. A splinted but ungrafted wound will contract rapidly, even after seven days, if the splints are removed. If the contractile process is allowed to begin, even splinting and split thickness grafting will not prevent it, though it can be slowed. Full thickness skin grafts, either free, pedicle, or rotation flaps, will markedly inhibit contraction, especially if active contraction has not yet commenced.

Lastly, contraction slows with smooth muscle relaxing agents and is halted by large doses of antiinflammatory steroids. Epithelization is also stopped by steroids, but in contrast to contraction, epithelization is restimulated by vitamin A. Therefore, we have three specific biochemical controls over the contraction process, steroids, antitubular drugs, and smooth muscle relaxants.

Traditionally, a sharp line has been drawn between "contracture" and "contraction." Certainly, scars do shorten, particularly if they often undergo reinjury. Unepithelized as well as epithelized wounds may shrink. In fact, shrinkage of wounds is commonly seen even after they seem to be healed. It is not always sure whether the mechanism is in the cell or merely due to shrinkage of scar collagen.

Since myofibroblasts have been found in open wounds, in Dupuytren's contracture, and others, the overlapping area between these two concepts will require detailed examination. This is because contraction can be inhibited by smooth muscle inhibitors and steroids. If contraction is what causes the early esophageal stricture (it certainly is not the motive power behind the chronic one), we should learn to be more alert to its early development in order to prevent it. Contracture can often be treated by local pressure and traction, but contraction is prevented by steroids, smooth muscle relaxants, and microtubular antagonists.

ENDOCRINOLOGY

Although much has been written on the endocrinology of repair, it seems fair to conclude that few of the usually defined endocrine substances have significant influence.

The major single exception is that cortisol and its congeners impair healing. Small dose steroid inhibition can be overcome with forced feeding, but large dose inhibition cannot. The effect of steroids is most pronounced if they are given before or within three days after injury and are thus able to suppress the inflammatory response. Poor repair is a common problem in Cushing's syndrome. The effect is within the wound and can be achieved by local steroid administration. The major mechanism appears to be through the exclusion of inflammatory cells, especially macrophages from the wound. If adequate doses of topical or systemic vitamin A are given, the effect can be mostly, but not entirely, overcome. Clean, primary repair usually goes to completion, albeit slowly, despite steroid administration. However, once the wound is open, the effects of steroids become vastly more troublesome.

Sex hormones are also wound-active. Estrogen depresses collagen synthesis and tensile strength mildly. Progesterone depresses them markedly. The combination of the two, as in most birth control pills, even more markedly retards repair. Progesterone increases neovascularization and oxygen supply. It also increases inflammation and therefore inhibits collagen synthesis. When estrogen is added, neovascularization is reduced to normal and repair is further decreased. Nevertheless, in most animals, females repair somewhat faster than males, and a pregnant or recently pregnant woman has extraordinary reparative powers.

Anabolic steroids, or male hormones, have long been touted as enhancers of repair. They have little practical value except that they share, with vitamin A, the power to counteract steroid retardation of repair, and can accelerate normal collagen synthesis in wounds, but only by a few percent.

Adrenocorticotropic hormone (ACTH), growth hormone, and thyroid hormone all have some influence on repair, but it seems minor in most instances. Some data suggest that aldosterone enhances repair. Insulin seems necessary for repair, if only in the sense that it is required to correct diabetic hyperglycemia. Diabetes, on the other hand, inhibits repair in many ways and is one of its most potent antagonists.

A number of substances increase fibroblast replication in culture including a platelet factor and a human, brain-derived fibroblast growth factor. Thrombin, insulin, and small doses of steroid seem to aid these growth factors. The clinical significance of these substances is uncertain.

CELLULAR INTERACTIONS IN THE WOUND; THE WOUND MODULE REVISITED

It seems helpful to visualize repair in terms of a functioning unit of tissue, termed here a "module." The basic concept is that macrophages, fibroblasts, and growing vascular tissue form a unit of interacting cells that support, regulate, stimulate, and nourish each other. The function of no one of these components can be fully understood in the absence of the others. Perhaps one might think of the module as the granule in granulation tissue or perhaps as the adhesion in peritoneal repair.

Figure 1.17 is a schematic diagram of tissue in which a wound has been made. The cut microvasculature has thrombosed and the initial bleeding has stopped. Platelets have been activated by collagen and thrombin and are already probably releasing mitogens.

One can now visualize the nutrition of a given point in the wound much as the nutrition of an orange seed after the orange has been cut in two through the seed in question and exposed to air. Whereas nutrition previously came from the sphere surrounding the seed, it now comes from a hemisphere. Whereas nutrition normally could be brought in from sources immediately adjacent, whatever nutrition that can reach the unfortunate seed after cutting and surface drying must do so by diffusion through damaged tissue. Now, leaving the analogy and returning to normal tissue, the vasculature that was once geared to the almost unvarying needs of connective tissue, or fascia, has thrombosed and is no longer adequate to meet the needs of exposure. Desiccation occurs rapidly. Furthermore, in the next few days, the injured area will become suffused with

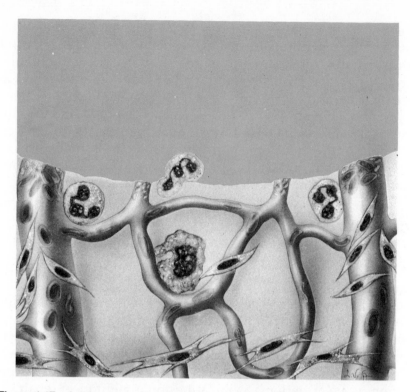

Figure 1.17 A schematic representation of the edge of the wound just after injury. Vessels have thrombosed and an inflammatory exudate, mostly polymorphonuclears, is appearing. Serum covers or fills the wound, and serum contains stimulators of cell replication at least partly made by platelets.

metabolically active white cells and then will become densely populated with metabolically active fibroblasts. Thus, at a time when connective tissue needs more nutrition than ever before in its life, its nutritional sources are least able to meet the need. Oxygen supply is inadequate, local P_{O_2} is low, and P_{CO_2} is high. Although, as discussed above, the exact signals are not known, it makes reasonable teleologic sense that an energy crisis has occurred, and emergency signals for increased nutrition are sent back to the nearest functioning vasculature (Fig. 1.18). This vasculature responds by sending capillary buds into the wounded area.

Now the symbiosis of the ecologic unit, the wound module, becomes apparent. The fibroblasts probably cannot migrate into the wounded area until the activated platelets and macrophages give the signal. The fibroblast is not actively encouraged to make collagen until lactate concentrates, and this lactate is probably largely formed by the macrophage. The signal for cell replication and collagen synthesis cannot be met unless oxygen, amino acids, glucose, trace metals, vitamins, and probably other elements are supplied by the vascular system, and most of these elements cannot diffuse over more than the shortest tissue distances. Hence, the fibroblast cannot respond to its stimulus until the vascular system has regenerated sufficiently to supply it. On the other hand, the vascular system cannot merely poke a vascular sprout into a space and then

Figure 1.18 Side view of the wound module as in a rabbit ear chamber. The P_{O_2} profile is shown above the tissue. Note the peaks over the vessels and the long gradient down to almost zero at the wound edge. Note the lactate gradient, high in the dead space and lower towards the vasculature. This demonstrates how the central wound remains hypoxic and acidotic despite the advancing vasculature.

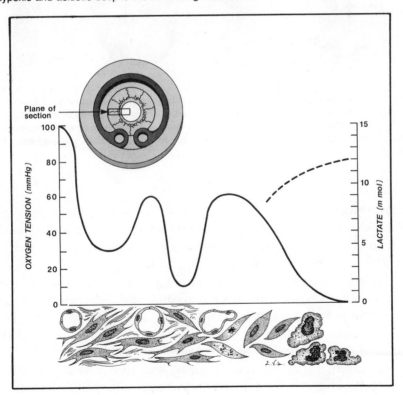

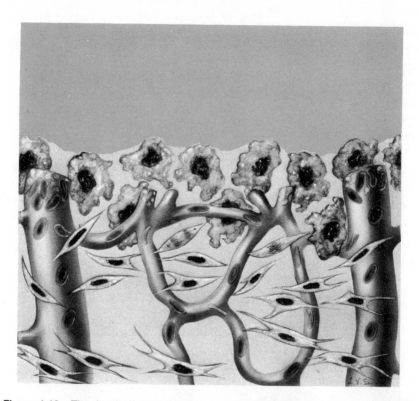

Figure 1.19 The developing "granulation tissue" now shows a more orderly arrangement of inflammatory response which is now predominantly macrophagic. Fibroblasts have appeared mostly from perivascular cells. Their mitoses are seen near the most distal functioning vessels. Endothelial capillary buds are appearing in the center of the preexisting capillary arcade. Macrophages are now in a position to stimulate angiogenesis and fibroplasia.

pump blood through it if there is no external support to prevent bursting. Hence, the lead fibroblast must struggle ahead with minimal nutrition until sufficient collagen gel is laid down to support the budding capillary (Fig. 1.19).

Once a new cycle of circulation has been established after two capillary buds, one from a higher and one from a lower pressure system, have met and fused, nutrition suddenly becomes more adequate to the mixture of macrophages and fibroblasts. The previously hypoxic fibroblast near the wound edge inherits a better food supply and can now make more collagen. The cell then provides a matrix by which the macrophage in the van of the advancing module can move ahead and fibroblasts can follow until the cells once again reach the limits of their supply lines where they again signal for a new vascular system. In watching granulation tissue grow, one has the feeling that each fibroblast is "born" into its "permanent" position. It performs its function in that spot while the vascular system and the rest of its "world" move past it. The new fibroblast is usually formed from a mitotic figure just distal to the most distal functioning capillary loop. The new fibroblast, therefore, is thrust into a hypoxic environment and is activated by it. As the vasculature moves by, the fibroblast, still in its same position, is given a more secure environment with greater energy supply and secretes more and more collagen into the

Figure 1.20   A new functioning capillary loop has been formed. The "wound module" is complete. Some of the old vasculature, now being in an area of lessened metabolic demand, is dropping out. Compare this idealized version with the photomicrograph in Figures 1.1 and 1.2.

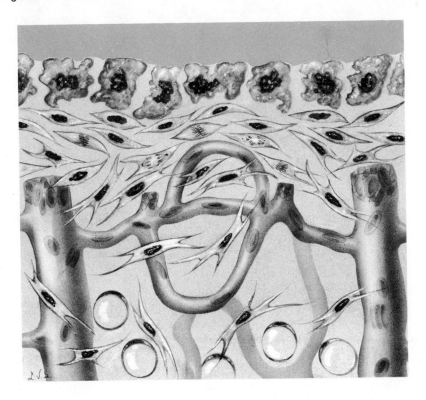

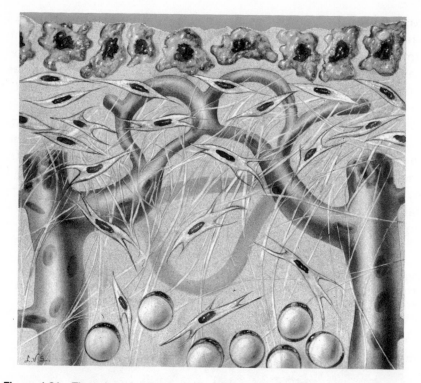

Figure 1.21 The edge of the wound has advanced, more new capillary loops have formed while those behind have dropped out. The supplying artery and vein are getting larger and larger. Compare this with Figure 1.2 and 1.22 which are an actual photographs of new vasculature advanced to about the same degree.

tissue spaces beside it. Meanwhile, the macrophage moves on (Fig. 1.20).

In uncomplicated repair, for instance the filling of an uninfected dead space, the fibroblast eventually disappears at the end of its life span. Much of the collagen that it had deposited to perform various vital functions has now been removed and replaced by fat (remodeling). As a result, the empty space made by the surgeon, first filled with tissue fluid, then with macrophages and early fibroblasts, then vessels and collagen, is left filled with fibrofatty tissue. The module moves across the dead space leaving behind it a kind of remodeled subcutaneous tissue of fat and collagen, unless the new tissue either remains inflamed or performs a mechanical function. In either of these

58

cases, the maturation to fatty tissue does not occur and the area remains tough and collagenous.

The evolution of the neovasculature is shown in the series of diagrams and in the photomicrograph of a rabbit ear chamber (Figs. 1.19–1.22). The advancing edge of granulation tissue is characteristically rich with microvasculature. As this portion of the tissue migrates into the dead space, the older microvasculature drops out leaving longer and larger stem vessels giving the effect of a grape arbor arising from the earth in a stout trunk growing ever upward into its smaller functioning branches.

In the primarily closed wound, this whole process is, of course, not necessary. In the first place, the tissue damage is usually less. If the wound edges are reunited well, their nutrition obviously reaches the center point from both sides of the wound. The coagulative process is followed by fibrinolysis, and some of the damaged vasculature is probably reopened to flow.

Figure 1.22 Actual photograph of a rabbit ear chamber. All the vessels shown are new since the ear chamber was empty at the time it was implanted. Note the large and long feeding vessels and the capillary arcades just beneath the edge of the wound. The slight "halo" just beyond the last functioning capillary is the van of the wound module. The dark area is the unfilled dead space. Note the new capillary loops to the left near the dead space—one predominates. *(Courtesy of Ian Silver, Professor of Comparative Pathology, Department of Pathology, University of Bristol, England.)*

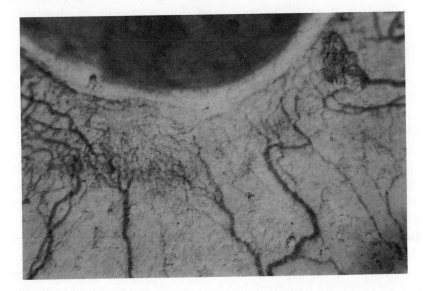

Although the mechanism is unknown, vessels reunite across the wound. With this mechanism available, the macrophage that reaches the center of the wound has relatively little debridement to do, and is exposed to desiccation and hypoxia for a relatively short period of time. Relatively few fibroblasts are needed to give support to already reasonably well supported microvasculature, and the process proceeds to completion with vastly less expenditure of energy.

This concept gives an interesting insight into certain clinical situations. Ischemic tissue in the foot of an arteriosclerotic patient may have enough vasculature to support itself, but once wounded it may not be able to support repair. Other, perhaps less ischemic tissue, will support primary repair, as in a transmetatarsal amputation. But if that suture line once opens and the underlying tissue is committed to heal by secondary intention, the energy available, while possibly able to support primary wound healing, cannot support the energy demands of secondary repair. Loss of the amputation stump then becomes inevitable.

If one keeps in mind the two polar situations, that of the granulating wound and that of the primarily closed wound, there should be relatively little doubt about how healing by delayed primary closure occurs. The wound is left open to air for about five days. The early wound module is usually forming by the fourth or fifth day when delayed primary closure is performed. When the wound edges are brought together, the layers of macrophages on each side fuse to form one, serving both sides. The growing capillary buds, instead of joining other sprouts from the same side, may find it more convenient to join sprouts from the other side. The microvasculature is thus formed and the wound has successfully come through its most ischemic, hypoxic, and vulnerable phase.

The diagrams of the wound module show the gradients of oxygen, lactate, and carbon dioxide occurring in the normally healing dead space (see Fig. 1.18) On inspection of these gradients, it should become apparent that the advancing edge of the healing wound is in a tenuous position. Cells have migrated out to the very limits of their ability to function. If the tenuous oxygen supply is interrupted or depressed, the cells that are at their survival limits may die. At the very least, they may temporarily lose function because of the extreme hypoxia.

The pathophysiology of variations in the blood gas environment will be discussed in the chapter on disorders of repair.

In examination of the metabolic gradients, the reader may find an apparent contradiction. I have stated that the greater the oxygen supply, the better the repair (or the lesser the oxygen supply the slower the repair). Yet I have said that hypoxia is an important stimulus. At first it seems that if more oxygen were added to this system, one would expect that the oxygen gradient into the wound space would be shifted upward, the most distal cells would be better supplied, and the lactate levels in the wound edge would fall, thus diminishing the stimulus to collagen formation. Conversely, if the oxygen content were to fall, lactate content would rise and the stimulus to collagen synthesis might increase.

The resolution is relatively simple. Fibroblasts, epidermal cells, and macrophages are facultative anaerobes. When more oxygen is supplied, they use it (as noted above). As a result, when excess oxygen is given, the peak P_{O_2} at the capillary nearest the wound edge is, in fact, elevated. However, the P_{O_2} at the wound edge is essentially unchanged because the excess oxygen has been consumed. The oxygen level in the wound space can be raised appreciably only if the capillary P_{O_2} is elevated to extreme levels reachable only by giving hyperbaric oxygen. Therefore, with the usual means of achieving hyperoxia, the essential hypoxia of the wound space is unchanged and the lactate "stimulus" remains. The extra oxygen may be used for several purposes, e.g., more efficient energy production, increased hydroxylation of proline and lysine, increased use by leukocytes.

If oxygen supply is diminished, cellular function is lost. Epidermal cells can survive but cannot migrate or divide. Even macrophages in the complete absence of oxygen begin to lose their cell membrane potential, their sodium and potassium pump mechanisms begin to fail; and they, together with the fibroblasts, begin to leak potassium and eventually may die. In the case of the fibroblast (see collagen above), molecular oxygen is required for hydroxylation of lysine and proline. Unless a significant number of prolines and lysines is hydroxylated, the collagen cannot leave the cell and lactate may accumulate. Unless more oxygen is supplied, collagen synthesis inevitably fails.

WOUND HEALING AS A MORE GENERAL PHENOMENON

Any surgeon who is familiar with pathology will have recognized by this time that the reparative process is not restricted to surgical wounds. It is seen in a wide variety of diseases, all of which are characterized by inflammation or interference with tissue nutrition, or both. The fibrosis seen in the healing surgical wound is not significantly different from the fibrosis in a developing atheroma, except that in the latter lipid deposition is somewhat more prominent. Menkin described wounds as granulomas, and he lumped them with such various diseases as rheumatic fever and reactions to foreign bodies. The fibrosis that obliterates the lung in organizing pneumonia contains the same fibroblasts and the same macrophages that are seen in surgical wounds, and the same can be said for scirrhous carcinomas. Though the discussion in this book is limited to management of the surgical wound, it is fascinating to consider how these observations apply to a wide variety of disease processes such as arteriosclerosis, arthritis, inflammatory immune processes, scirrhous carcinomas, strictures, scleroderma, and others. If one examines this perspective, the mitogens secreted by the activated platelet and macrophage begin to assume an impressively important position in human biology and disease.

SUMMARY

Consideration of the basic mechanisms of wound healing underscores the vital principle of surgery that tissue must be respected and must be handled gently. The more damage done to a wound edge, the more microvasculature remains to be regenerated, the more ischemic tissue must be debrided, and the larger the gaps that must be bridged by epithelium, vessel, and fiber. Furthermore, dead tissue is easily infected. Fibroblasts and macrophages are not the only cells that must exist in the tenuous wound environment. The polymorphonuclear leukocyte, though playing no essential role in repair, must monitor the area, ingesting and killing the contaminating bacteria. As will be developed later, not only repair, but resistance to infection, depends on this environment.

The surgeon might, at first, have difficulty accepting the concept of the exquisite dependence of repair and resistance to infection on tissue perfusion, oxygenation, and nutrition.

However, he should remember that one of the oldest observations in surgery is that tissues with poor blood supply not only heal poorly but are also easily infected. Starved patients heal poorly. These are established surgical facts. Thus it is not the principle but *the degree* to which the principle governs that is hard to accept. Experimental fact says that the basic principle is operative in proportion to the degree of perfusion or nutrition deficit *starting from normal*. Biologically, this concept is more acceptable than one necessitating postulation of a "magic" dividing line which occurs at some mysterious distance between the normal and the observably pathologic.

Thus, if the surgeon wants optimal repair, he has to aim for optimal physiologic conditions. The better the condition of the patient, the better the condition of the wound. "A little" hypovolemia, "a little" hypoxia, "a little" malnutrition, "a little" antiinflammatory steroid take their toll. Only a full understanding of the process of repair can aid the surgeon in avoiding its disorders.

BIBLIOGRAPHY

Each reference in this selected bibliography has been chosen on the basis of its appropriateness for the beginning student of wound management. Many references were included not just because they are current, but also because their own bibliographies will lead the interested student into the more detailed pertinent literature. Others were chosen because they will direct the reader to the major recent books and compendia.

Cellular Aspects of Repair

Branemark PI: Capillary form and function: The microcirculation of granulation tissue. Bibl Anat 4:9, 1965

Gospodarowicz D, Moran JS: Stimulation of division of sparse and confluent 3T3 cell populations by a fibroblast growth factor, dexamethasone, and insulin. Proc Nat Acad Sci 71 (11):4584, 1974

Harington JS: Fibrogenesis. Environ Health Persp 9:271, 1974

Hunt TK, Ehrlich HP, Garcia JA, Dunphy, JE: Effect of vitamin A on reversing the inhibitory effect of cortisone on healing of open wounds in animals and man. Ann Surg 170:633, 1969

Leibovich SJ, Ross R: The role of macrophages in wound repair. Am J Pathol 78:71, 1975

Levene CI, Heslop J: The synthesis of collagen by cultured pig aortic endothelium and its possible role in the pathogenesis of the fibrous atherosclerotic plaque. J Molec Med 2:145, 1977

McLean AEM, Ahmed K, Judah JD: Cellular permeability and the reaction to injury. Ann NY Acad Sci 116:986, 1964

Ross R, Odland G: Fine structure observations of human skin wounds and fibrinogenesis. In Dunphy JE, Van Winkle W Jr (eds): Repair and Regeneration. New York, McGraw-Hill, 1969

Schoefl GI: Studies on inflammation, III. Growing capillaries; their structure and permeability. Virchows Arch Pathol Anat 337:99, 1963

Spector WG, Lykke WJ: The cellular evolution of inflammatory granulomata. J Pathol Bact 92:103, 1966

Stephens FO, Dunphy JE, Hunt TK: Effect of delayed administration of corticosteroids on wound contraction. Ann Surg 173:214, 1971

Vassalli J, Hamilton J, Reich E: Macrophage plasminogen activator: modulation of enzyme production by anti-inflammatory steroids, mitotic inhibitors, and cyclic nucleotides. Cell 8:271, 1976

Weeks JR: Prostaglandins. Ann Rev Pharmacol 12:317, 1972

Zweifach BW, Grant L, McCluskey RT (eds): The Inflammatory Process, 2nd ed. New York, Academic Press, 1973–74

Physiology of Repair

Ehrlich HP, Grislis G, Hunt TK: Metabolic and circulatory contributions to oxygen gradients in wounds. Surgery 72:578, 1972

Heughan C, Grislis G, Hunt TK: The effect of anemia on wound healing. Ann Surg 179:163, 1974

Hunt TK: Physiology of repair. In Gibson T, van der Meulen JC (eds): Wound Healing. 1st International Symposium on Wound Healing, Rotterdam, April, 1974. Montreux, Switzerland, Foundation for International Cooperation in the Medical Sciences, 1975

Hunt TK, Pai MP: Effect of varying ambient oxygen tensions on wound metabolism and collagen synthesis. Surg Gynecol Obstet 135:561, 1972

Niinikoski, J: Oxygen and wound healing. Clin Plast Surg 4:361, 1977

Niinikoski J, Hunt TK, Dunphy JE: Oxygen supply in healing tissue. Am J Surg 123:247, 1972

Remensnyder JP, Majno G: Oxygen gradients in healing wounds. Am J Pathol 52:301, 1968

Silver IA: In Pikkarainen J, (ed): Biology of the Fibroblast, Sigrid Juselius Foundation Symposium. London, Academic Press, 1974

Epithelization

Im, MJC, Hoopes JE: Energy metabolism in healing skin wounds. J Surg Res 10:459, 1970

Johnson FR, McMinn RM: The cytology of wound healing of body surfaces in mammals. Biol Rev 35:364, 1952

Rovee DT, Kurowsky CA, Labun J, Downes AM: Effect of local wound environment on epidermal healing. In Maibach HI, Rovee DT (eds): Epidermal Wound Healing. Chicago, Year Book Medical Publishers, 1972

Silver IA: Oxygen tension and epithelization. In Maibach HI, Rovee DT (eds): Epidermal Wound Healing. Chicago, Year Book Medical Publishers, 1972

Wound Contraction

Abercrombie M, Flint MH, and James DW: Collagen formation and wound contraction during repair of small excised wounds in the skin of rats. J Embryol Exp Morph 2:264, 1954

Guber S, Rudolph R: The myofibroblast. Surg Gynecol Obstet 146:649, 1978

Montandon D, D'Andiran G, Gabbiani G: The mechanism of wound contraction and epithelization. Clin Plast Surg 4:325, 1977 (Note: The most recent and extensive review but brief and easy reading).

Rudolph R, Woodward M: Spatial orientation of microtubules in contractile fibroblasts in vivo. Anat Rec 191:169, 1978

Ryan GB, Cliff W Jr, Gabbiani G, et al: Myofibroblasts in human granulation tissue. Human Pathol 5:55, 1974

Stone PA, Madden JW: Effect of primary and delayed split skin grafting on wound contraction. Surg Forum 25:41, 1974

Van Winkle W, Jr: Wound contraction. Surg Gynecol Obstet 125:131, 1967

Collagen Structure and Synthesis

Bailey AJ, Sims TJ, LeLons M, Bazin S: Collagen polymorphism in experimental granulation tissue. Biochem Biophys Res Comm 66:1160, 1975

Barnes MJ: Function of ascorbic acid in collagen metabolism. Ann NY Acad Sci 258:264, 1975

Bauer EA, Eisen AZ, Jeffrey JJ: Regulation of vertebrate collagenase activity in vitro and in vivo. J Invest Dermatol 59:50, 1972

Chung E, Keels EM, Miller EJ: Isolation and characterization of the cyanogen bromide peptides from the (111) chain of human collagen. Proc Nat Acad Sci 70:3521, 1973

Comstock JP, Undenfriend S: Effect of lactate on collagen proline hydroxylase activity in cultured L-929 fibroblasts. Proc Nat Acad Sci 66(2):552, 1970

Gay S, Miller EJ, Fischer G: Collagen in the Physiology and Pathology of Connective Tissue. New York, Springer-Verlag. 1978. Note: The most current reference on collagen in pathologic conditions.

Gould BS: Ascorbic acid-independent and ascorbic acid-dependent collagen-forming mechanisms. Ann NY Acad Sci 92(1):168, 1961

Hawley PR, Faulk WP, Hunt TK, Dunphy JE: Collagenase activity in the gastro-intestinal tract. Br J Surg 57:896, 1970

Hodge AJ, Schmitt FO: The charge profile of the tropocollagen macromolecule and the packing arrangement in native type collagen fibrils. Proc Nat Acad Sci 186, 1960

Ireland RL Kang AJ, Igarasli S, Gross J: Isolation of two distinct collagens from chick cartilage. Biochemistry 9:4993, 1970

Kefalides NA: Isolation of a collagen from basement membrane containing three identical α chains. Biochem Biophys Res Comm 45:226, 1971

Kivirikko KI, Prockop DJ: Enzymatic hydroxylation of proline and lysine in protocollagen. Proc Nat Acad Sci 57:782, 1967

Levene CI, Bates CJ: The effect of hypoxia on collagen synthesis in cultured 3T6 fibroblasts and its relationship to the mode of action of ascorbate. Biochim Biophys Acta 444:446, 1976

Monson JM, Bornstein P: Identification of a disulfide-linked procollagen as the biosynthetic precursor of chick-bone collagen. Proc Nat Acad Sci 70:3521, 1973

Nimni ME: Collagen: its structure and function in normal and pathological connective tissues. Semin Arthritis Rheum 4(2):95, 1974

Page RC, Benditt EPA: A molecular defect in lathyritic collagen. Proc Soc Exp Biol Med 124:459, 1967

Tanzer ML: Crosslinking of collagen. Science 180:561, 1973

Van Winkle W Jr: The fibroblast in wound healing. Surg Gynecol Obstet 124:369, 1967

Viljanto J: Biochemical basis of tensile strength in wound healing. Acta Chir Scandinav Suppl 333, 1964

Miscellaneous

Brunius V: Wound healing impairment from sutures. Acta Chir Scandinav (Suppl) 395, 1968

Chvapil M: Pharmacology of fibrosis: definitions, limits, and perspectives. Life Sciences 16:1345, 1975

Ehrlich HP, Hunt TK: Effects of cortisone and vitamin A on wound healing. Ann Surg 167:324, 1968

Hunt TK, Hawley PR: Surgical judgment and colonic anastomoses. Dis. Colon Rectum 12:167, 1969

Oegema TR, Laidlaw J, Hascall VC, Dziewiatkowski DD: The effect of proteoglycans on the formation of fibrils from collagen solutions. Arch Biochem Biophys 170:698, 1975

Pareira MD, Serkes KD: Prediction of wound disruption by use of the healing ridge. Surg. Gynecol Obstet 115:72, 1962

Smahel J: The healing of skin grafts. Clin Plast Surg 4:409, 1977

General and Reviews

Gibson T, van der Meulen JC (eds): Wound Healing. 1st International Symposium on Wound Healing, Rotterdam, April, 1974. Montreux, Switzerland, Foundation for International Cooperation in the Medical Sciences, 1975 (note: A recent compendium of current research).

Kulonen E, Pikkarainen J (eds): Biology of fibroblast, Fourth Sigrid Juselius Foundation Symposium, Turku, Finland, August 1973. New York, Academic Press, 1973 (note: A truly excellent compendium of various specialized topics in collagen chemistry and wound healing).

Majno G: The Healing Hand. Man in the Ancient World. Cambridge, Ma., Harvard University Press, 1975 (note: An elegant history of man and his wounds).

McMinn RMH: Tissue Repair. London, Academic Press, 1969. (note: Especially strong on the biologic and comparative aspects).

Peacock EE Jr, Van Winkle W Jr: Surgery and Biology of Wound Repair. Philadelphia, Saunders, 1970

Rogers BO (consultant), Montandon D (ed): Clinics in Plastic Surgery. An International Quarter. Symposium on Wound Healing, vol 4, no 3. Philadelphia, Saunders, 1977 (note: A recent compendium of reviews of specific topics. Has excellent sections on epithelization, contraction, oxygen, and skin grafts).

Schilling JA: Wound healing. Physiol Rev 48:374, 1968

2
DISORDERS OF REPAIR AND THEIR MANAGEMENT
Thomas K. Hunt

The general surgeon thinks of disorders of repair in terms of wound dehiscence, anastomotic leaks, or wound infection. The plastic surgeon thinks of them as hypertrophic scar, keloid formation, and contracture. Urologists' and gastroenterologists' concerns are strictures of the esophagus, duodenum, ureter, urethra, and obstruction of the bowel due to adhesions. All of these belong to the same spectrum of disorder that, in a broader view, includes occlusion of arteries due to arteriosclerosis, deformation of heart valves due to valvulitis, and scar or stricture of the trachea due to injury or prolonged intubation. This grouping of seemingly diverse diseases may seem strange at first because many of them are best known for their ultimate result and others for their anatomic location. However, a scar is a scar whether its cause is a club, a knife, or an immune or chemical reaction—whether its location is the skin, a joint, or the vascular endothelium (Fig. 2.1.).

Some of the above examples, one will note, while truly *disorders of repair* are not necessarily *disordered* repair. In practice, it is difficult to decide just what normal repair is. What is abnormal is often confused with what simply is undesirable. The often reported belief that repair cannot be improved beyond a predetermined norm loses meaning because the predetermined norm cannot be defined. For instance, the general surgeon desires strong union of soft tissue in an acceptable time. The hand surgeon wants union of tendons, but union is useless unless the healed tendon can glide and flex within its sheath. The neurosurgeon repairing a peripheral nerve wants as little connective tissue repair as possible. Each of these surgeons has his or her own ways of modifying results of repair. Some attempt to modify repair with microscopic surgical technique, others with immobilization, still others with physical therapy, nutrition, suppressive steroids, traction, or pressure.

Methods of modifying repair will undoubtedly multiply as knowledge of its mechanisms increases. However, many of the mysteries of repair have already been investigated, and this section is dedicated to expanding the clinical use of the substantial body of data on disordered repair that is available now.

In the previous section, normal repair was described as a sequence so tightly coordinated that anything that prevents, exaggerates, or delays any part of the sequence will also modify subsequent events. Therefore, we will consider disorders of

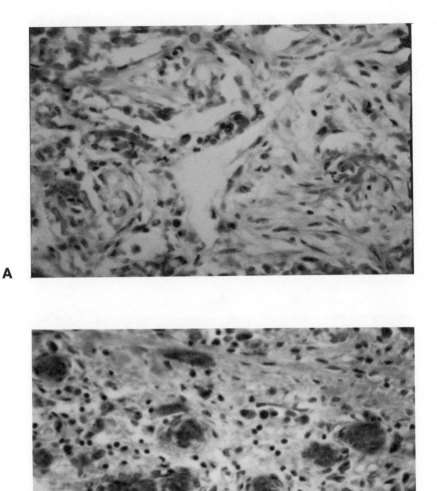

Figure 2.1 Scar tissue in disease states. **A.** Lung in organizing bacterial pneumonia. **B.** Heart with coronary thrombosis.

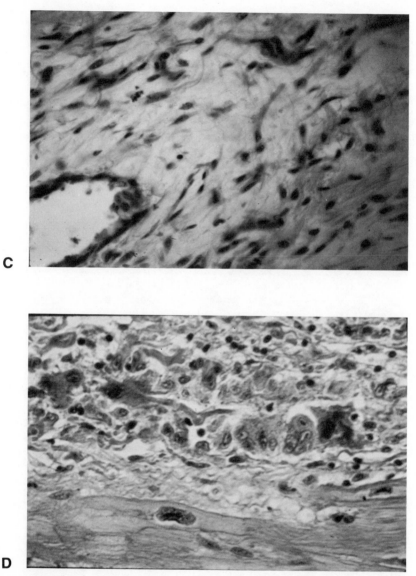

Figure 2.1 Scar tissue in disease states (contd.) **C.** Omentum in advanced peritonitis. **D.** Heart with rheumatic fever. Note that all these diverse diseases illustrate the same elements of scar.

repair in the same sequence in which the normal process was described. The reader should keep in mind that one surgeon's healing is another's scar. Therefore, in some circumstances the surgeon may wish to avoid some of the disorders mentioned, but in other circumstances the surgeon may actually wish to induce them.

THE INJURY

The character of the injury has a great deal to do with the subsequent repair. For example, chemical or immunologic "injury," when continuing to occur in a target tissue, may continue to stimulate collagen deposition. Scar gradually adds to scar, and aging scar shrinks. The foreign body that stimulates an inflammatory response will continue to excite scar formation until that foreign body is either removed by the phagocytes or by the surgeon. Perhaps the most vivid medical example is progressive pulmonary fibrosis due to inhalation of asbestos fibers (asbestosis).

Injuries heal slowly when destruction of local blood supply is a primary feature. The burn wound is such an example. During the first 48 hours after a burn injury, local vessels occlude and the area of necrosis deepens. The demarcation point between live and dead tissue is determined as much by ischemia as by thermal exchange. Because of this ischemic state, subsequent repair cannot possibly keep the pace of repair that follows a lesser injury, because to repair skin requires more nutrition than is needed to keep it alive. Healing of a burn must await neovascularization; and initiation of burn repair, therefore, is slow. For instance, if identical small third degree burns are made in an animal and one is completely excised, the excised wound will heal faster, even though it is the deeper wound at the onset.

The severity of injury influences the speed of repair. For instance, if wire mesh cylinders are implanted in animals to excite reparative ingrowth of connective tissue, the rate at which new tissue grows into each cylinder slows when another injury, such as severe leg contusion, is added.

Hemorrhage of 13 percent of blood volume incurred at the time of wounding slows repair if replacement is delayed an hour, but not if reinfusion is immediate.

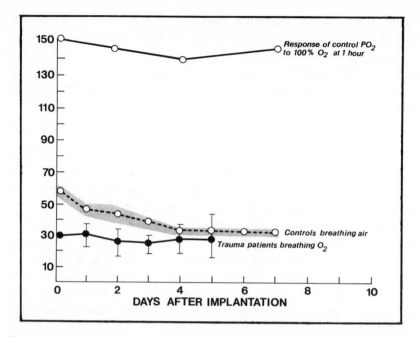

Figure 2.2 Oxygen supply in test wounds in severe trauma victims as compared to identical test wounds in normal volunteers. Note that trauma victims had low wound P_{O_2} despite oxygen breathing. The upper line represents the response of normal subjects to 100% oxygen breathing.

Repair suffers after massive injury for a number of reasons: the endocrine response to the injury is exaggerated; the catabolic response to injury is magnified; oxygen becomes less available to the injured tissue, even though cardiac output and oxygen-carrying capacity of the red cell are increased (Fig. 2.2).

An episode of shock at any time during healing, from the moment of injury onward, has the potential to delay repair. This relates the whole concept of the "sick cell" to wound healing. Injury is not only a phenomenon of tissue. It involves cells, and cells can and do suffer sublethal injury. The anatomic defects, mitochondrial loss, disruption of membranes, and so on, have been documented on many occasions. During the period of recovery, oxidative metabolism, cell membrane function, and protein synthesis must be impaired. How repair occurs within the cell is almost a total mystery. The clinical task of ensuring acceptable repair in a multiple trauma victim is vastly more difficult than in a patient with a clean elective operation.

COAGULATION AND HEMOSTASIS

The first event that follows physical injury is blood coagulation. Coagulation, of course, has its homeostatic value. In addition, as noted in the first chapter, several of the components of coagulation, namely platelets, plasminogen activator, fibrin, and thrombin, may facilitate fibroplasia and neovascularization. These proteins probably can exert their salutory effects without the accumulation of excessive blood clot within the wound.

Surgeons have had an almost pathologic fear of blood clot within wounds for many years. Halstead performed experiments showing that blood clot within tissue retains some resistance to infection and is not *necessarily* a problem in itself unless it is accompanied by significant bacterial contamination. However, blood clot in wounds is often undesirable. It is a barrier between tissue surfaces. It forces wounds to heal by secondary intention when, without clot, they may have healed primarily. Unfortunately, large clots are not simply resorbed. Much of a large clot must be replaced, i.e., "organized" by wound tissue. Therefore, large clots or excessive infiltrations of blood into tissue often lead to hard induration in wounds that may persist for many months. Blood *clot* is not a stimulator of repair as once was held by orthopedic surgeons, however. Bone ends that are held together so tightly that no hematoma can possibly enter heal better than those which are allowed to collect a blood clot.

Though blood in wounds retains some ability to suppress infection, its presence will add virulence to some infections. Injection of normally subinfective doses of *E. coli* into the subcutaneum and peritoneum become fatal infections if accompanied by injection of whole blood or hemoglobin. The hemoglobin seems to interfere with leukocyte chemotaxis and/or phagocytosis.

INFLAMMATORY RESPONSE

If no inflammation whatsoever occurs, the reparative sequence goes no further. If too little occurs, subsequent repair is slow. If too much inflammation occurs, repair may be prolonged since excessive numbers of inflammatory cells competing with fibroblasts for vital nutrition may slow repair; and excessive, continuing low grade inflammation usually leads to excessive scar.

Steroid Hormones

The human inflammatory response is extremely sensitive to steroid hormones. Any antiinflammatory steroid will suppress repair if the administration is begun at or before the time of wounding or within the first two or three days thereafter. Polymorphs and macrophages fail to enter the wound. Therefore, the signal for fibroplasia is presumably suppressed, fibroblasts fail to appear, and the wound remains indolent. The signals for neovascularization also seem to fail, thus diminishing energy sources.

In practice, steroids alone rarely bring repair to a complete standstill unless given in very large doses. Primarily closed wounds in the renal transplant patient taking steroids usually heal in a reasonable time. However, if the wound is left open, or falls open, the steroid effect becomes vastly more significant. We frequently see transplant patients who are healing a primarily closed surgical wound satisfactorily, but at the same time cannot heal an open wound such as one from an intravascular shunt or an avulsion of skin. As noted before, the open wound requires more circulation and more energy expenditure for healing than the primarily closed wound.

Antiinflammatory steroids started four or five days after injury, when inflammation is already well developed, inhibit repair considerably less than steroids started just after wounding. Therefore, when necessary, it is possible to allow the inflammatory process to begin and to delay administration of needed steroids until after the fourth or fifth day. Though primary repair can be protected by this means, contraction and epithelization of open wounds will be delayed no matter when steroids are started.

The highly antiinflammatory steroid hormones are more detrimental to repair than steroids such as cortisol that have a lesser antiinflammatory effect. Certainly, when given in equivalent salt-retaining doses, the antiinflammatory steroids are far more detrimental to human repair than cortisol. Therefore, whenever it is possible, and whenever one wishes rapid, strong repair, the surgeon should substitute physiologic doses of cortisol for the more antiinflammatory steroids. Cortisol dosage can be reduced following the operation, and normal repair can be expected. However, patients with severe Cushing's syndrome, in which the long-term catabolic effects of steroids have weakened the connective tissue, will still have problems with repair because of inadequate strength of the uninjured tissue.

Antiinflammatory steroids also increase the likelihood of wound infection by interfering with the migration of phagocytes into the wound. This is a serious problem. Furthermore, steroids inhibit the clinical signs of infection, often allowing it to progress undetected.

The replacement dose of cortisol to support a postoperative patient is usually 100 mg cortisol phosphate intravenously or intramuscularly every 8 hours. The second day it is usually 50 mg every 8 hours. Thereafter, the doses are usually adjusted to the needs of the individual. At this level, there is little or no effect on the healing wound. Every normal postoperative patient receives approximately these amounts from endogenous sources.

Vitamin A and Anabolic Steroids

If antiinflammatory steroids cannot be stopped, or if they have already suppressed the reparative process, some repair can be stimulated by administering vitamin A or so-called anabolic steroids. These agents can restimulate a suppressed inflammatory reaction. How they do so is unknown, but they are thought to reverse the stabilizing effect of steroids on lysozomal and cell membranes. Vitamin A is also an excellent immune adjuvant. In the laboratory both humoral- and cell-mediated immune mechanisms retarded by steroids have been restimulated by vitamin A.

Therefore, although there is little documented clinical experience to draw from, and the effect is not proved in humans, a surgeon should probably be careful about using systemic vitamin A when there is a vital need for steroid suppression of inflammation. For instance, one could safely give large doses of systemic vitamin A to a patient with chronic rheumatoid arthritis in order to prepare him for a surgical procedure. A single reactivation of arthritis may not be significant in the total ill-

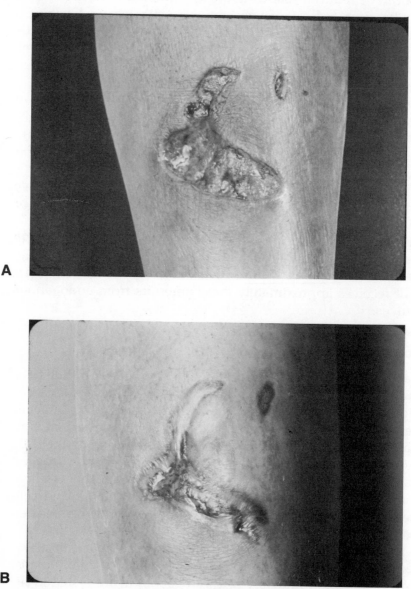

Figure 2.3 Photographs of a leg wound in a 20-year-old girl with lupus nephritis taking prednisone. **A.** At 16 days, no healing can be seen. **B** was taken a week later after seven days of topical vitamin A therapy. Note that closure is all due to epithelization and not to contraction.

78

ness. On the other hand, the addition of large doses of vitamin A to a patient holding tenuously to a vital kidney transplant could possibly tip the scales in favor of rejection. In such a case, the use of topical vitamin A has been very helpful. Little of the vitamin is absorbed when applied topically, and there is little or no evidence that exacerbations of inflammatory processes occur when topical vitamin A is used over small portions of the body (Fig. 2.3).

The optimum dose of vitamin A for this purpose is unknown. The largest dose recommended by the Food and Drug Administration is 25,000 Units per day. This dose, given for a few weeks, is safe and has seemed effective. Topical vitamin A is usually supplied in concentrations of about 1000 U/g and may be applied about three times a day, although, again the optimal dosage is unknown. Since zinc is necessary to mobilize vitamin A from the liver and since steroid therapy depresses serum zinc, some surgeons have adopted the practice of giving zinc as well as vitamin A in therapy of steroid-retarded repair. There is no proof of efficacy, however.

The effect of antiinflammatory steroids extends to the epithelial cell as well as to the inflammatory cell and fibroblast. Both epithelization and contraction are inhibited by steroids. In fact, both of these processes can be *stopped* by antiinflammatory steroids, *no matter when the steroid is given.*

Vitamin A and anabolic steroids will restimulate epithelization, but do not restimulate steroid-retarded contraction. There may be, in this slight inconsistency, a premise that one can prevent stricture of the esophagus or trachea by giving steroids, while making it possible to epithelize the open lesion with concomitant administration of vitamin A. This concept has not yet been tested.

Other Antiinflammatory Compounds

Other antiinflammatory compounds also suppress repair, though their effects are of borderline clinical significance. Careful studies on animals have shown that aspirin, phenylbutazone, and vitamin E inhibit inflammation and this effect can be reversed by vitamin A or anabolic steroids. Aspirin also increases the likelihood of wound hematoma. It seems likely that this effect is mediated through its antiplatelet activity.

79

Doses of aspirin as small as about 2 g per day will interfere with platelet function, but much larger doses are necessary to inhibit repair perceptibly.

Toxic doses of alkylators, such as nitrogen mustard, can inhibit the inflammatory response and thus delay the appearance of fibroblasts, collagen synthesis, and contraction. In this case, the major effect is on the bone marrow.

Azathioprine, an inhibitor of cellular immunity, seems not to inhibit repair.

PHAGOCYTE FUNCTION

One of the fundamental properties of a healing wound is its resistance to infection. Almost all wounds are contaminated, yet relatively few become infected. Nevertheless, a disproportionately large number of human infections begin in injured tissue. Disruption of the epithelial barrier allows entry to a variety of bacteria, yet the wound falls prey only to an exclusive group.

The magnitude of the contamination is important, but the condition of the wound is probably just as important. The well-made and well-tended surgical wound is relatively resistant to infection. A wound well made in healthy tissue can resist many more contaminating organisms than a poorly made wound, especially one in a compromised tissue or host.

Wounds possess an innate, or natural, immunity. In the past few decades, this natural immunity has emerged as the *principal* means by which the wound survives a microbial challenge. In fact, the wound possesses an extensive armamentarium of natural defense mechanisms that contribute to its overall resistance to infection. Furthermore, this natural immunity can be temporarily elevated or depressed. Experience with leukopenic patients has illustrated the critical role played by phagocytic leukocytes. In addition, several neutrophil functional deficiency states, which increase susceptibility to wound infection, have been recognized (see Table 2.1).

The aim of this section is to trace the antibacterial activity of the leukocyte as it functions in the wound and as its function may be affected by the wound.

Table 2.1 Table of Leukocyte Disorders

Disorders of chemotaxis and mobility	"Lazy" leukocyte syndrome
	Diabetes mellitus (hyperglycemia)
	Corticosteroid therapy
	Ethanolism
	Certain types of sepsis
	Hyperosmolar syndromes
	Acquired complement deficiencies
	Sarcoidosis
Disorders of opsonization	Rheumatoid arthritis
	Ethanolism
	Acute glomerulonephritis
	Burns
	Sickle cell disease
	Multiple myeloma
Defective granule function	Myelogenous leukemia
	Chédiak-Higashi syndrome
	Neutrophil pyruvate kinase deficiency
Depression of oxidative killing	Chronic granulomatous disease
	Wounded tissue
	Tissue hypoxia (sickle cell disease)
	G-6-PD deficiency (rare)
	Myeloperoxidase deficiency

Margination, Migration, and Chemotaxis

As soon as the wound is made, leukocytes of all varieties marginate, i.e., stick to the endothelium of small vessels. They slip through the leaky barrier between endothelial cells, attracted by any of a number of substances ranging from products of macrophages, to bacterial metabolites, and complement factors. After the cells leave the circulation and squeeze through tiny orifices, they migrate long distances through damaged tissue and arrive in a cleanly incised wound in good functioning order, not detectably changed from their fellow leukocytes still in circulation. Antiinflammatory steroids and uncontrolled diabetes suppress this chemotaxis and migration.

Recognition and Opsonization

Having arrived in the wound, phagocytes must recognize their natural prey. Phagocytes cannot ingest many organisms unless the organisms are first exposed to either serum or specific antibody. Substances in serum that attach to microorganisms and facilitate ingestion by phagocytes are referred to as opsonins. The best understood opsonic substances are in the complement system. The opsonic molecules on the bacterial surface fix the bacterium to the cell wall of the phagocyte through an interaction with receptor molecules on its surface. There is conflicting evidence on opsonic activity of fluid taken from human wounds. Opsonins for staphylococci are the same in serum and wound fluid. Wound fluid opsonins for *E. coli*, however, appear to be depressed. No others have been tested.

Figure 2.4   Electron microscopic view of a polymorpho-nuclear leukocyte (granulocyte) in the act of ingesting a bacterium. Note the close approximation of granulocyte cell membrane to the bacterium. This "approximation" is aided by opsonins. *(Photograph courtesy of Dorothy Bainton M.D., Associate Professor of Pathology, University of California, San Francisco School of Medicine)*

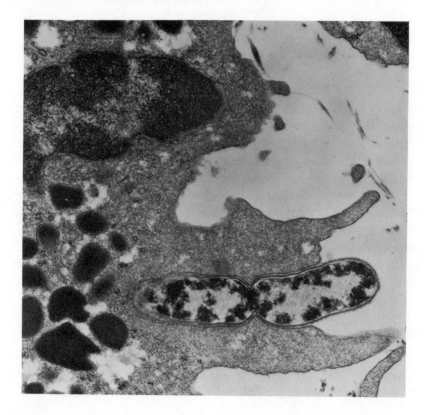

Ingestion

Once the phagocyte fixes the bacterium to its surface, its pseudopodia extend around the bacterium, eventually engulfing it (Fig. 2.4). In the process, the external cell membrane of the phagocyte invaginates to form the intracellular phagocytic vacuole or phagosome. The requisite energy can be derived from anaerobic metabolism, a fact which becomes more important as the process develops. It can occur in hypoxia, but is suppressed in uncontrolled diabetes, perhaps due to lack of energy production.

Degranulation and Microbial Killing

Nonoxidative Killing During the process of degranulation, enzyme-containing cytoplasmic granules (often called lysosomes) migrate through the cytosol toward the developing phagosome. The granule membranes fuse with the phagosomal membrane, spilling their acid hydrolases, phosphatases, highly cationic esterases, lysozyme, myeloperoxidase, and a variety of other enzymes into the digestive vacuole and onto the microbe. Enzymes escape, or are secreted, into the extracellular wound fluid as well (Fig. 2.5). Several of the granule proteins and enzymes, including lactoferin, lysozyme, and cationic esterases, have antimicrobial activity directed against certain organisms either in the phagosomes or in the extracellular fluid. Granular enzymes, therefore, soon appear in extracellular wound fluid. Myeloperoxidase and lysozyme, for instance, are highly concentrated in human wound fluid by the first postoperative day. Lysozyme can hydrolyze the protein capsules of pneumococci. Much of the innate resistance of wounds to infection may be attributable to these substances.

Oxidative Killing All of the above systems are effective in the absence of oxygen. However, complex mammalian organisms have developed an additional extremely important system of bacterial killing which selectively uses oxygen. An outline of the major features of this system is shown in Figure 2.6. The

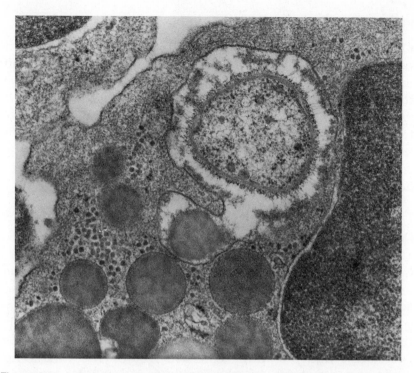

Figure 2.5 A granulocyte in the process of "degranulating." The members of the granule and the phagosome fuse like soap bubbles coalescing. The granules contain a variety of hydrolytic enzymes. See Figure 2.6. *(Photograph courtesy of Dorothy Bainton, M.D. Associate Professor of Pathology, University of California School of Medicine, San Francisco)*

hypoxic wound environment would seem to impair it.

Coincident with ingestion, the normal phagocyte exhibits an increase of oxygen consumption as much as 20 times greater than its basal rate. Some of the oxygen consumed in this respiratory burst is enzymatically reduced by a single electron to form superoxide (abbreviated O_2^-). Superoxide is an unstable molecule that has demonstrated bactericidal activity against certain strict anaerobes not equipped with superoxide dismutase (which changes O_2^- to H_2O_2). Superoxide is rapidly reduced to hydrogen peroxide in the phagosome. Hydrogen peroxide itself kills certain organisms, and in the presence of myeloperoxidase (MPO) and halide ions, the antimicrobial activity of hydrogen peroxide is greatly amplified. Other high-

84

energy derivatives such as hydroxyl radicals and singlet oxygen are formed during phagocytosis and may play a role in microbial killing as well.

The significance of this respiratory burst has only recently been recognized due to discovery of a rare but important inheritable disorder called chronic granulomatous disease (CGD). The phagocytes of children with CGD do not exhibit the increased oxygen consumption and these children are unduly susceptible to such aerobic organisms as *S. aureus, Serratia marcescens, Candida albicans, Salmonella, Pseudomonas* and some other gram-negative organisms. Cells from children with CGD do not have the primary oxidase necessary to reduce oxygen to the previously described microbicidal radicals, and therefore these cells can ingest microorganisms but cannot kill some of them.

Figure 2.6 A general, schematic diagram of the oxidative microbial killing mechanism. Most of the reduced, "active" forms of oxygen are microbicidal to certain organisms. Chronic granulomatous disease is due to an inherited absence of the primary oxidase. Note that the absence of oxygen would mimic the absence of the enzyme. The NADPH is regenerated through the hexose monophosphate shunt (HMPS). The HMPS is defective in patients with G-6-PD deficiency, and these patients are unusually susceptible to infection as well.

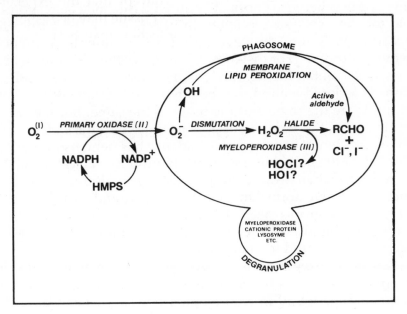

Normal leukocytes in the absence of oxygen exhibit a microbicidal defect resembling that seen in CGD. This is to be expected since the absence of the primary oxidase must be equalled by the absence of its substrate, oxygen. Obviously, without oxygen superoxide cannot be made. This may account for the particular sensitivity of wounded tissue to infection by a limited group of microorganisms. The group of organisms that typically causes infections in children with chronic granulomatous disease includes most of the common wound pathogens, except for the anaerobes. Anaerobes are killed by the nonoxidative mechanism. However, while clostridia, bacteroides, and other anaerobes are not protected from leukocyte killing in the absence of oxygen, they do grow more rapidly and produce their toxins far better in an anaerobic environment. Thus the vast majority of the common wound pathogens share one common property—they survive in a hypoxic environment. The hypoxic nature of wounds thus seems also to determine their pattern of infectibility.

That wounds in ischemic tissue are easily infected is one of the first principles of surgery. That oxygen deficiency may be the first of many possible causes of infectibility is easily integrated into clinical experience. The concept that the expected low Po_2 in otherwise "normal" injured tissue may be responsible for the usual susceptibility to infection may be harder to accept. We know, however, that environments influence wound infection. For instance, the open healing wound, while inevitably contaminated, rarely is the source of invasive infection. The closed wound, on the other hand, frequently is. The wounds are the same and the tissue is the same, but the environments of the wound surfaces in these examples are vastly different. Recent experimental evidence has demonstrated that the size of the inoculum necessary to produce clinical infection is reduced when wound oxygen tension is decreased and is increased above normal in some types of wounds when wound oxygen tension increases. Thus, there is a direct relationship between wound Po_2, the size of the inoculum, and the resistance of the wound to infection (see Fig. 2.7).

Leukocyte oxygen consumption and, presumably, peroxide production are progressively depressed as Po_2 falls into the normal range found in wounded tissue. Trauma at a distance

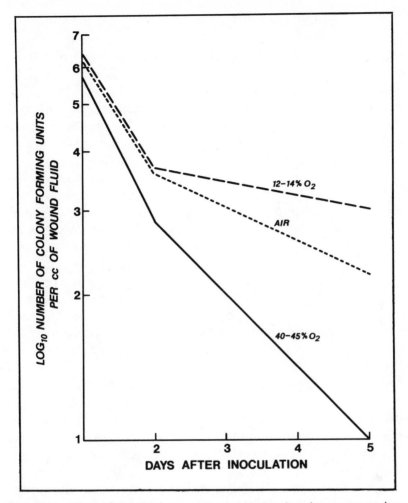

Figure 2.7 Killing of Staph 502-A in wounds of rabbits kept in various oxygen environments.

from the wound lowers wound space Po_2, and also increases susceptibility to infection. In the test tube, human leukocytes kill certain organisms more than twice as fast in air-equilibrated environments ($Po_2 = 150$) as in nitrogen ($Po_2 < 5$).

These observations, as spelled out in the language of the biochemist and physiologist, are extraordinarily important to the surgeon. Both white cell and fibroblast function are depressed by hypoxia. Wounds in hypoxic tissue heal poorly *and* become infected. This is obviously true in the arteriosclerotic extremity; and if one looks for it, it is equally true in the hypovolemic and hypoxic patient. The surgeon can enhance the natural resistance in wounds by maintaining good blood volume and adequate arterial oxygen tension. In animals, natural resistance can be increased above "normal" by maintaining slight arterial hyperoxia, up to about 40 percent to 50 percent oxygen in the breathing mixture, but this concept requires confirmation in humans. Even more, however, this effect directs attention to the technique of making wounds. Ischemic tissue, produced by hacking strokes of the knife, resists infection poorly. Tissues desiccated by cautery or dried by prolonged exposure to air cannot be perfused and are excessively infectible. Tissue strangulated by too many, too large, or too tight sutures become infected easily, even if contaminated by a minimal number of organisms. The state of the microcirculation, as left in the wound by the operating surgeon, not only determines how rapidly the wound will heal—perhaps whether it will heal at all—but also determines whether it will be able to resist the inevitable bacterial contamination.

The Achilles heel of the wound, the weak spot of antibacterial defenses, is the subcutaneous tissue. The vast majority of infections and instances of nonhealing occur there. The skin reflects the state of the subcutaneous microcirculation. As a patient becomes hypovolemic, vasoconstriction appears first in the skin. If perfusion is poor, the diligent surgeon can find it and correct it. We use a systematic examination of the pre- and postoperative patient to assess perfusion. Perfusion of the wound will be adequate if: the capillary return over the central forehead is less than 1.5 seconds; if eye turgor is normal (the standard is the examiner's eye); if mucous membranes are moist and the patient is not excessively thirsty; if the skin near the wound is warm; if the skin over the knees (where the earliest signs of vasoconstriction can be seen or felt) is only barely perceptibly cooler than the thighs and calves; if pulse and blood pressure are normal; if urine volume is adequate (this is one of the least sensitive measurements); and if the patient can stand from a recumbent position without perspiring or paling, and without a major drop of blood pressure or rise in pulse.

We have tested this examination against measurement of Po_2 in human wounds and have found the two to correlate. The only major exception is the multiple injury patient. Although wound Po2 can be kept at its highest in this patient by maintaining good clinical indices of perfusion using these tests as a guide to fluid volume replacement, wound Po2 can rarely be elevated to normal in the first four days after injury. Occasionally, sophisticated management of cardiac output and lung function can achieve near normal wound Po2. See Chapter 3 for other aspects of host resistance to infection, both normal and disturbed.

The Foreign Body and Sutures

Certain foreign bodies potentiate infection. Some are less dangerous than others. The degree of potentiation parallels the tendency to incite an inflammatory response. Figure 2.8 shows the Po2 of a wound surrounding a relatively well-tolerated foreign body. One can speculate that a microbe caught in the interstices of a porous substance, in a Po2 of zero, occupies a protected position, even more so if the space it occupies is too small to allow a leukocyte room for pursuit. Po2 around a Teflon, Silastic, or nonreactive metal implant remains relatively high, and the smooth surfaces allow no haven for bacteria.

Some foreign bodies cause such an extreme, acute inflammation that repair for a short distance around them is inhibited. They encyst in a fibrous pocket filled with leukocytes. They may cause extensive scar formation. Those foreign bodies that are smooth-surfaced (no pores large enough to accept bacteria) and do not stimulate an inflammatory reaction are well tolerated by tissue and increase infection risk minimally. From what is known of inflammatory reactions and topography of materials, it would be expected that catgut and polyfilament sutures are infectible and nylon, wire, polypropylene, and polyethylene monofilament sutures are resistant. Experimental and clinical results support this expectation.

Sutures are foreign bodies. Those which cause inflammation (catgut, cotton, silk, synthetic absorbables, and multifilament plastics, in about that order of inflammatory potential) also tend to be ejected from the wound. Deep sutures of catgut or synthetic absorbables will usually "dissolve" before they are ejected. Silk, cotton, and multifilament plastic do not dissolve

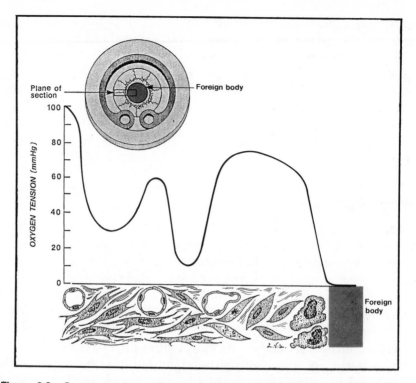

Figure 2.8 Oxygen tension profile of a well-healed rabbit ear chamber wound which contains a well-tolerated foreign body. Note that Po2 is essentially zero on the surface of the foreign substance. Po2 would start falling considerably further from the foreign body if it were to excite a chronic inflammatory reaction.

rapidly, though silk and cotton are absorbable sutures in the long run. Thus, when they incite severe inflammation through infection or immune reaction, they tend to form suture sinuses.

Choosing suture material is one of the "arts" of surgery. Fortunately, the decision is not *always* important. Wire is durable and inert but often painful to both the surgeon and the patient. Monofilament plastics are durable, usually comfortable, and inert; but none yet developed ties as easily as silk or cotton. Vascular anastomoses require plastic sutures. Anastomoses done with silk tend to attract platelets and cause local clotting. Furthermore, in the long-term anastomoses may become aneurysmal as silk sutures absorb.

The way sutures are used is frequently more important than the nature of the material used. The best surgeon can often compensate for the worst suture, and the worst surgeon can generally defeat the best suture. Specific uses of sutures will be described in other chapters.

Tape should be used to close skin whenever it is technically possible. It has proved effective in preventing infection, especially in contaminated wounds. If the wound is "wet" with blood, and tape will not stick, sutures for a day or two followed by replacement of sutures with tape give about the same protection. Skin staples may offer many of the same advantages although they have not been tested in this regard. Wounds closed with tapes and subcuticular sutures are more resistant to infection than those closed with traditional suture techniques.

Surgeon versus Granulocyte

In reality, the granulocyte and macrophage are both scavengers of wound debris and killers of microbes. They "clean up" after the surgeon. Unfortunately, each cell has a limited capacity for phagocytosis. We have demonstrated in our laboratory that if the cell expends that limited capacity to ingest dead fat, for instance, its microbicidal capacity is diminished. The surgeon has the power to minimize the dead tissue that must be ingested, and thus he has in his hands a major means of preventing infection.

NEOVASCULARIZATION

If neovascularization does not occur, the wound cannot heal. The chief known inhibitors of neovascularization are antiinflammatory steroids. Patients with severe regional vascular compromise also appear to have a poor neovascular response.

Irradiation of experimental wounds, started at or shortly after the moment of wounding, prevents cell differentiation and multiplication. Thus it suppresses the replication of vascular endothelial cells and prevents capillary budding.

Neovascularization is influenced by estrogen and progesterone. Progesterone excess seems to enhance it. Estrogen excess alone seems to inhibit it, but estrogen–progesterone combinations increase the vascularity of experimental wounds. Patients with zinc deficiency appear to have poor neovascular response, though this has not been studied. Specific inhibitors or stimulators of neovascularization have not been identified.

THE FIBROBLAST AND COLLAGEN SYNTHESIS

Disorders centering about fibroblast functions are the best known disorders of repair. (see Figs. 1.6–1.11 and 2.10–2.15.)

Fibroblast Proliferation

If the inflammatory response is suppressed by steroids, the fibroblastic response is diminished. Consequently, collagen synthesis in the new wound is retarded. However, steroids have little direct effect on fibroblasts; and when they are started the fourth or fifth day after wounding, collagen deposition is not changed.

Once the precursors of the fibroblast receive the proper signal, they reproduce. The burst of mitoses is seen on the second to fifth day. Antimitotic agents such as radiation, vinblastine, colchicine, and nitrogen mustard (alkylators), if given during this time, are wound inhibitors since they prevent cell division. Such antimetabolites as 5-fluorouracil, and antibiotics such as actinomycin D, are also detrimental for essentially the same reasons. All these drugs can be given once, on the day of wounding, with little harm to repair unless severe marrow depression occurs. From the second day until adequate tensile strength has developed (normally 7 to 10 days) wound repair is sensitive to antimitotics; but these drugs can again be given with relative safety as soon as a healing ridge is present in primarily closed wounds, or as soon as an open wound is epithelized.

Repair is retarded if a dose of nitrogen mustard large enough to prevent the normal inflammatory response is given. This effect is at least partly countered by anabolic steroids. The literature on chemotherapeutics and their effects on repair is confusing and often contradictory. Large doses, especially given early, can be deleterious; but judicious doses, kept below marrow suppression levels, are probably well tolerated on the day of wounding or by about the 10th day in a well-healing wound.

Radiation Radiation therapy, particularly through its long-term effects, presents a difficult obstacle to repair. As little as

92

250 R will retard neovascularization and contraction in an open animal wound. As with steroid hormones, however, there is a time frame. A small radiation dose (about 250 R) given 24 hours before wounding has little effect on repair. The effect of this dose then increases until it reaches a peak when the radiation is given at 36 hours after wounding. By five to seven days the effect is again considerably reduced. Radiation presumably inhibits the differentiation and the multiplication of the "stem" cells into fibroblasts or endothelial cells into proliferating vascular buds.

Also, as in the example of steroid effect, radiation is far more deleterious to an open wound than to a closed one. A securely healing wound with complete epithelization and no hidden serum or blood collection can safely receive radiotherapy, probably as early as one week postoperatively. However, if aggressive radiotherapy is given in the area of a wound space filled with pus or serum and the collection is opened later, the resulting space may not heal without special treatment.

Thus, it appears that the stem cell at rest is relatively immune to radiation. The differentiating or multiplying cell is more susceptible. One would expect, then, that repair of a wound made some time after radiation is stopped might occur relatively normally. This is quite true and has been observed in both animals and man. The usual delay period has been four to eight weeks, at which time the severe inflammation of radiation is subsiding and blood supply is still good.

As more time passes, however, irradiated tissue loses its blood flow. The typical long-term effects of irradiation develop. The skin hardens and becomes pigmented and shiny. Intimal proliferation slowly closes blood and lymph vessels, and abnormal vessels are seen as telangiectasia in the injured skin. Obviously, not all irradiated skin develops the maximal radiation change, and the risk of poor repair at this stage is proportional to the visible damage done to the local circulation. Once again, the basic principle is illustrated: ischemic tissue heals poorly and is susceptible to infection.

Open ulcers in tissues severely damaged by radiation offer a challenge to the surgeon. Debridements are followed by surface necrosis and more debridements. Tissue fails to bleed when cut. Exposed irradiated tissue often has insufficient blood

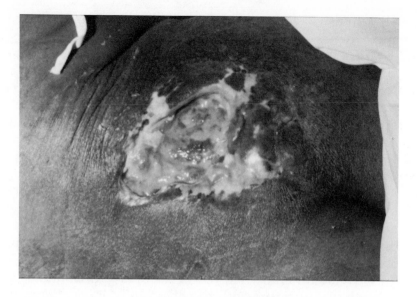

Figure 2.9 This radiation ulcer had not healed in 17 years. Though treatment with antibiotics, oxygen, xenografts and, finally, autografts took about 10 weeks, the wound has remained closed.

supply to withstand exposure without further necrosis. However, the tissue can often be saved by meticulous dressing with homograft or xenograft skin, starting immediately after adequate debridement. If 40 percent oxygen is breathed for most of the day during a few weeks of meticulous dressing, new capillaries can be seen growing into the hyalinized, radiated tissue. Skin autografts often will "take" on such tissue. Alternatively, new circulation can be brought in by operating to create pedicle flaps of skin or muscle. Recently, pedicle grafts of omentum have been used to fill large tissue defects once infection has been controlled and dead tissue has been removed (Fig. 2.9).

Even more recently, intermittent hyperbaric oxygen therapy has been used with some success. Daily exposure to hyperbaric oxygen for 30 to 60 days at 3 atmospheres pressure has been reported to allow spontaneous closure of even osteoradionecroses. The use of oxygen for this purpose seems rational since the basic defect seems to be microvascular insufficiency.

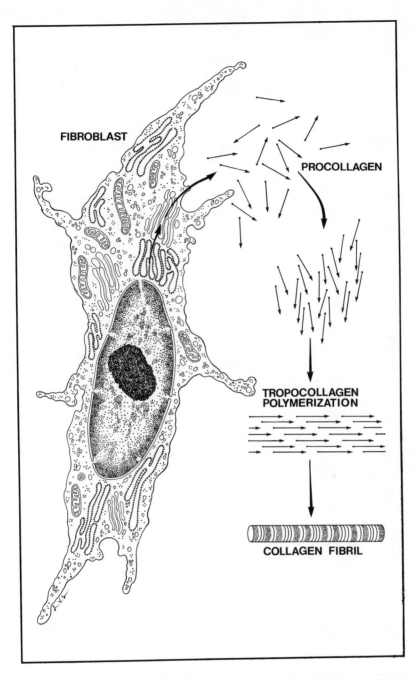

Figure 2.10 Diagrammatic representation of steps in collagen synthesis from translation to secretion. Not shown is the cleavage of the registration peptide which occurs in the extracellular space before final polymerization.

Ascorbic Acid

Little is known about the phase of collagen synthesis during which the amino acid chain is assembled. Just after it is assembled, however, several important processes occur. Hydroxylation of proline and lysine in the molecule is a particularly important step. The responsible enzymes are prolyl and lysyl hydroxylases. Their substrate is oxygen, and cofactors are ascorbic acid, ferric iron, and alpha-ketoglutarate. Without ascorbate, the collagen molecule can be synthesized up to but not beyond the point of proline and lysine hydroxylation (Fig. 2.10). If hydroxylation does not occur, collagen precursors tend to accumulate in large vacuoles within the fibroblast. Collagen turnover is unbalanced; that is, collagen synthesis is inhibited but lysis continues. Therefore, the first clinical effects of scurvy are usually purpura, from breaking unsupported small vessels (especially in the gingiva), or failure of new wounds to heal. The excessive rate of collagen turnover in wounds remains above that of normal skin for at least six months after injury. During this time, the wound is susceptible to scorbutic "paralysis" of collagen synthesis. In severe scurvy, apparently well-healed wounds have been reported to have ruptured.

Scorbutic wound failure responds with astonishing rapidity to the administration of vitamin C (large doses given by IV route are the most effective). Although this cause of wound failure was once common, it is rarely seen today in America and Europe. (see Fig. 2.11).

Oxygen

There are two ways in which oxygen deficiency may affect collagen synthesis. First hypoxia diminishes energy production. Several molecules of ATP are needed to insert each amino acid into the collagen chain. The energy requirement of ATP synthesis could be met by glycolytic or anaerobic metabolism in a hypoxic circumstance, but before much collagen could be made, a severe acidosis would occur. Certainly, total loss of oxidative metabolism should severely limit the rate of collagen synthesis. Second, as explained in the previous section, atmospheric oxygen is the substrate for hydroxylation, and no hy-

96

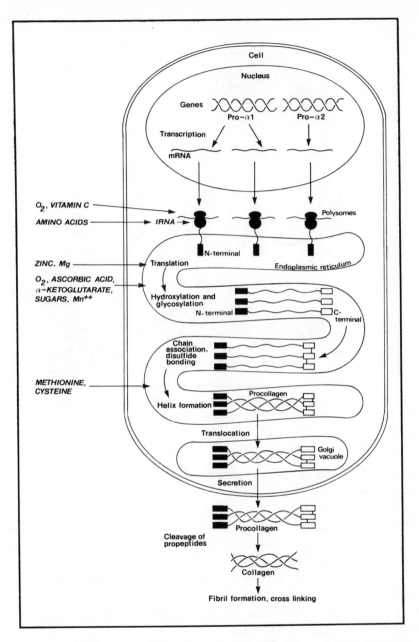

Figure 2.11 Diagrammatic representation of steps in collagen synthesis from translation to secretion. Note the cleavage of the registration peptide (the rectangles at the ends of the molecule) that occurs in the extracellular space before final polymerization. Important nutrients at certain steps are noted on the left.

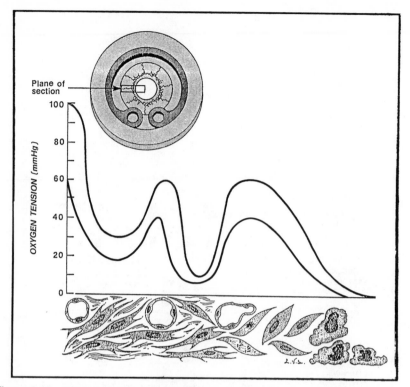

Figure 2.12 Wound chamber showing effects of systemic arterial hypoxia (lower line) as opposed to normal oxygen tension (upper line).

droxylation can occur without it. Without hydroxylation, collagen synthesis and excretion stop.

At moderately low Po_2, one of these mechanisms or the other, or both, could be the limiting factor in collagen synthesis. As Po_2 approaches zero, both mechanisms must be important. The equilibrium constant for prolyl hydoxylase suggests that hydroxylation should slow below about 20 torr. Many fibroblasts in the wound exist in tensions below this. Theoretically, therefore, any decrement of oxygen supply below normal will slow collagen synthesis.

Figures 2.12 and 2.13 show some of the dynamics of wound oxygen tension in rabbit ear chamber wounds in animals made hypoxic or hypovolemic. Of the two, hypovolemia is the most damaging. Figure 2.14 shows the vascular pattern of a normal

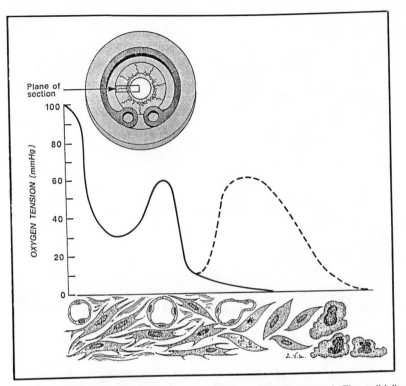

Figure 2.13 Oxygen tension profile of a rabbit ear chamber wound. The solid line represents the profile in hypovolemia, as opposed to normovolemia represented by the dashed line. The distal-most capillary shuts down as a result of volume loss, and the fragile leading edge of the wound literally becomes *an*oxic. In contrast, low arterial P_{O_2} just depresses the P_{O_2}—more at the peaks than the low points. For view of vasoconstriction due to hypovolemia, see Figure 2.14.

wound and the same field photographed after a loss of more than 20 percent of the total blood volume. Obviously, blood flow is diminished.

Anemia

Anemia is commonly, and often mistakenly, thought to affect repair. The implication is that it does so through interfering with oxygen transport to the wound. Numerous investigators have studied the relationship of anemia to wound healing because the clinical observations have excited debate. Their re-

99

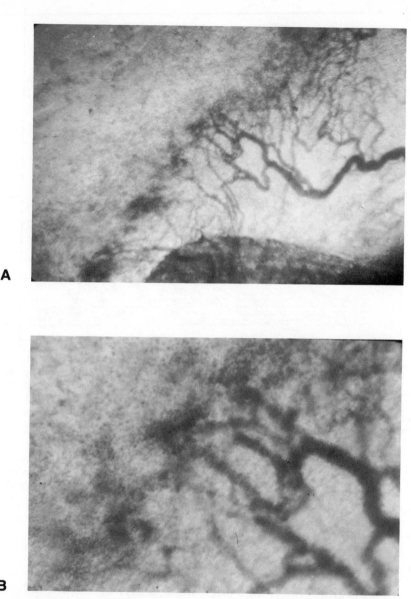

Figure 2.14 Photomicrographs of a rabbit ear chamber wound seen from the top. **C** and **D** photographs were taken of the same field as the **A** and **B** after about 20 percent of the blood volume had been removed. For the oxygen profile view of a similar wound model, see Figure 2.13.

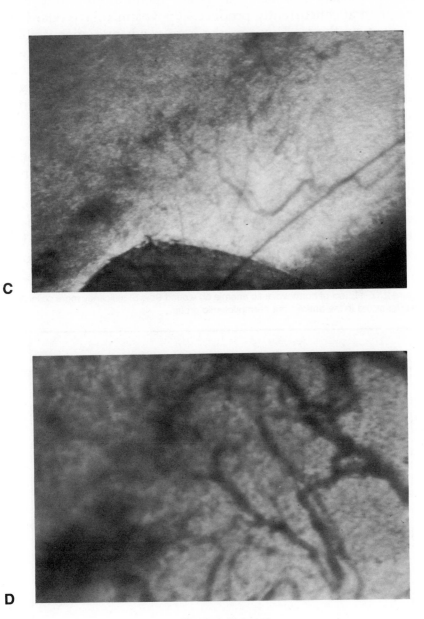

C

D

Figure 2.14 (cont.)

sults are easily summarized: Those methods of producing anemia that concurrently produce hypovolemia have retarded collagen synthesis. Those methods of producing anemia that do not produce hypovolemia have not affected repair until red cell mass falls to extremely low levels. In normal animals, if the blood volume is normal, the packed red cell volume must go below 15 percent before wound strength in primarily healing wounds is retarded. In recent tests of dead-space wounds in normal animals, a packed cell volume of 30 percent with normal blood volume was found more suitable for repair than one of 40 percent in terms of total collagen deposition in the wound (Fig. 2.15).

On ward rounds, this debate tends to degenerate to irrational levels, and a reasonable perspective must be kept. The statement that anemia is irrelevant to repair cannot be defended in every clinical case. There is no doubt that if cardiac function

Figure 2.15 Effect of normovolemic anemia on wound PO_2. Significantly more collagen was deposited in the anemic but normovolemic group.

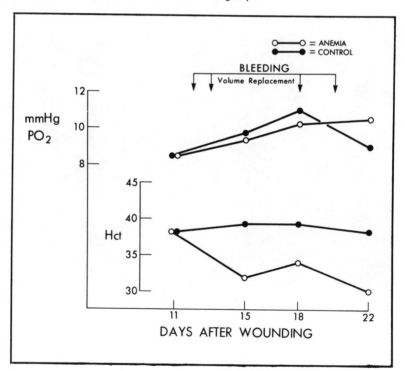

depends upon the degree of anemia, as it will in some patients with arteriosclerosis, the well being of the wound will also depend upon the degree of that anemia. If the wound in question is in a diabetic foot, cell volume may well be important. On the other hand, if an anemic patient can maintain a normal blood volume, if he can mount an increase in cardiac output to accommodate to his anemia and his surgical problem, if his 2,3,DPG levels can compensate, and if his circulatory system is in sufficiently good condition to allow the increases of blood flow in the region of the wound and those vital structures that feed it, his anemia is unimportant to his wounds and need not be corrected until packed cell volumes reach quite low levels. These conditions apply to the majority of surgical patients, and blood transfusions to "aid healing" should be given relatively rarely.

PHARMACOLOGIC INHIBITORS
OF COLLAGEN SYNTHESIS AND FIBER FORMATION

Collagen synthesis and fiber formation can be inhibited by drugs. To our conventional eye, this might seem a liability. Seen from the perspective of a sufferer from excessive scar formation, however, it may become a major advantage.

Chemotherapeutics

Inhibitors of protein synthesis, such as actinomycin D and 5-fluorouracil, will inhibit repair during the period of maximum cellular response; namely, the 2nd to 10th day in a primarily healing wound. The effect of these drugs depends mostly on the ability to prevent synthesis of nuclear protein, and somewhat less on their ability to impair protein synthesis in the cytoplasm. Therefore, such drugs given in moderation are rarely clinically important to the wound, unless they are given during the initial period of cell replication and early collagen synthesis.

Inhibitors of Proline
and Lysine Hydroxylation

Theoretically, one can supply the fibroblast with an amino acid similar to proline that meets the structural characteristics for inclusion in the polypeptide chain, but which is not subsequently hydroxylated. A number of molecules have met these requirements, including those in which the number four carbon position—the only one normally hydroxylated—is missing, is in the wrong configuration (i.e., cis vs. trans), or is already occupied by another substance (See Chap. 1). In cell culture, one can produce collagen that presumably cannot be extruded from the cell and possibly cannot be fully cross-linked. So far, however, attempts to modify the physical properties of the healing wound through this means have failed or are impractical due to toxicity of the agent.

Alternatively, hydroxylation of proline and lysine can be inhibited. α,α-dipyridyl complexes iron which is a necessary cofactor in this reaction. Large doses are toxic, and small doses are under evaluation.

Inhibitors of Intracellular Collagen Transport

Colchicine, an agent that interferes with microtubule function and arrests mitoses in metaphase, slows collagen transport from the cell to the extracellular space. In wound healing studies, colchicine suppresses epithelization, markedly retards contraction, but does not affect tensile strength (i.e., collagen deposition). Vinblastine has similar effects.

Inhibitors of Collagen Cross-Linking

Attempts to understand and thereby prevent the cross-linking of normal extracellular collagen have shown some promise as inhibitors of scar formation. Figure 2.16 shows the steps in collagen polymerization at which cross-linking can be prevented. Chronologically, the first is at the cleavage of the terminal, or registration, peptides. There is at least one enzyme responsible for this step, and a disease due to genetic absence of that enzyme has been described. In cattle the condition is called dermatosparaxis and is usually lethal. The affected calves often have skin so soft that it can be wiped away by the examiner's hand.

The next important step in collagen cross-linking is the formation of lysine-to-lysine intermolecular covalent bonds. There are several enzymes responsible for this step. The first enzyme, lysyl hydroxylase, like prolyl hydroxylase, is inhibited by lack of ascorbic acid, iron, or oxygen as noted above. The second enzyme, lysyl oxidase, converts the hydroxyl group to an aldol and initiates the lysine-lysine linkage (see Fig. 2.16). A family with a genetic disposition to a deficiency of the enzyme has been discovered. The children suffer from structural failure and usually die of the inexorable consequences of curvature of the spine, subluxation of joints, and other manifestations. Attempts to fuse bones or stiffen them with prostheses have failed. The disease has recently been tentatively called Ehlers-Danlos type V (see section on disorders of the collagen fiber).

Lysyl oxidase is also inhibited by B-aminoproprionitrile (BAPN). This effect was found by veterinarians searching for the cause of connective tissue and wound failure in cattle. Animals ingesting sweet peas called *Lathyrus odoratus* developed knock-knees, aortic aneurysms, dislocated lenses, and other signs of connective tissue "failure." The active principal was found to be BAPN. Recently, this compound has been used to prevent tendon adhesions in animals. It has also been used to prevent esophageal strictures after lye burns in dogs. The first human experiments were plagued by toxicity, and a second generation of human experiments is in progress. If "nontoxic" doses of this compound could be used to soften areas of rapid collagen turnover, a significant clinical breakthrough in diseases of scar tissue might be achieved. Undoubtedly, related compounds with similar properties remain to be discovered.

The third step in the collagen cross-linking process is inhibited by penicillamine, a metabolic by-product of penicillin. Penicillamine complexes the oxidized lysine at the aldol stage, preventing the aldol condensation. As a result, cross-linking is prevented (Fig. 2.16). Penicillamine weakens new scars and could conceivably cause approximately the same result as BAPN, except that extremely large doses are required. Penicillamine, in relatively lower doses, is used in the treatment of Wilson's disease, but its potential to modify scars has not been systematically exploited. Theoretically, very large doses of penicillin could result in accumulation of enough penicillamine to inhibit the gain of tensile strength in wounds. By extrapolation from rat data, the dose required in the human would be over 100 million units per day.

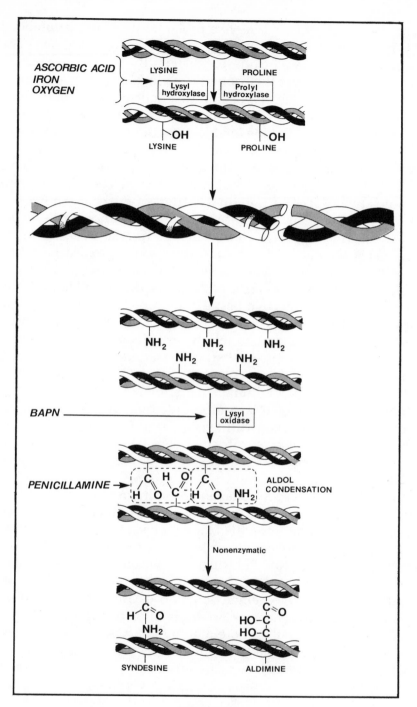

Figure 2.16

It may become possible to control undesirable scarring pharmacologically. The clinical potential is enormous. No one agent has yet proved totally effective, but from our investigator's vantage point, it seems as if we are close to clinical use of pharmacologic inhibitors as we gain a better understanding of the scarring mechanism.

DISEASES RESULTING IN POOR COLLAGEN ACCUMULATION

The medical conditions that most commonly affect repair, besides steroid hormone excess, are diabetes, malnutrition, and infection.

These and a number of other diseases interfere with the deposition and accumulation of collagen, for reasons that are still obscure. (The words "deposition" and "accumulation" are used in this context because it is not always clear whether fibroblast function, collagen synthesis, collagen excretion, or collagen lysis is the major problem.)

Diabetes

Diabetes strikes close to many mechanisms of repair. Diabetics heal poorly; and, when their diabetes is out of control, their wounds are especially liable to infection. Infection worsens the diabetes, and the vicious cycle of diabetes→infection→poor healing→worsening diabetes, once established, tends to continue.

Several general explanations for these effects of diabetes have been offered:

1. Diabetic microvascular disease interferes with blood flow and oxygen distribution; and, as noted above, white cell defense and fibroblast function are poor in hypoxic wounded tissue. The addition of major diabetic vascular occlusion limits regional blood flow and exaggerates the hypoxia. If regional coronary flow is compromised by diabe-

---

Figure 2.16 Schematic diagram of the extracellular assembly of collagen fibrils. Remember that the molecules align in the "quarter stagger" as shown in Figure 2.10. The various manipulable steps in collagen secretion and cross-linking are shown.

tic arteriosclerosis, the heart may not be able to elevate cardiac output in response to major inflammation or injury. Thus, the important mechanisms that compensate for injury, blood volume loss, anemia, and infection may be eliminated.

2. Diabetic neuropathy impairs sensation. Peripheral parts are thus repeatedly injured, because the patient cannot sense the injury. Ulcers develop at the sites of repeated injury. Even the best, or most normal, repair cannot overcome frequent abrasions, contusions, or ischemia due to pressure.

Though the above-mentioned mechanisms are undoubtedly present, they do not explain the entire diabetic lesion in repair. Even in the absence of microvascular disease or neuropathy, insulin deficiency interferes with collagen deposition in wounds. Hyperglycemia seems to change collagen synthesis from Type I collagen toward Type III collagen in cell culture and changes the proportion of noncollagenous protein synthesized by the fibroblast. This may be the basis of such diverse complications of diabetes as cataracts, Kimmelstiel–Wilson syndrome (basement membrane), and arteriosclerosis. However, its significance to wound healing is not yet known. Insulin deficiency must exaggerate the regional energy deficiency in the wound caused by the microcirculatory defect of injury. Obviously, failure of glucose to enter the cells of the wound module will interfere with anaerobic as well as aerobic metabolism, and uncontrolled diabetes could be expected to be detrimental to repair. Recent studies have shown that insulin levels in wound extracellular fluid are about one-third those of blood. Furthermore, the insulin that finally manages to reach the wound through the long diffusion distances may be lysed, presumably by hydrolytic enzymes. Recent evidence suggests that insulin is broken down more rapidly in early wounds than in relatively mature ones. It would appear that the inflammatory reaction which is so important to the lysis of foreign and damaged proteins in early wounds may take its toll in insulin as well.

However, insulin is far more important to the early wound than it is to the more mature one. Wounds in untreated streptozotocin-induced diabetic rats heal very poorly even before the microangiopathy of diabetes develops. We created dead space wounds in diabetic animals, and measured collagen deposition on the 20th day. When insulin therapy was begun 10 days after the wound was made, collagen deposition was only slightly improved over that seen in untreated diabetic controls. On the other hand, if the insulin was given during the first 10 days, and none was given in the remaining 10 days, healing was almost the same as in normal, nondiabetic controls. The possible explanations for these finds are many, but the surgical lesson would seem to be clear. Close control of blood sugar with both insulin and glucose is important, especially in the early postoperative period.

The diabetic leukocyte is also at a disadvantage. The well-controlled, adult-onset diabetic seems normally resistant to infection. The diabetic out of control is not. Studies of white cells, suspended in serum taken from diabetic patients who were out of control, have shown major deficits in margination (adherence) of white cells to the vascular membranes, migration to the site of injury, in phagocytosis, and in bacterial killing. Leukocytes from hyperglycemic but not ketotic diabetics showed the same abnormalities, but controlling the diabetes tended to reverse these deficits toward normal. Only intracellular killing remained relatively impaired. The mechanisms for these changes are yet unclear. However, once again, the surgical lesson seems clear. Resistance to infection is greater when blood sugar is well controlled. Humoral and cellular immunity in diabetes has not been well investigated. Current data suggests that humoral antibody responses are muted in juvenile-onset diabetics. The problem is undoubtedly worse in patients whose obesity is out of control.

At the moment, a few facts are available that lead surgeons to believe that both hyperglycemia and insulin deficiency interfere with the function of the cells of the wound module. Since the concepts of energy production would seem to be particularly important to wound healing and resistance to infection, it would seem that the most prudent course in the control of diabetes in the surgical patient would be to assure that both insulin and glucose supplies are maintained.

The mild diabetic undergoing a minor, clean operation has always been and probably will continue to be well managed by restricting the glucose intake somewhat and decreasing the administered insulin. However, the more severe diabetic undergoing a major operation, especially a contaminated operation, faces a high complication rate. Recent advances in control of diabetes have shown that when insulin is given by constant infusion, even severe diabetic crises can be controlled with the use of amazingly small amounts. Therefore, in severe diabetics it would seem prudent to obtain control of diabetes for perhaps 24 hours before operation through the constant infusion of approximately one unit of crystalline insulin per hour, with appropriate infusions of glucose. This insulin dosage, with glucose, can be continued in the postoperative period with little risk. Insulin levels can be maintained in the physiologic range, insulin receptors on the cells can be saturated, and energy metabolism can be maintained at its best achievable level.

One of the most severe challenges to wound healing is the combination of steroid hormone excess and diabetes as is often seen in Cushing's syndrome and in renal transplant patients. Experiments have shown that adrenocorticosteroids exaggerate the diabetes and that both interfere with the growth of fibroblasts. The observation applies to both adult onset and juvenile onset diabetics. In this circumstance, the constant infusion of insulin in postoperative care has been especially useful, although our experience has not yet absolutely proved efficacy in terms of reduced wound complications.

Infection

Minor infections, even those that are not in the wound, interfere with repair. While this effect is clinically evident, its mechanism is entirely unknown. An infection in the wound may stop the progress of repair.

The net result of infection often is to increase the synthesis and deposition of collagen in the tissue surrounding the infection. In this case, however, though collagen deposition may be increased, the pattern of deposition is often undesirable. On the one hand, union of the wound may not occur, and on the other, hypertrophic scar may result.

The mechanism of the increased deposition is thought to occur through stimulation of macrophages by organisms or their toxins. Obviously, to achieve normal repair, infection, either in the wound or away from it, must be controlled.

Malnutrition

The detrimental effect of malnutrition on wound healing has been known for centuries. Understanding the effect of nutrition is now so clinically important that Chapter 5 in this volume is devoted entirely to the subject.

Jaundice

Strong clinical impression suggests that healing is retarded in jaundiced patients. Very little research has been done, but what there is supports clinical experience. Patients with liver failure have many reasons for disordered repair including, among others, hypovolemia, hypoalbuminemia, edema, renal failure, and malnutrition. Obstructive jaundice seems to retard angiogenesis and rate of gain of tensile strength in the abdominal wound in animals.

Uremia

Uremic patients and uremic animals are liable to wound dehiscence. Though this observation has been made several times, research into the mechanism has been limited.

Wound strength and total collagen deposition into the wound are diminished by uremia and the decrement is proportional to the degree of uremia. The amount of granulation tissue in open wounds is similarly depressed.

Some studies indicate that high concentrations of urea interfere with polymerization of collagen, but the concentrations of urea studied were considerably higher than would be encountered even in the most severely uremic patient. Other studies indicate that serum from uremic patients and animals suppresses growth and replication of fibroblasts in culture. There seems to be a wound "toxin" in uremic serum.

The most recent study suggests that collagen synthesis and wound strength relate more precisely to malnutrition and weight loss than to degree of uremia. Certainly, one of the major clinical observations made following the introduction of intravenous nutritional therapy was that open wounds in uremics, unhealable by old standards, would respond to nutritional therapy.

Though the mechanism by which uremia retards repair is unknown, the treatment appears to be relatively effective. Wounds made in patients undergoing careful dialysis without excessive anticoagulation will heal well especially if aggressive attention has been made to the correction of nutritional deficiencies. Nevertheless, it is probably wise to accept that uremia, even the best treated uremia, still represents a risk to wound healing. Therefore, the best surgical technique, and closures of major wounds with widely placed nonabsorbable sutures are probably still important.

DISORDERS OF THE BALANCE OF COLLAGEN SYNTHESIS AND LYSIS

Keloids

Keloids are large, firm masses of scar-like tissue that originate in wounds such as burns, incisions, insect bites, or even vaccinations and acne. They grow beyond the original wound, sometimes reaching prodigious size. The overlying epithelium tends to be darker than normal for the given host. Some people

Figure 2.17 Keloid in a burn scar. Some of this keloid, particularly the radiating edges, looks like hypertrophic scar. *(Photograph courtesy of Stephen H. Miller, M.D., The Milton S. Hershey Medical Center, Pennsylvania State University.)*

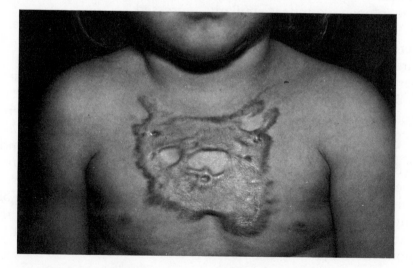

are "keloid formers," i.e., they tend to develop multiple keloids, even from trivial wounds. In general, the tendency to form keloids grows with increasing skin pigmentation. Keloids most commonly occur in the area between the ears and the waist, and out the arms to the elbow (Fig. 2.17).

On cut section, keloids consist of firm, pink or white tissue. The microscopic appearance is of thick, homogenous, eosinophilic bands of collagen admixed with thinner collagen fibers and fibroblasts. The cellularity (fibroblasts, monocytes, and vessels) is not as great as in an active, early dermal scar, and the overlying epidermal structures are usually thin or atrophic. Keloids may be confused with *Dermatofibrosarcoma protuberans*, but they have little or no malignant potential themselves.

Collagen synthesis in keloids is greater than that in neighboring normal skin. Thus, keloids would seem simply a disease of uncontrolled collagen synthesis, were not collagen lysis also elevated. The balance between lysis and synthesis must be upset, with synthesis (obviously) the greater of the two by a small margin. The etiology is thought by some to relate to tension on the wound, while others feel it depends on melanocyte-stimulating hormone (MSH). The latter theory fits the clinical facts well, i.e., keloids occur in darker skinned patients, rarely occur on the palms and soles where melanocytes are rare, and tend to occur during puberty and pregnancy when MSH is stimulated. Corticoids tend to suppress MSH. Several investigators have noted increased immunoproteins in keloids and feel that immune mechanisms may be causal (data as yet unpublished).

Steroid injections may cure small keloids by accelerating collagen lysis. Larger lesions can be excised, the wound grafted if necessary, and irradiated during the first few days or weeks.* Alternatively, the wound edges can be injected with steroids at the first sign of recurrence. Surgical treatment of large keloids is often discouraging. Excisions require skin grafts or flaps for closure, and the resulting large wounds may form new and larger lesions. Lastly, keloids may respond to local pressure maintained for four to six months.

---

*The author has removed one carcinoma of the thyroid about 30 years after a keloid of the neck was irradiated.

Hypertrophic Scar

Hypertrophic scars are bulky scars that stay within the boundaries of the wound. At the extremes, keloids and hypertrophic scars are easily distinguished. There is an overlap of features, however, and often a distinction cannot be made between them. Both tend to occur in wounds that are deep enough to involve the reticular dermis. Hypertrophic scars tend to be less bulky, less aggressive, and less rigid than keloids. They tend to occur more often around joints and areas of motion and tension. Whereas keloids enlarge and rarely resolve spontaneously, hypertrophic scars tend to evolve to a peak size and often regress over a period of months or years. Unfortunately, in the later stages they may contract, drawing delicate eyelids with them or restricting joint motion.

Histologic features of hypertrophic scars are somewhat similar to those of keloids. However, in hypertrophic scars, the large collagenous bands tend to occur in whorls, centering about clusters of cells and small vessels. Some of the central cells are macrophages, others are fibroblasts and myofibroblasts.

In certain cultures, hypertrophic scars are considered decorative. Practitioners encourage them by cutting patterns in skin with sticks and crude iron knives, and rubbing the open wounds with local medicaments usually containing foreign bodies (Fig. 2.18).

In our culture, however, hypertrophic scarring can be one of the major problems of clinical surgery. It is the bane of the burn patient and the enemy of the reconstructive surgeon. Determination of its cause(s) and development of techniques or drugs that might control it are among the highest priorities of surgical research. Two major theories of origin have been presented. One is that hypertrophy is a response to tension along or across the scar. Tension tends to promote collagen deposition and lessen lysis. Tension leading to continued reinjury with subsequent recurrent inflammation may also increase the tendency of scar to contract. Release of tension by such methods as Z-plasty or skin graft is often effective treatment for hypertrophy.

The second major theory of the origin of hypertrophic scars is

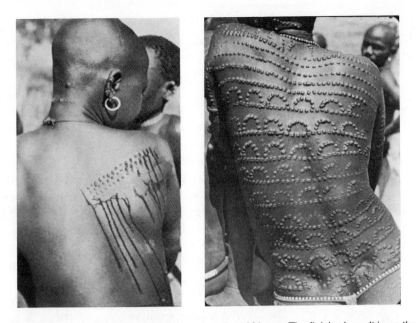

Figure 2.18 Hypertrophic scar being produced on Africans. The finished result is on the right. *(Photograph by Oskar Luz.)*

that there is continued inflammation or infection serving as a constant stimulus to connective tissue formation. Certainly, anything that continues to activate macrophages at the center of the whorls could explain the changes of hypertrophic scar. In favor of this explanation is the tendency of such scars to resolve in time and the fact that hypertrophic scars are sometimes effectively treated with excision and replacement with skin graft. Both explanations seem plausible, and it is also possible that hypertrophic scarring may be the result of a number of causes.

Application of pressure and traction may prevent or reverse hypertrophic scarring. Firm pressure at about capillary pressure level (about 22 mm Hg) causes diminution of mass by collagen lysis, probably by retarding synthesis due to diminished circulation. External or skeletal traction can increase the excursion of a joint spectacularly if the treatment is begun while the scar is still "active," i.e., in the first 6 to 12 months when collagen lysis and replacement are well above normal.

Splinting can maintain position achieved by traction, but to be truly effective, splinting and pressure should be continued day and night for 4 to 6 months. Considerable imagination may have to be exercised to achieve effective (and nondamaging) therapy. The aid of a brace expert is often essential.

Injection with fluorinated highly antiinflammatory steroids is effective for small scars. Injection can be done with a tuberculin syringe (preferably with a fused-on needle since injection pressures are high) or with a high pressure jet.

If the scar is under tension, skin grafts or Z- or W-plasties are the preferred treatment for moderate or large contractures. Skin grafts should be thin (about 0.008 in) so that hypertrophic scars or keloids will not arise in donor sites. Postoperatively, the wounds can be treated with radiation, steroids, splints, or pressure as noted above. Often, if operation can be delayed for a year after injury, a scar may regress spontaneously.

Incisions that cross isotonic low tension lines (often called Langer's lines) at right angles often become hypertrophic. Clinically, it is important to design incisions that cross these lines at oblique angles, even to the extent of using S-shaped incisions. Alternatively, preventive Z-plasties can be used. Scars placed across lines in which skin hollows are present, such as below the eye or lower lip, to the side of the nose, or in the neck, have a particular tendency to shorten, obliterating the hollow and restricting the normal motion of the skin. "S" incisions, or even parallel incisions running with the low tension lines, are very useful.

Contraction and Contracture

"Contraction" and "contracture" are two sharply different words that have overlapping biologic backgrounds. "Contraction" is a biologic process in which open wounds shrink. It can be inhibited by skin grafts with a thick dermal component. The motive force of contraction, the force that moves normal tissue at the edge of the wound toward its center, is thought to originate in myofilaments within so-called myofibroblasts. Contraction is often considered a normal and benign process.

"Contracture" is a word that specifically implies loss of motion of tissue or loss of excursion of a joint. It may occur as a

116

result of *contraction* or as a result of excessive scar formation with shortening due to collagenous cross-linking. The concept of *contracture* usually implies obvious scar formation.

Literature before about 1960 often fails to distinguish between these two terms. Since then, a sharper discrimination has been made, but the tendency to distinguish between the two concepts may have gone a little too far.

The usual concept of scar shrinkage leading to *contracture* is that it is due to a progressive intermolecular cross-linking of scar collagen with a net progressive shortening. First, an excess of collagen is deposited as in all scars. Patients tend to protect the tender, healing scar. They hold the underlying joint (scar) in the shortest comfortable position, tending not to stretch it because stretching causes pain. Scar collagen molecules then tend to cross-link and fix the scar in the shortened, resting position (see Chap. 1, Fig. 1.11). Perhaps a case could be made to call this mechanism "fibrocontracture."

The above explanation does not preclude *contraction* of myofibroblasts as part of the shortening force. For instance, Dupuytren's *contracture* is aptly named. It is, of course, an excessive deposition of scar-like nodules and bands of collagen along the palms and fingers which gradually shorten causing loss of motion of the involved fingers. Myofibroblasts have been identified in the nodules of Dupuytren's *contracture*. This is probably an example, then, of the motive force of *contraction* probably participating in the process of *contracture*. Myofibroblasts are also seen in the plantar aponeurosis *contracture* of Lederhose's disease, in Peyronie's syndrome, in idiopathic carpal tunnel syndrome, in trigger tenosynovitis, in hepatic cirrhosis, and in contracting muscles taken from patients with ischemic *contractures*.

Further overlapping of the two concepts can be seen in wounds of the face. When true contraction occurs, skin must move inward toward the center of the wound. Skin does not generate anew for this purpose; it is pulled into place from its original position. *Contraction*, therefore, occurs best in loose, stretchable skin. In areas such as the scalp or shin, the force of the contracting myofibroblast is matched by the normal skin tensions, and *contraction* is not as pronounced. However, contraction of a large wound of the face can lead to a stretching of the skin so that contraction of a wound of the cheek, for instance, can limit the motion of an eyelid. In this case, the concept of *contracture* is, again, evoked through the process of *contraction*.

The question then arises, does *contraction* contribute to that form of *contracture*, called stricture, that closes tubular organs such as the esophagus where there is little normal tissue tension but also little tissue to stretch into the wound? It would be useful for this question to be answered because *contraction* can be so easily prevented with thick split skin grafts, antiinflammatory adrenocortical steroids, colchicine, and vinblastine. Long-acting smooth muscle relaxants slow contraction but only temporarily. It remains a tantalizing possibility that stricture of the esophagus, for instance, occurring after a burn or anastomosis of the esophagus could be prevented or treated with the use of any of these agents. No rigorous proof in the human is available, but clinical experience indicates that injection of steroids into stricturing esophagus and trachea has therapeutic benefit, especially when combined with dilatation. In several extremely difficult cases, we have used systemic steroids to potentiate the effects of esophageal or tracheal dilatation with considerable success (see Appendix B, case report #9, p. 162).

The treatment of contracture of a joint is the same as that outlined in the section on hypertrophic scar. If adequate traction—a few pounds of constant traction is enough—is placed on a relatively young *contractured* wound, the scar will stretch. The same effect can be obtained, though more slowly, with serial stretching and fixation in a stretched position with casts and splints. Usually, even an old *contracture* can be stretched out in a few days if adequate traction is applied. If, at the same time, local pressure is applied, the mass of a hypertrophic scar can be diminished. The pressure dressing will also tend to hold the scar in the elongated position. It is often necessary to excise and graft an old contractured wound as after a burn of the neck. After such a procedure it makes good clinical sense to splint the part in the extended position until the tendency to shrink is gone, which is in about four to six months. One may have to use specifically constructed splints to "train" the scar just as the orthodontist "trains" the growth of the jaw in children. Once the contracture has stopped advancing, thick skin grafts can be used to keep it at bay.

Predicting the Clinical Balance between Synthesis and Lysis

That wound healing is a race between synthesis and lysis of connective tissue protein is one of the most clinically useful concepts ever developed in wound healing theory. By understanding the basics of the wound healing process, and by knowing those factors that aid it and those that detract from it, the surgeon is now prepared to make an assessment of "wound risk." One of the lessons of surgical judgment is that if a risk is anticipated, the surgeon often can put himself in a better position to prevent or treat it. For instance, every surgeon is familiar with assessing pulmonary risk. If it is severe, the risk is minimized if the patient is more vigorously supported postoperatively with respiratory therapy, intensive care, and so on. The same can be done for wound risk. The patient with a precarious anastomosis can be nourished, oxygenated, have the blood volume repaired, can be given antibiotics, can have the anastomosis bypassed or defunctionalized, and so on. All of these measures are far more effective when done in anticipation of trouble rather than for the correction of an established problem.

In the last chapter, the concept of competition between synthesis and lysis was developed. In the first few weeks after injury, collagen synthesis exceeds lysis and wound mass increases. Thereafter, normally, lysis becomes ascendant and the scar changes its architecture, becomes more pliable, and loses mass. This balance is delicate, and acceleration of lysis or deceleration of synthesis, or both, may make the difference between normal healing or no healing at all (see Chap. 1, Figs. 1.9, 1.10).

The surgeon often must make decisions based on the concept of how a wound will fare in the postoperative period. In certain cases, heavy abdominal closures may have to be used to avoid almost certain dehiscence if lesser techniques were to be used. Colostomies may have to be made to prevent leaks from high-risk colon anastomoses. Operations for cure of intestinal fistulae may have to be postponed until circumstances unfavorable to healing are corrected. The surgeon may find a pertinent guide to making these decisions in Table 2.2, in which factors that decrease collagen synthesis or deposition are compiled with factors that favor collagen lysis.

Table 2.2

Factors that decrease collagen synthesis
  Preoperative
    Starvation (protein depletion)
    Steroids
    Infection
    Associated injuries
    Hypoxia
    Radiation Injury
    Uremia
    Diabetes
    Advanced Age

  Operative
    Tissue injury
    Poor blood supply
    Poor apposition of surrounding tissues (pelvic anastomosis)

  Postoperative
    Starvation
    Hypovolemia
    Hypoxia
    Drugs—e.g., actinomycin, 5-FU, methotrexate, etc.

Factors that increase collagen lysis (all are active before and after operation)
    Starvation
    Severe Trauma
    Inflammation
    Infection
    Steroids

It is tempting to place a numerical value on each factor and to suggest that precautions against failure of wound healing be initiated when the sum reaches a certain point. However, most of these factors (e.g., starvation and diabetes) occur in various degrees, so a precise quantification cannot be made. A few illustrative examples might nonetheless be helpful. A patient with an intestinal fistula, who has lost 20 percent of his normal weight, is taking large daily doses of an antiinflammatory steroid, has an actively draining abscess, and is suffering from immune pneumonia, would have little chance of a successful closure of the fistula. However, if the starvation could be corrected, if the steroids could be omitted and converted to adrenal replacement doses of cortisol, or counteracted with vitamin A, the prognosis would be far better. (For this purpose, "starvation" means protein depletion or acute weight loss of more than about 15 to 20 percent). If the infection could be well drained, and if any hypoxia attendant upon the immune pneumonia could be easily corrected, such a patient would almost certainly undergo the operation successfully.

More simply, a diabetic out of control, with active peritonitis due to diverticulitis and perforation, cannot be expected to undergo sigmoid resection with successful reanastomosis. The anastomosis would almost certainly leak. Trauma surgeons have learned to avoid primary colon closures or anastomoses if there are other significant injuries to endanger healing of the colon suture line. On the other hand, one may be free to close a colon injury if it is small, if it is out of the pelvis, if contamination is light, and if there are no other injuries or medical conditions as noted in Table 2.2.

Atrophic Scar

Occasionally, the wound healing process seems to stop prematurely and when such scars are exposed to tension, they tend to stretch and become thin. This phenomenon is probably similar to that of stretch marks occurring after pregnancy or in Cushing's syndrome. In fact, the microscopic appearances of stretch marks and atrophic scars are similar. It occurs more often in women, and seems to depend on an individual predilection to atrophy and thinning. The mechanism is unknown. It seems not to be related to suturing technique. If the patient has other stretched scars, one can predict stretching after future operations unless the incisions are made in very loose skin along lines of tension. In a sense, atrophic scars are the opposite pole of the hypertrophic scar. Both can occur as a result of tension. Overaggressive treatment with intralesional steroids may produce atrophic scar. Atrophic scars are sometimes attributable to one of the Ehler-Danlos syndromes and are then most frequently apparent over the knees or shins.

Carcinoid Syndrome and Others

In the past few decades, surgeons have learned to recognize such diseases as retroperitoneal fibrosis, pleuropulmonary fibrosis, and endocardial fibrosis. One disease that is beginning to become significant to our knowledge of repair is the fibrotic carcinoid syndrome. The "carcinoid syndrome" is a "shorthand" term for a class of problems resulting from release of excessive 5-hydroxytryptamine, a powerful vasoconstrictor, from argentaffin cells in carcinoid tumors. Patients with this disease develop hyperperistalsis, diarrhea, and bronchoconstriction. These tumors also release bradykinin after catecholamine stimulation. Bradykinin is a vasodilator and produces the flushes that characterize the syndrome. The tumors may also produce prostaglandins that can be either vasoconstrictors or vasodilators. Patients with so-called carcinoid tumors of the abdomen may develop severe, retroperitoneal scarring. One of the particularly vexing late manifestations of the disease is repeated intestinal cramps and apparent obstructions, which are due partly to the severity of the fibrotic reaction and partly to the release of smooth muscle-stimulating amines. In this condition, retroperitoneal fibrosis (sometimes containing tumor cells) may lead to obstruction of the ureters, bile duct, duodenum, or even major blood vessels. When the malignant carcinoid has metastasized to the liver or lungs, subendocardial fibrosis, fibrotic valvular lesions in the heart, and pleuropulmonary fibrosis may become significant clinical problems.

Carcinoid has been related to Riedel's struma and sclerosing cholangitis. It is not known why fibrosis and the carcinoid syndrome are related, though there are a few clues. There is a critical need for serotonin (5-hydroxytryptamine) during fibroblast proliferation. Prolonged ischemia due to vasoconstriction might be expected to lead to proliferation of fibroblasts and collagen. Endothelial injury due to vasoconstriction may injure the local vessels and cause platelet aggregation and subsequent fibrosis. Serotonin also seems to stimulate collagen production in granulation tissue, but the mechanism is unknown. When released slowly in the cornea, both serotonin and bradykinin produce angiogenesis and scar. Macrophages are a part of the cellular reaction.

A "variant" of the fibrotic carcinoid syndrome is produced by methysergide which is used as a preventive for migraine. This drug is a serotonin antagonist that binds and holds tightly to receptor sites for serotonin. Methysergide, a semisynthetic ergot alkaloid, is a vasoconstrictor itself and prevents the vasodilation of the migraine. Therefore, it is not surprising that methysergide may have effects that mimic those of serotonin.

122

The association of the two compounds in the fibrotic syndrome suggests that the vasoconstrictive effect is somehow the basis of this unusual deposition of connective tissue. About 10 percent of patients taking methysergide develop some type of adverse effect, usually after one to two years of therapy. Among these effects are vascular insufficiency involving the coronary, carotid, brachial, femoral, iliac, and mesenteric vessels, retroperitoneal fibrosis, pleuropulmonary fibrosis, fibrotic thickening of cardiac valves, and mitral regurgitation. Fibrotic lesions usually regress after the drug is stopped.

"Idiopathic retroperitoneal fibrosis" has also been reported. It is usually seen as a thick plaque of scar tissue centering about the L4-L5 level, often reaching from the renal pelvis to the brim of the bony pelvis. Its earliest sign is medial displacement of the ureters at the L4-L5 level. Most cases are now thought to be due to methysergide or carcinoid syndrome, but sickle cell anemia and several infectious etiologies have also been implicated. Practolol, an experimental compound related to propranolol but retaining some vasoconstrictive properties, also has been implicated in retroperitoneal fibrotic disease.

All of these syndromes have the same pathology—an initial inflammatory lesion followed by replacement with relatively acellular connective tissue. Treatment is to withdraw related drugs and to add steroids if necessary. If renal, intestinal, or vascular problems persist, surgical lysis of the obstructed structures is often necessary.

Pharmacologic Agents

There are other "wound-active" pharmacologic agents whose main effect seems to disturb the balance of collagen synthesis and lysis. In effect, this may just be a "miscellaneous" category in which the actual mechanism of drug effect is unknown.

Serotonin, methysergide, practolol, and others have been discussed above. The mechanism of their effect is unknown, and it is particularly intriguing to speculate why their effects have anatomic specificity for the retroperitoneum, the heart, and the blood vessels.

Diphenylhydantoin Long-term use of diphenylhydantoin often leads to gingival hyperplasia. Other hypertrophic connective tissue problems have been attributed to it, including thickening of the skull and leonine facies, a feature of the serotonin syndrome as well. Even a variant of retroperitoneal fibrosis has been ascribed to diphenylhydantoin. Several investigators have shown that large doses of diphenylhydantoin will increase the rate of gain of tensile strength in wounds of skin and bone in animals. However, others have shown that it affects several aspects of repair including both collagen synthesis and lysis. No single clear hypothesis for its mechanism has emerged. Its various effects are dose- and time-dependent.

Sex Hormones and Antifertility Agents   A number of authors have reported differences in healing capacities between the sexes. In general, females seem to heal and regenerate somewhat better, and pregnancy seems to accentuate the difference. Despite the excellent blood flow in the abdomen and pelvis, however, infection in caesarian section wounds are discouragingly common, and often are due to anaerobes such as Bacteroides. Recently, in animals, estrogen-progesterone combinations, as used in antifertility agents, have been shown to delay the healing process largely by interfering with neovascularization and oxygen supply. Strangely, progesterone alone does not affect repair although it increases neovascularization. We have not noted a clinical problem due to antifertility agents, but we might recall the difficulty experienced in proving that these agents increase the risk of intravascular thrombosis.

Pentazocine   Pentazocine, a commonly used narcotic, produces an extreme response at injection sites in chronic users. (No such effects have been reported with oral use.) Injected subcutaneous tissue may become "rock hard" and injected muscles may become fibrotic and useless. Once again, there is no explanation except that the lesions show an inflammatory response.

Arteriosclerosis

The occurrence of endocardial and endothelial fibrosis suggests some similarity between drug-induced lesions and arteriosclerosis. In effect, atheromata are scars, some of which contain lipids. These scars are undoubtedly the result of fibroblastic activity. Fibroblasts with myofibrils are probably involved, since these "hybrid" cells are found in the lesions. Arteriosclerosis is indistinguishable from wound healing in arteries. The major questions to be asked are: what is the source of the injury, and what are the initial events that mediate the reparative process?

Current evidence suggests that any event which can injure the endothelium can bring forth the characteristic response. "Injuries" due to immune complexes, mechanical irritation, radiation, vasoconstrictors, and toxic molecules have been studied. For instance, homocystine, which concentrates in the blood and urine of patients lacking homocystine synthetase, is toxic to the vascular endothelium. The first reaction to the injury appears to be platelet aggregation. In homocystinuria, platelet survival times are low and arteriosclerosis is frequent. As noted before, platelets mixed with thrombin stimulate fibroblast replication. A growing understanding of the relationships among endothelial injury, platelet aggregation and activation, and fibroplasia in arteries is one of the exciting current developments in medical research.

DISORDERS OF THE COLLAGEN FIBER
Ehlers–Danlos Syndrome (Soft Collagen Syndromes)

The hyphenated name refers to the two discoverers who, at the turn of the century, described several forms of inherited diseases expressed as incompetent connective tissue. The eponym is now often used as an umbrella term for newly discovered diseases characterized by connective tissue failure, or "soft collagen" syndromes. Seven forms have now been described, and this probably does not yet exhaust the heterogenicity of the group. Diseases placed in this category may or may not have anything more in common than unduly fragile connective tissue.

The forms of the Ehlers–Danlos syndrome vary from a minor thinning and softening of skin to almost total failure of mechanical properties of collagen in which skin tears, arteries rupture, joints dislocate, corneas dislocate, and so forth. The now "classical" tabulation is shown in Table 2.3. When possible, the genetic disorder which has subsequently been found to account for the subtype is also shown.

Table 2.3 Forms of the Ehlers–Danlos Syndrome

Type	Name	Clinical Features	Genetics	Biochemical Defect
I	Gravis	Classic features, all severe	Autosomal dominant	Unknown
II	Mitis	Classic features, all mild	Autosomal dominant	Unknown
III	Benign hypermobile	Generalized marked joint hypermobility without skeletal deformity; skin features minimal	Autosomal dominant	Unknown
IV	Ecchymotic, arterial, or Sack–Barabas	Severe bruisability; thin skin; rupture of bowel and large arteries; joint laxity limited to fingers	?	Defect in synthesis of type III collagen
V	X-linked	Stretchable skin, joint hypermobility minimal; skin fragility and bruisability variable	X-linked recessive	Unknown
VI	Ocular	Scoliosis severe; skin features moderate; blindness from retinal detachment or ocular rupture	Autosomal recessive	Deficiency of lysyl hydroxylase
VII	Arthrochalasis multiplex congenita; dermatosparaxis	Short stature; severe joint laxity with congenital dislocations; moderate skin stretchability and bruisability	Autosomal recessive	Deficiency of procollagen peptidase

The "classic features" are thin, lax skin with unusually visible veins; hyperextensible joints; so-called onion skin scars of thin, silvery, atrophic epithelium seen especially over the knees and shins; and molluscoid skin tumors. The history includes dislocations, multiple breaks of the skin, and easy bruisability. Other less common manifestations include cardiac valve incompetence. Gastrointestinal perforations and hemorrhage, hiatus hernia, eventration of the diaphragm, intestinal diverticulae, and rectal prolapse are among the gastrointestinal manifestations. Postoperative bleeding and suture line disruption are fairly frequent complications of operation.

The surgical importance of the soft-collagen syndromes is not fully known. There have been attempts to link it with recurrences of hernias, and the author has seen hernia recurrence in patients with Ehlers-Danlos syndrome (see Appendix B, p. 161), but the extent to which these syndromes contribute to the overall number of recurrent hernias must be fairly small. In my practice, in which I look for these problems, I have seen 15 or 20 patients who have objective evidence of "soft collagen." Any patient who has had obvious failure of repair, for instance, a recurrence of a hernia (especially a child), and who is not obese should be examined for features of a soft collagen disorder. If any suspicion arises, a coagulopathy should be sought as well since, for reasons unknown, the two often coexist. In general, the surgical problems will be proportional to the severity of the connective tissue abnormality. By no means, however, are these patients all inoperable.

Type I (Gravis) may become a surgical problem. Skin is easily broken; orthopedic problems are common; hematomas are frequent; coagulation problems are common. Repair is poor, and special care should be taken to allow for it. It is the author's impression that wound contraction is very poor. Tissue is soft and fragile, and one sometimes feels he is trying to sew buttons to ice cream. Hernias are probably best repaired with the aid of plastic mesh.

Type II (Mitis) is rarely a surgical problem. These patients have done well after both elective and emergent operations.

Type III is not usually considered a surgical problem. Obviously, however, surgical repair of joint dislocations is likely to be futile.

Type IV, the ecchymotic or vascular type, is a serious, often insurmountable surgical problem. Only a few patients in whom this syndrome has expressed itself as spontaneous arterial tears have been operated successfully. Sutures cut through arteries, and vascular repair in the usual sense is often impossible. Females face a real mortality risk in childbirth.

Types V, VI, and VII also present real surgical problems. In Type VII multiple attempts at correction of scolioses have been made without reported success.

Marfan's Syndrome

This disease has been personified by Abraham Lincoln who is thought to have had it. It is characterized by tall, lanky habitus and arachnodactyly. Seriously affected patients suffer from lax ligaments, dissecting aneurysms, myopia and dislocated lenses, pectus excavatum, and scoliosis. Repair of the aneurysms is plagued by soft connective tissue and by sutures cutting through tissue. Nevertheless, surgical correction of "stable" aneurysms is usually successful. Correction of dissecting aneurysms is less often successful. No biochemical etiology is known, but generation of the disease has been traced to genetic origins. As an autosomal dominant with variable degrees of expression, there is some overlapping with homocystinuria.

Homocystinuria

Homocystinuria is an inborn error of metabolism due to a defect in cystathione synthetase that is autosomoly recessive and is characterized by an excess of homocystine in the urine.

Ocular problems are common, especially ectopia lentis. Arterial and venous thromboses are common, and as noted elsewhere, arteriosclerosis is greatly accelerated in this disease, presumably due to a toxic effect of the homocystine on platelet function with subsequent massive accumulation of platelets on the arterial intima. Both venous and arterial thromboses are common. Mild skeletal deformities are fairly common.

Treatment is usually vitamin B_6 in pharmacologic doses. Folic acid may be added. Operations are not generally a problem in these patients except for the problem occasioned by arterial and venous insufficiency. Obviously, anticoagulants or platelet aggregation inhibitors are probably indicated for postoperative care after major operations.

Cutis Laxa

This is the so-called India-Rubber-Man disease. It is a heritable disease in which the skin is thick, easily stretched, and hangs in pendulous folds. It is continually confused with Ehlers-Danlos syndrome (Type V); and, in fact, Ehlers and Danlos both diagnosed their first patients as having cutis laxa. Hernias are fairly common, but repair is usually successful. Plastic mesh is probably desirable to bolster repair. Plastic revision of the pendulous folds of skin is useful, and healing is usually normal though subcutaneous hematomas often occur. On the other hand, the pendulous folds often recur as the skin continues to stretch.

The basic disease is one of elastic tissue. Histologic examinations of skin frequently shows fragmentation of elastic fibers. The biochemical background is unknown.

Osteogenesis Imperfecta

Osteogenesis imperfecta is a soft connective tissue syndrome in which bony manifestations predominate. Blue sclerae constitute one of the hallmarks of this syndrome. Hernias are fairly common. Thin skin is characteristic and subcutaneous hemorrhages occur after minor injuries. Occasional cases of valvular regurgitation have been reported.

The fundamental defect for this syndrome is unknown, but it is presumed to be in the maturation of the collagen fiber. Some data suggest that the collagen molecule is faulty, but most data indicate that fiber formation is at fault.

Though widened scars have frequently been reported, healing is not usually a problem in this syndrome. In fact, orthopedic operations are often life and function saving.

Pseudoxanthoma Elasticum

Pseudoxanthoma elasticum (PXE) is a heritable disorder, probably of the elastic fiber. Its major manifestations occur in the skin, the eye, and the cardiovascular system. Visible skin changes usually begin to occur in the second decade; and they include fatty streaks and creases in areas of wear and tear, such as the neck, face, axilla and elbows. Angioid streaks of the retina are diagnostic. Plastic surgery for the skin lesions is practicable. However, the condition tends to progress.

Changes in the blood vessels are usually in the elastica laminae. Hemorrhage is probably the most common complaint related to the disease. Hemorrhage may occur in the skin or in the gastrointestinal tract where it frequently mandates operation. Bleeding may also originate in the uterus, urinary tract, and the eye.

Disorders of healing are not a part of PXE, and the patients are operable.

Others

There are other diseases of connective tissue, particularly the mucopolysaccharidoses that now should be called "disorders of proteoglycans." The defect in these syndromes is genetically expressed through enzyme deficiency, but the connective tissue abnormalities are secondary to developmental abnormalities occasioned by the abnormal patterns of proteoglycans. Healing is not generally a problem. Hernias are common in these diseases and can be repaired successfully.

There now can be little doubt that many other types of soft collagen syndromes will be found. We have had experience with a number of patients exhibiting connective tissue failure. Recurrent hernias coupled with frequent dislocations, degenerative lumbar disc disease, failures of spinal fusions, and frequent bleeding without coagulation defects make a strong case for a soft collagen syndrome.

We have seen other patients with recurrent hernias who have only soft velvety skin and highly soluble collagen. In most cases, we have been able to repair the hernia definitively. In most cases we have used mesh reinforcement of the repair.

These diseases are rare. The vast majority of recurrent hernias are due to infections and technical errors. The surgeon should not use this category of diseases to excuse faulty technique. But when faced with a patient who, in addition to his recurrent hernia, also has had multiple ruptured discs, dislocations, and failure of bony fusion, the surgeon might pause to wonder if the tissues can be effectively joined with ordinary techniques or if they can be joined at all.

A summary of known defects in collagen fiber formation is given in Table 2.4.

Table 2.4 Source, Nature, and Examples of Collagen Defects

Site	Manifestations
Defects in structure of the collagen molecule	
Amino acid sequences determined by mRNA	None known
Post-mRNA synthesis of hydroxyproline and hydroxylysine	Ehlers–Danlos syndrome (EDS-VI), scurvy*
Post mRNA additions of galactose to hydroxylysyl residues	None known
Removal of the NH_2-terminal extension from the precursor form	EDS-VII, dermatosparaxis in cattle and sheep
Defects in structure of the collagen fiber	
Cross-link formation	EDS-V, lathyrism in animals, homocystinuria,* D-penicillamine-induced changes in skin, Marfan's syndrome
Interaction with other components of connective tissue	None known
Rate of collagen synthesis or degradation	
Collagen synthesis, gene deletion, or transcriptional defect causing lack of Type III synthesis.	EDS-IV
Change in rate of synthesis	Progressive systemic sclerosis*; inflammatory state of rheumatoid arthritis*; fibrosis* as in scars, keloids, pulmonary fibrosis, hepatic cirrhosis, etc.; some hormonal disturbances*
Change in rate of degradation	Pannicular invasion of cartilage in rheumatoid arthritis*; some hormonal disturbances*

*Probably secondary defects.

EPITHELIZATION

Epithelization is rarely a problem in primarily closed wounds. Occasionally, epithelium may even bridge an otherwise non-healing wound. However, epithelization is not an isolated process. As epithelium covers an open wound, capillary circulation recedes, granulation tissue shrinks, and fibroblasts tend to disappear under it. Hypertrophic scar and keloid are the major exceptions.

The newest epithelium, when it is only a few cells thick and lies on the surface, derives its liquid and solid nutrition from beneath, but may use some oxygen from the atmosphere around it. Adding oxygen to the atmosphere often will speed the rate of travel and maturation. Occasionally, added oxygen may encourage epithelization when it seems to be totally stalled.

Nutritional requirements seem to be about the same as for other reparative cells. Epithelization proceeds slowly in the starved patient, but this may just be an expression of the fact that epithelium will not cover atrophic or hypertrophic (edematous) granulation tissue.

The early reparative epithelia are obviously fragile (see Chap. 1, Fig. 1.13). Dressings applied wet and removed when dry (so-called wet-to-dry dressings) often adhere to and then remove each few hours' epithelial growth. Epithelization around joints or on constantly flexed skin may need the aid of splints to prevent cracking and allow coverage.

When epithelization is active, a hypertrophic epithelium is usually seen at the wound edge where squames may build up and flake off. "Frustrated" epithelization often can be detected when this hypertrophic edge occurs with little evidence of advancement of epithelium over the wound. This is a clue that local conditions are inadequate and epithelization can be improved by such measures as removing harsh dressing substances, splinting, resting, controlling local infection, improving hydration, or increasing oxygen supply.

Excess antiinflammatory steroids may stop epithelization at any stage. It is usually restored by locally administered vitamin A despite the continued presence of the steroid. Continued high levels of cortisol, as in Cushing's disease, will impair epithelization—again, this can be countered with vitamin A.

Since mitosis is active as long as epithelization is occurring, most cancer chemotherapeutics in adequate doses will stop or slow epithelization. This happens regularly when dosage is high enough to cause "toxicity." Radiation of epithelizing wounds will temporarily stop epithelization. It will resume slowly at the end of the treatment unless very large surface doses are given. It is generally best not to radiate uncovered wounds, but all radiotherapists have seen ulcerated neoplasms heal to complete epithelial coverage after irradiation.

WOUND COMPLICATIONS
Wound Pain and Hypesthesia

Wound pain is the most common complaint of surgical patients. When retention sutures are used, wound pain may be localized to one or more particular spots. Usually the patient can be told that the pain will diminish in time. If a painful area persists, it may be due to a small stitch abscess, an irritating heavy plastic or wire stitch, a neuroma, or a hernia.

Neuromas usually cause discrete tender spots and, when irritated, cause radiating pain. They can be removed easily under local anesthesia. Unfortunately, the pain, or at least the complaints of pain, tend to recur.

Irritating sutures can be removed, often under local anesthesia. Relief of pain is dramatic. Hernias usually become larger and the diagnosis becomes apparent as time passes.

Hypesthesia, due to nerve damage, is the next most common complaint. The patient can be assured that he will become accustomed to the hypesthesia, and sensation will improve somewhat. After several months, patients rarely are concerned about hypesthesia. Sensation returns even into free skin grafts months after placement. Most persistant hypesthesia results from destruction of nerve trunks.

Hemorrhage

Wound hemorrhage occurs most frequently in patients with hypertension or coagulation defects and is generally associated with trauma and massive transfusion. Other frequent contributing causes are aspirin ingestion, thrombocytopenia, reactive hypertension after anesthesia, excessive motion, retching, and cough. A wound hematoma is almost always the result of surgically controllable bleeding. The diffuse oozing from the wound that accompanies coagulation defects usually is associated with bleeding into a body cavity as well, and is rarely accompanied by hematoma formation. The treatment for an expanding wound hematoma is to reopen the wound under sterile conditions in order to locate and ligate the bleeding vessel. The blood clot should then be removed. Procrastination leads to continued bleeding, hard and painful hematomas, and possible wound infection. A significant hematoma should rarely be allowed to go without reexploration and evacuation. A hematoma left to resorb may persist for many months. Unless there is definite proof of infection, one should resuture wounds from which hematomas have been evacuated.

Patients operated on while taking therapeutic doses of anticoagulants face a high wound risk. Patients receiving small prophylactic doses of heparin (5000 units every 8 to 12 hours) face a lesser but still definite risk. Patients taking aspirin seem to face a definite added risk. Dextran-70 (about 10 ml per kg at operation and then every second day) seems to give the least risk.

Serum Collections

Serum collections occur most frequently in undermined skin wounds such as those done for mastectomy and in wounds in obese patients where there is a large potential dead space. The exact etiology is not known, though factors such as excessive motion, operations that cut many lymphatics, and inflammation due to poor surgical technique have all been incriminated.

The fluid in these spaces is not simply serum. It is poor in oxygen, gamma globulin, and alpha globulin while it has excess hydrogen ion and carbon dioxide. It reflects the metabolism of the wound. In the early dead space, when the wound is less than 10 days old, it contains large quantities of cationic protein, myeloperoxidase, and other phagocyte products. As a result, the fluid has a natural resistance to infection. Some organisms will live and multiply better in serum than in wound fluid. However, this natural resistance is easily overcome if there is a foreign body in the wound. As the wound ages, the white cell population decreases, macrophages predominate. This fluid from human and animal wounds, when tested in the laboratory, causes replication of fibroblasts and neovascularization. Antibiotics introduced into the bloodstream will equilibrate between wound space and blood.

The risk of infection after an aspiration of a serum collection with a sterile hypodermic syringe is small. Aspiration is a reasonable management method of small collections of less than 10 or 20 ml. However, large collections almost always recur after aspiration. The treatment of choice is then drainage, unless an important foreign body lies within. To drain a collection, a stab wound is made and a small drain inserted. With the dead space obliterated, the healing wound is highly resistant to infection. The drain can be removed in a few days in most cases.

Dehiscence, Wound Separation, Burst Abdomen

Dehiscence is a major complication, especially in wounds of the abdomen, chest, and joints. It represents failure of the wound to gain sufficient strength to withstand stresses placed upon it. The separation may occur when overwhelming force breaks sutures, when absorbable sutures dissolve too quickly, or when tight sutures cut through tissue. The latter is by far the most common. The most frequent technical errors leading to dehiscence are (1) placing sutures too close to the wound edge and (2) tying sutures so tightly that they cut through the strangulated tissue before significant repair can begin. The strangulated tissue is, of course, also infectible.

Surgeons rarely, of their own volition, choose sutures of inherently inadequate strength. However, absorbable sutures lose strength independent of the time pattern of the patient's repair. Numerous studies done in animals and man have demonstrated increased dehiscence rates when absorbable sutures are used for closing abdominal wounds. Even so, some surgeons (presumably those who read less) still use this material. Unfortunately, hospital audits have shown that a few surgeons consistently produce the most dehiscences.

If the surgeon had perfect foresight, dehiscence would be unheard of. A closure that will not dehisce can be chosen if necessary. The choice of suture material and closure technique must take into account the individual patient and type of operation. The infection-prone, aged patient with cough or pulmonary insufficiency, the hypoproteinemic, the hypertensive, and the hypovolemic patients are all at risk, and their incisions should be closed accordingly (see Tables 2.2 and 2.3). Fascial closures of catgut are probably never indicated. Synthetic ab-

135

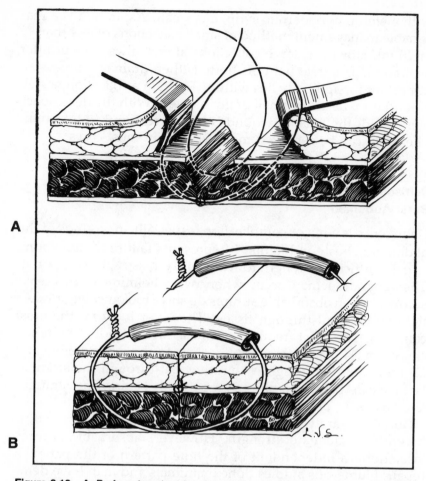

Figure 2.19 **A.** Preferred method for closure of a wound which is likely to dehisce. **B.** Preferred closure of a dehiscent wound. The skin might be lightly packed open if infection is present. *(From Dunphy JE, Way LW, (eds): Current Surgical Diagnosis and Treatment, 3rd ed., 1977. Courtesy of Lange Medical Publications.)*

sorbable sutures are more acceptable, but these sutures must be used thoughtfully. One probably ought not to use them in a large abdominal wound in a patient who cannot be expected to heal at a normal rate.

Almost all dehiscences occur by the fifth to eighth post-operative day in patients who have not yet developed a cutaneous healing ridge, and about half are associated with infection. When a healing ridge can be detected, i.e., induration beneath the skin extending to about 1 cm on each side of the wound, the surgeon can confidently remove retention sutures, since the risk of separation has passed.

Dehiscence of abdominal wounds is usually preceded by a sudden serosanguineous drainage. Dehiscence, of course, may lead to evisceration. In the management of dehiscence, the surgeon has two alternatives: (1) pack the wound until healing occurs and accept the inevitable hernia that follows, or (2) remove the entire old closure, and replace it with widely spaced #22 to #24 wire twisted over "bolsters" to prevent unnecessary cutting of the skin (Fig. 2.19). Twisting the wire is important since the closure may have to be adjusted to compensate for edema or shrinkage of the wound edge. Tied wire or plastic sutures cannot be adjusted (without special devices), and hang as taut bands across any open space, ready to erode into a loop of intestine. The mass wire suture closure can also be used to prevent dehiscence in the high-risk patient. It should not be used for all patients because it is painful and carries a risk of wires eroding into deeper structures.

Closure technique is important to prevent dehiscence. The most secure closure for *general* abdominal use is buried wire (#28 to #30) or monofilament plastic (0 to 00) placed 1 to 2 cm back from the wound edge and a little less distance apart. The sutures encompass fascia, but should be extraperitoneal if possible. Although there is some debate, either simple or so-called far-far—near-near (figure of 8) sutures can be used (Fig. 2.20). With this closure, dehiscence rates should fall below 0.5 percent. Several prospective blind studies and many retrospective studies support this choice.

Dehiscence of chest wounds also is sometimes heralded by serosanguineous drainage, and often by paradoxic respiratory movement of the skin of the incision. Resuture is usually the only alternative, and heavy sutures, placed around nearby ribs or sternum, should be employed. Joint wound dehiscence is usually found in the deep tissues and may be undetected for long periods. This type of dehiscence is usually caused by use of absorbable sutures that are too small in size.

Unless a dehiscence is clearly a mechanical or technical problem, a defect of repair should be suspected, identified, and treated.

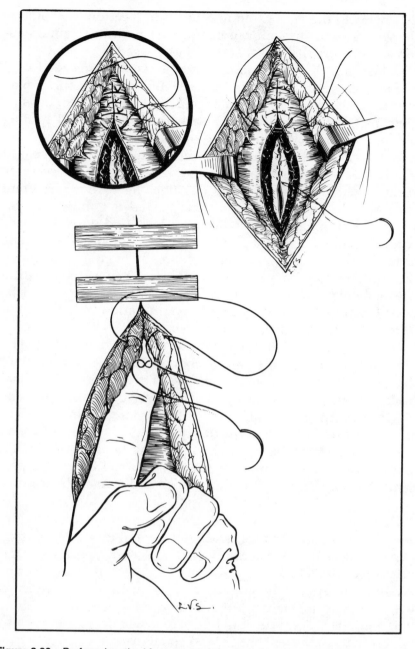

Figure 2.20 Preferred method for general abdominal closure in a patient at moderately high risk of dehiscence. *(From Dunphy JE, Way LW, (eds): Current Surgical Diagnosis and Treatment, 3rd ed., 1977. Courtesy of Lange Medical Publications).*

Suture Sinus

Sinus tracts form when suture sites become infected, and the infection makes its way to the surface. Appearance of a small abscess in or near the wound a few weeks or more after operation usually indicates that a foreign body or suture will be found within. As long as the suture remains, the sinus will persist. Gentle exploration with an ordinary crochet hook frequently removes the suture. If a suture cannot be removed easily, waiting a few weeks for spontaneous ejection may be a wise course. However, few patients should have to tolerate a draining sinus for many weeks or months. If the sinus persists, it is best to open the entire affected portion of the wound, remove all suture material that can be found, and leave the wound open. This should be done under local anesthesia and in good light with adequate equipment. Occasionally, we see bowel fistulae as a consequence of careless, blind cutting of deep tissues to remove a hidden suture. Suture sinuses are seen most with silk, cotton, and heavy multifilament plastic. They are found least with wire and plastic monofilament sutures.

Incisional Hernia

Incisional hernias represent a failure of fusion, or a weakness of the eventual fusion, of the sides of wounds. Most are caused by technical errors in closure, in conjunction with patient problems such as severe obesity, infection, or prior dehiscence.

To some extent, incisional hernias represent deep dehiscences or separations of wounds. This cannot explain the clinical problem entirely, since every experienced general surgeon has seen incisional hernias in which there were satellite hernias in retention suture holes. Furthermore, hernias often follow infections where, with skin open, the surgeon can see that the closure is intact. Yet in a year or so a hernia is seen. In this case, infection has probably increased the rate and scope of collagen turnover thereby "weakening" the tissue. The scar collagen gradually complies to stretching, just as it complies to traction, and hernia results, especially in the obese patient.

A surgeon's incidence of hernia in primarily healed abdominal wounds should be no higher than 1 or 2 percent. Herniation is rare in flank and chest wounds. After wound infection, the incidence of abdominal hernia rises to about 10 percent. After dehiscence and closure, the incidence rises to over 30 percent.

Attempts have been made to equate incisional hernias with defects of collagen cross-linking but, though the individual and unusual problem may have defective collagen at its roots, the problem more commonly is one of surgical technique. Many scholarly papers demonstrate that one type of incision leads to more or fewer hernias than another. Yet, in the last analysis, excluding operations on the excessively obese, if one avoids infections, and uses good surgical technique, it is possible to use almost any incision with a low order of hernia formation. Just as the worst surgeon can defeat the best suture, so can he defeat the best-designed incision. This is not to say that one should use any incision that one pleases. It does say that hernia is usually a "surgeon problem" not dependent on the type of incision.

Experience with patients who have had intestinal bypass procedures shows that obese patients tend to form incisional hernias. We have never successfully (i.e., for more than a few months) repaired a preexisting incisional hernia in a patient who was 100 percent or more over ideal weight.

In our experience, ventral hernias in obese patients begin to become permanently reparable when the patients have lost about 30 percent of their maximum weight. We refuse to repair uncomplicated incisional hernias in seriously obese patients. We tell the patient that he has a responsibility in his illness and that we will not accept responsibility until he loses weight. Unfortunately, few patients comply.

When a hernia develops in an infected wound, the surgeon has a difficult problem. There is undoubtedly a rapid turnover of collagen in the vicinity of this inflamed hernia for six months to a year, and within this time repair is liable to failure. Most experienced surgeons will wait a year or more after the last visible sign of infection is gone before they will attempt such a repair. Antibiotics specific to the old infection should be started a few days before repair and should be continued for a few days after repair. Operations done through old infected wounds frequently become reinfected with the same organism, presumably from spores encysted within the tissue. Furthermore, one regularly encounters old sutures buried in small pockets of pus that frequently yield viable bacteria.

The basic principle of incisional hernia repair is to close normal tissue to normal tissue without undue tension. The hard and scarred hernia ring feels as if it will give a lasting repair. Unfortunately, though this tissue seems hard, it is brittle, and its scarred architecture is not suitable for holding sutures successfully in the long run. Sutures tend to tear out in the early stages, and the scarred fascia stretches around the sutures in the long run leaving the sutures atop a soft bulge of hernia sac.

The palpable and symptomatic incisional hernia is rarely the only one present. Usually, if there is one sac, there are others. Each should be located and included in the repair. Reclosure under tension invites recurrence. Relaxing incisions in surrounding fascia should be used liberally, but care should be taken to avoid devascularizing the wound.

It is sometimes necessary to use a plastic mesh to close the hernia or to reinforce a weak repair. The current material of choice is commercially available polypropylene mesh. Before plastic mesh is used, the surgeon should become familiar with the various techniques that can enhance its value. The major objectives with mesh repairs are (1) to anchor the mesh to normal fascia and (2) to try to construct a layer of tissue (of peritoneum) beneath the mesh so that satellite hernias around the edges of the mesh will not occur. There is much difference of opinion about how liberally one should use plastic mesh. Currently the differences cannot be adjudicated scientifically.

Cancer

"Marjolin's ulcer" refers to a squamous cell carcinoma that has developed in an old burn wound usually in one that healed slowly and was not skin grafted. Ulcerated keloids are especially prone to develop malignant changes, particularly those due to burns or associated with chronic ulceration or chronic sinus tract as seen near a draining osteomyelitis. Any ulcer in a wound that has not healed over a period of months should be suspected of being malignant. Any persistent ulcer in a wound more than a few years old should be assumed to be a possible malignancy, and biopsy should be done.

The mechanism of the malignant change is unknown. However, under the constant stimulation of the wound, the epidermal cell is kept in a state of rapid turnover and is then, presumably, more susceptible to genetic damage. On the other hand, sarcomatous change of the mesenchymal component of the wound is extremely rare and may not even exist.

Adhesions

While surgeons regard adhesions as a disorder, they are usually, in fact, an expression of normal repair. Though adhesions are now the most common cause of intestinal obstruction, it is probably safe to say that adhesions have saved more ischemic bowels from perforation and more precarious anastomoses from leaks than they have caused intestinal obstructions.

An adhesion represents an assembly of wound modules. In their formative stages, each carries a capillary loop; and in their adult form, they carry visible vessels literally parasitizing circulation from surrounding tissues to what otherwise would be ischemic tissue (see the section on tendon repair).

A number of years ago, it was widely believed that adhesions could not spring from an intact peritoneum. This view never fit observable fact, but for years it has had surgeons stitching, pulling, tearing peritoneum to cover defects that theoretically might have caused adhesions. Literally all of a considerable body of evidence states the contrary. Adhesions are far more likely to spring to ischemic peritoneal flaps than they are to areas simply devoid of mesothelium. In fact, mesothelium regenerates extremely rapidly, though no one knows the origin of the cells or any of the mechanisms. Closure of peritoneal defects invites adhesions, as several investigators have now shown. Numerous drugs and other substances have been placed in the peritoneal cavity to suppress adhesions, but most have made the problem worse.

This is not to say, however, that adhesions are inevitable or even always desirable. There are many causes for them, most of which we can easily do without. Talc glove lubricant was the first substance found to cause adhesions. Talc (silicate) is, of course, the most potent stimulant of macrophages known. Its successor, starch powder, though an improvement, is not free of problems. While a small amount can be resorbed from the

142

peritoneal cavity, a large amount causes granulomas. Even the small amount that is tolerated by the "normal" peritoneal cavity participates in granuloma and adhesion formation in the presence of peritoneal injury.

Extensive studies of tissue obtained at laparotomy when adhesions are found showed foreign body granulomas in over half the patients. Talc was found most often; but in addition, gauze, starch, suture material, and digestive tract contents were also found. Some feel that the normal peritoneum disperses these substances, and that abnormal peritoneum cannot. Therefore, it is thought that they collect in the areas of injury.

As in other examples of "healing," fibrin is often prominent in injured peritoneum. Fibrin polymer also causes angiogenesis when implanted in the cornea. The thought that excessive fibrin collection, as in peritonitis, may account for some adhesions is an intriguing one that seems to fit the clinical facts. Attempts to control excessive fibrin deposition may eventually prove to have some value clinically.

Many attempts have been made to prevent adhesions. Those which are directed against the healing process would seem to be doomed to failure since effective suppression of repair will have unacceptable side effects. Experience has tended to confirm this pessimistic view. Antiinflammatory steroids as well as fluorouracil in high doses, for instance, can prevent adhesions, but the cost in poor wound healing and infections is high. At lower doses, they are not effective; however, measures taken to avoid unnecessary peritoneal injury will be rewarded. Prevention of drying, intestinal spills, and unnecessary trauma will minimize adhesions. Similarly, prevention of foreign body implantation is predictably desirable. Washing or wiping starch powder from gloves, using as little suture material as possible, and so forth, are important. Lastly, since ischemic tissue has such potential to cause adhesions, adequate debridement and surgical judgment of tissue perfusion are important. Once again, good surgical technique seems to be the surgeon's most important ally.

Often forgotten in the literature is the tendency for the "adhesive process" to regress. In fact, adhesions follow the same rules as does the skin wound. They reach a peak density and vascularity at some point (usually, we guess, at two to four weeks) and then tend to disappear. The fate of intestinal plication procedures employing multiple sutures to cause "educated" adhesions to hold the bowel in a functional position and prevent further obstructions is a good example. The author has occasionally done them and had some opportunity to inspect the result years later. In some cases, almost no adhesions could be found. Similarly, we have seen patients in whom a dense adhesive process literally prevented correction of gastroesophageal or pelvic problems. However, a year later, it was possible to try again and succeed without much difficulty since the adhesive process had receded. Many surgeons fear reoperative surgery, but it is often not as difficult as anticipated, if enough time has elapsed.

If not enough time has passed, reoperations may be difficult, indeed. A common illustration is the gastrectomy patient who had the intestinal tract opened for awhile only to develop a painless but complete intestinal obstruction at about two weeks after the operation. If one reoperates then, adhesions can be formidable. We have seen patients whose obstruction, apparently due to extensive periintestinal fibrin deposition, could not be corrected surgically at two to three weeks. In time, however, with adequate parenteral nutrition, the process resolved, and the patients are well without further operation.

At the present time, the best means of preventing adhesions is to avoid unnecessary injury, avoid implantation of unnecessary foreign body, avoid or remove ischemic tissue, use omentum or mesentery to provide needed collateral, and avoid closure of peritoneal defects if any tissue tension or ischemia is likely to be incurred. Pharmacologic control or intraperitoneal infiltration of drugs or plastics is not now feasible.

THE NONHEALING WOUND

One of the most troublesome problems a surgeon faces is failure of a wound to heal. The most common problems are ulcers, pressure sores (so-called bed sores), and wounds on the lower leg. One reason for the difficulty in treatment is the problem of differential diagnosis. Table 2.5 lists causes the author and editors have encountered. There may be others.

Though the literature on this subject is highly complex, the principles of approach tend to simplify the problem. First,

Table 2.5 Reasons for the Failure of Wounds to Heal

Cancer
    Basal cell
    Leukemia
    Melanoma
    Squamous cell
    Others

Chronic Trauma
    Factitious ulcer
    Hyperactive child (erosion or biting)
    Peripheral neuropathy
    Poor hygiene
    Proximal nerve injury or degeneration
    Pruritus (jaundice, leukemia, etc.)

Drug Therapy (See Appendix A)

Infectious
    Anaerobic infections (such as Meleney's ulcer)
    Diabetes (relates to many of the above)
    Fungus
    Leprosy
    Other specific infections due to rare bacteria, parasites, or protozoa
    Syphilis
    Tuberculosis
    Tularemia
    White cell disorder (See Table 2.1)

Nutritional (See Table 2.2)
    Crohn's disease
    Felty's syndrome with thrombocytopenia
    Immune pyoderma gangrenosa
    Other autoimmune disease (see Vascular Disorders)
    Ulcerative colitis

Radiation

Vascular Disorders
    Arterial ischemia
    Arteriosclerosis
    Arteriovenous fistulae (congenital or traumatic)
    Diabetes
    Hypertensive arteritis
    Immunologic arteritis
    Pressure sores
    Sickle cell anemia
    Postphlebitic syndrome
    Varicose or incompetent veins

etiology should be found. Most patients will have vascular disease, neuropathy, or will be taking steroids. If there is any doubt, however, biopsy or excise the wound for histology (including acid-fast and fungus stains) and for culture. A swab culture of the wound surface is almost useless. Cultures are done on excised tissue, and a sample is saved for anaerobic culture.

There are many ulcerative diseases due to rare infectious organisms. The diagnosis is usually made by persistent attempts to culture, and often by repeated biopsy and use of special strains.

Blood tests such as blood counts and smear, glucose, and bilirubin are done. Hemoglobin electrophoresis and G-6-PD assay in black patients are also done. Neuropathy, lues, and so on should be examined for. If the problem is an ulcer on the foot, the patient's shoes should be examined for quality, abnormal wear, irritating points, and so on. A full history and physical examination followed with sigmoidoscopy or other gastrointestinal studies if necessary should be done.

If the cause is still not apparent, tests of white cell function may be worth doing. If no cause is still apparent, a behavioral disorder is possible. If the patient is a child, infectious diseases or hyperactive disorders become likely causes.

Probably the best treatment also helps in the diagnosis. One should consider immobilizing the area with bed rest, a cast, or other protection that the patient cannot manipulate. This will usually sort out the patient with factitious disease. Immobilization is the single most useful treatment in any case. Unna's paste boot, which contains zinc oxide, is often a good compromise for immobilization and protection of extremity ulcers.

If hospitalization becomes necessary, the best treatments are usually full rest with immobilization in splints, and wet or moist dressings changed two or more times daily and not allowed to dry. The limb is elevated for venous and infectious disorders and depressed slightly for arterial problems. Debridement to viable tissue should be done and specimens sent for culture. Skin dressings of porcine skin, homologous skin, or placental membranes protect the ulcer from drying and tend to conserve energy in patients with vascular insufficiency. Skin dressings should be used only over viable, relatively clean surfaces. They should be changed every 12 to 24 hours if they do not remain tightly adherent to the surface of the wound. When a porcine or homologous skin dressing "takes" enough in a few days to cause bleeding when it is removed, a take of an autograft is ensured.

The oxygen supply should be increased however necessary, whether the means be arterial or venous operation, breathed or local oxygen, pulmonary or cardiac care. If necrosis is advancing, however, simply increasing breathed or local oxygen is useless.

Nutrition may need improvement. Zinc has been mentioned often in treatment of chronic leg ulcer. Serum zinc levels are usually below 100 mg percent if zinc deficiency is a factor. The exact role of zinc in treatment of the chronic ulcer is unclear. Most nonhealing ulcers due to nutritional problems are healed by a more general approach to correcting malnutrition.

Specific antibiotics should be used to control infections. Chronic ulcers rarely respond to antibiotics alone unless they are due to such diseases as tuberculosis, syphilis, tularemia, and certain others. Debridement is necessary and antibiotics are probably most useful when started just before the wound is to be closed. This gives the least opportunity for superinfection.

The importance of detecting diabetes cannot be emphasized enough. Ulcers due to diabetes are often underestimated, and may be the only sign of widespread, deeper gangrene.

Neuropathic ulcers will usually heal when adequately protected, and preventing reoccurrence may become the major problem. Foot care and special protective splints may be essential.

Treatment of autoimmune disease may put the surgeon in the odd position of treating poor healing with steroids. If immune arteritis is a major feature of the disease, steroids may be effective. Leg ulcers are common accompaniments of erythema nodosum. Though it is not recorded to date, we have seen healing of chronic ulcers following splenectomy and correction of the thrombocytopenia of Felty's syndrome. Pyoderma gangrenosa secondary to ulcerative colitis usually responds only to steroids or colectomy.

Factitious ulcers are usually on the dorsum of the hand or on the leg. Biopsies may show foreign body reactions. Other clues include the sharp, curved edge of the wound made with the fingernail or other sharp instruments. Rigorous protection of factitious ulcers will always heal them.

If isologous skin grafts can eventually be placed, slight hyperoxia is helpful in ensuring complete take. The patient should not be allowed up for at least a week after skin grafting. Leg ulcers may require longer immobilization.* Some large ulcers will require pedicle graft coverage, and some, especially neurotrophic ulcers, may require excision of underlying bony prominences to prevent recurrence. Often excision of avascular scar is the quickest route to successful grafting.

SUMMARY

Both as surgeons and physicians, we routinely accept the great gift of "normal" repair. In accepting this gift, however, we accept many of its disorders as well. Perhaps the "dreamers" who have read this chapter will recognize a few useful patterns emerging with our advancing understanding. Were it within our charter, it would easily have been possible to elaborate attractive theories accounting for many disorders of repair: theories that have not been checked, theories that could not be checked on the basis of present knowledge, and theories that would undoubtedly turn out to be overly simplistic when their time came for critical examination. Yet, we certainly hope that the interested reader will find in some of these all too random observations room for the exercise of his or her own imagination.

We hope that the reader has gained an appreciation of repair. Although repair almost always occurs within limits currently acceptable to the practicing surgeon, we hope that the surgeon will not necessarily be satisfied with these results, any more than Lister and Paré were satisfied with the accepted norms in their times. Furthermore, we hope that we have given the reader a brief glimpse of what could occur were repair not quite as dependable as it is. The major lesson is that repair is still a delicate and easily confounded "ecosystem" in which unthinking meddling may have, and often has had, disastrous consequences. The lessons of history and science clearly show that

---

*Some experts require the patient to have as long as three weeks bed rest after grafting of a stubborn leg ulcer.

repair often requires aid, and that it frequently responds to modification, whether it be planned modification or just carelessness. If anything has been accomplished by this chapter, it is, we hope, that the surgeon will no longer assume blindly that the wound will do well for him. We hope, instead, that the surgeon's means of giving aid to the wound has been increased.

We still find that the major contribution the surgeon makes to the healing of wounds is in technical skill. If the surgeon is gentle, clean, uses cautery, and sutures with appropriate restraint; if the surgeon does not "fuss" with tissue, picking it up and dropping it; does not rub it, dry it, or kill it with clamps, then both the surgeon and the patient will be rewarded.

Surgeons are working in expanding horizons. We are "testing" the limits of repair daily with more extensive procedures, more excursions into contaminated or infected tissue, more placement of foreign bodies, more pharmacologic obstacles. In these conditions, we can expect wound problems and can anticipate that we must engage ourselves actively in their prevention and solution.

These first two chapters have begun the process of describing how to anticipate, avoid, and solve wound problems. The next chapter deals with the background of host resistance to infection and how to support it.

APPENDIX A

Drugs That Affect Repair

Drug	Effect
Anabolic steroids	Accelerate steroid-retarded repair
	May slightly accelerate normal collagen deposition
Anticoagulants	Hematoma formation
Antiinflammatory steroids	Suppress inflammation
	Suppress protein synthesis
	Suppress contraction
	Suppress epithelization
Aspirin	Suppresses inflammation
β-aminoproprionitrile (BAPN)	Suppresses collagen cross-linking
Chemotherapeutics	Arrest cell replication
	Suppress inflammation
	Suppress protein synthesis
Colchicine	Arrests cell replication
	May suppress collagen transport and contraction
Diphenyl hydantoin	Causes hypertrophic scar for unknown reasons; may affect both collagen synthesis and lysis
Methysergide	Causes excess scarring for unknown reasons
Oxygen	Excess speeds epithelization and collagen synthesis; deficit slows both processes
Penicillamine	Prevents collagen cross-linking
Penicillin	Liberates penicillamine
Pentazocine	When injected may cause extreme fibrosis
Radiation	Suppresses cell replication
	Destroys blood supply due to endarteritis
Sex hormones and antifertility agents	Variable effect. Some inhibition of angiogenesis
Vitamin A	Restores steroid-retarded inflammation
	Has own effect (unknown) as a nutrient
Zinc	Depletion may retard collagen synthesis and epithelization; excess does not accelerate them
	Questionable whether effect is pharmacologic or nutritional

APPENDIX B

Case Reports Illustrating Some Disorders of Repair

Case Report No. 1

A 48-year-old male was referred for treatment of a nonhealing wound at the lower tip of the right scapula. A large liposarcoma had been removed about six months before. The area had been irradiated (over 6000 R) starting a few weeks after the operation. A large serum collection had appeared and was opened. This produced a large undermined nonhealing wound. All attempts to treat it failed. The ulcer was extremely painful.

A trial attempt was made to treat the exposed part of the ulcer with chronic breathing of 40 percent oxygen combined with serial xenografting (porcine) until removal of the xenografts caused bleeding. An isograft was then placed and was successful. With this knowledge, we then excised the entire undermined area. The base was found covered with a hyaline substance resembling cartilage and containing almost no blood vessels. The whole ulcer was immediately covered with xenograft. Despite the graft coverage, a few areas became necrotic and required redebridement. The tip of the scapula was avascular and was removed. Chronic 40 percent oxygen breathing and specific antibiotics (for bacteria recovered from debrided tissue) were continued (Fig. 2.21).

After several weeks, we could see neovascularization forming in the hyaline "tissue," and eventually bleeding occurred when the xenografts were changed. The surface of the wound beneath the grafts became sterile to swab and biopsy culture. Autografts were placed and "took." After each grafting, xenograft or autograft, the patient noted lessening of pain.

The patient was discharged with his ulcer completely covered. On his way home he was involved in an auto accident in which a rib fracture "compounded" into the radiated area, through the new skin grafts. The ends required debridement

151

because of pain when they rubbed together. The ends became dried, did not heal, and after a few months became actively infected. The two affected ribs were surgically debrided to the pleura. Lung could be seen gliding beneath. Despite xenograft coverage, the pleura became necrotic, infected, and sloughed, exposing collapsed lung. A large plastic shield was made and sealed to the skin. Suction was applied and oxygen was "bled" into the space through a needle valve. With this treatment, the lung expanded and sealed to the pleura around the periphery of the radiation-damaged tissue. This left a "collar button" wound with a central hole and a space between lung and radiated parietal pleura. Oxygen treatment and xenografting were continued until these surfaces became vascularized and bled on removal of xenografts left for several (no longer than four) days.

Through a right subcostal incision, the patient's omentum was released from the greater curvature of the stomach and a "pedicle flap" of omentum was placed on the left gastroepiploic vessels. This pedicle was led subcutaneously through the beds of the two affected ribs, into the pleural space, and arranged so as to fill the hole. The result is shown in Fig. 2.21. Five days later the omentum was skin grafted. The patient was again discharged well.

Subsequently, a new area of bone necrosis medial to the excised area appeared. It was not actively infected, but the patient was referred for hyperbaric oxygen therapy in an effort to make the necrotic bone "sequester." The therapy was successful. Only a local sequestrectomy was needed.

COMMENT It proved to be a mistake to radiate this surgical wound while a "dead space" remained. The movable scapula probably kept this wound open beneath the skin.

This was an extremely difficult case. Obviously, much attention was given to diet, immobilization when necessary, blood volume, and so on. This problem probably would have been fatal if it had not been treated aggressively. Infection would eventually have reached the radiated spinal column.

The pain in the wound seemed to be "ischemic." It responded dramatically to skin grafting. The area is now painless. The neovascularization stimulated by the hyperoxia is

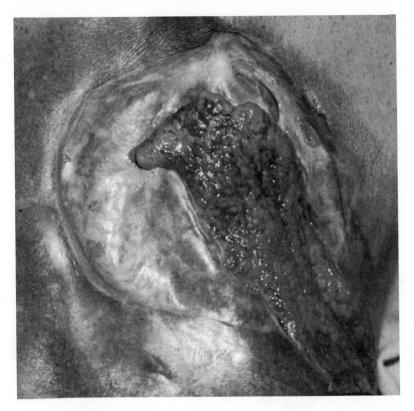

Figure 2.21 Radiation ulcer of case report #1. The granular tissue is the pedicle omental graft. The lighter recessed tissue is where skin grafts have taken to open wound. A few new vessels can be seen. The surrounding dark area is radiation damaged skin.

now receding somewhat; nevertheless, new vessels as large as 1 mm can be seen through the grafted skin.

Case Report No. 2

A 76-year-old woman consulted a surgeon about a large ulcer in her right shoulder. It was approximately 25 cm in diameter, and the muscles of the back could be seen in its base. She said it had been there for several months. She reported radiation therapy to that side of the chest 20 years before for breast cancer. The lesion had a foul odor, and there were several large and nontender nodes in the supraclavicular fossa. The surgeon admitted the patient to the hospital and began antibiotics and local dressings. When the lesion did not improve in a week, he asked for further consultation.

When we first saw the patient, thickening of the edges of the ulcer was apparent, and the nodes were fixed in the base of the neck. A biopsy of the ulcer showed squamous cell carcinoma. Treatment with chemotherapeutics was begun.

COMMENT Radiation damage is not always expressed as ischemia. This malignancy looked enough like a necrotic ulcer to make the confusion understandable.

Case Report No. 3

A 50-year-old woman with a long history of lupus erythematosus was admitted two weeks after a pyloroplasty and vagotomy were done for upper gastrointestinal bleeding. The immediate problem was an open and nonhealing operative wound.

The patient had been taking 6 to 10 mg dexamethasone per day for a number of years. She had had cerebritis, moderate renal failure, arthritis, and pleuropericarditis. At the time of admission, these manifestations, with the exception of the pleuropericarditis, were quiescent.

Using local vitamin A on the wound, granulation tissue became evident within about a week. The wound characteristically did not contract, but instead epithelized, leaving a broad atrophic scar.

Several weeks after admission, during an onset of lupus, she developed mild gastrointestinal hemorrhage. A five-day course of oral vitamin A was begun, together with the appropriate antacid therapy, and within a week all traces of blood in the stool had disappeared.

The patient recovered from this incident and was discharged. A few months later, she was readmitted with exsanguinating upper gastrointestinal hemorrhage. An emergency operation was performed, and a deep duodenal ulcer was found with a vessel bleeding at its base. The vessel was ligated, a vagotomy was completed, and the operation was terminated because, through most of it, the patient had been in shock. A number of small abscesses around old multifilament sutures and a small

154

intraperitoneal abscess were encountered and evacuated. Pseudomonas were cultured. In the postoperative period, intensive pulmonary care and attention to blood volume were emphasized. Large doses of vitamin A were applied topically to the subcutaneous portions of the wound, which had been left open. Erythema and granulation tissue appeared within an appropriate time. Throughout this, the dexamethasone dose remained at about 8 mg per day.

Unfortunately, high gastric acid production persisted despite both operations, and local radiotherapy to the stomach was begun. Approximately two months after the completion of radiotherapy, the patient complained of severe upper abdominal pain, and a gastrointestinal series revealed three large penetrating gastric ulcers. There seemed little alternative to an operation.

The patient was hospitalized and was given forced alimentation. She weighed only 85 lb, and it was impossible to decrease the dexamethasone below 8 mg per day. She was given 25,000 units of vitamin A for a week prior to the operation. The patient would not stop smoking and vigorous pulmonary therapy was begun. At the time of the operation, she had gained approximately 7 lb and her pulmonary function had improved. Antibiotics specific to the old infections found in the wound were begun the day before the operation and were continued for a week thereafter. A difficult total gastrectomy (due to ulcers deeply penetrating the liver and pancreas) with esophagojejunostomy and Roux-en-Y jejunojejunostomy was done. No abscesses were encountered. Despite the fact that the dexamethasone had to be continued, the wound healed primarily. After a short problem with atelectasis, the patient's pulmonary function was kept relatively normal in the intensive care unit and her arterial Po_2 was kept between 150 and 200 torr. Approximately three weeks after the operation, the patient was discharged and had no further problems with gastrointestinal bleeding, pain, or abdominal sepsis until her death three years later from cerebritis.

COMMENT It would seem fair to say that a few years ago this surgical feat could not have been accomplished. Obviously, all the strategy in the management of the patient focused on the esophagojejunostomy. If it had failed, the chances for recovery were slim.

Case Report No. 4

This 21-year-old woman had scleroderma for many years. She had lost several fingers and toes to ischemic necrosis. She had been taking prednisone for several years in dosages of about 20 to 40 mg per day.

In January, she developed severe pneumonia and spent an unknown time lying prone on the floor, with her knees resting on a heater. In hospital, the pneumonia gradually cleared with antibiotics. Prednisone was continued. However, the tissue over one knee became necrotic and sloughed to the bone. A small ulcer developed on the other side. A series of treatments to the wounds began with topical enzymes, antibiotics, splinting and skin autografts. The smaller ulcer gradually healed; but the larger one, now 4 cm in diameter, remained totally unhealed and unhealing with unchanged periosteum visible in its base. By May (four months later), the attending physicians felt that the tissue was too ischemic to heal and made plans to discharge the patient.

When we first saw the patient in May, the wound was clean and uninflamed but also not necrotic. Local dressings with vitamin A were recommended, but the physicians in charge gave 25,000 to 50,000 units of vitamin A orally per day while continuing the local therapy. This was kept up for about three weeks. Within five days, there was enough inflammation around the wound to cause comment by the nurses that the wound was infected (a normal response to vitamin A). Fibrin appeared on its surface and the deep (2 cm) hole started to fill in and epithelize. Mask oxygen therapy (40 percent O_2) for about 10 hours daily was started. Within four weeks the cavity was filled and a small autograft was placed and healed. However, despite the discontinuance of the systemic vitamin A a few weeks before, an episode of arthritis occurred which required raising the dose of steroids for eventual control. Nevertheless, the wound did well and the patient is now at home. We suspect that local therapy with vitamin A would have been adequate for this patient. With it, the arthritis might not have reoccurred.

156

Case Report No. 5

A 50-year-old man asked to have a repair of his abdominal incisional hernia. The hernia had appeared after an operation to control bleeding from a peptic ulcer. His right subcostal incision had suddenly dehisced on the seventh postoperative day. A mass closure was done, and the hernia gradually appeared as a diffuse weakness in the next six months. An attempt to repair the hernia failed in the first six months. His surgeon, a man of excellent reputation, referred the patient to a leading academic surgeon who again repaired the hernia. The wound dehisced in the recovery room. At the reclosure, the sutures were intact and had pulled through the tissue. A diffuse weakness appeared slowly after the reclosure.

The patient reported that he had had three excisions of ruptured intervertebral disks, and two attempts at lumbar fusions which had failed. Several family members, all male, had repeated dislocated joints and ruptured intervertebral disks.

On physical examination, there was a large diffuse weakness (hernia) of the abdominal incisional area. A small McBurney incision (made at age 10) showed no evidence of herniation. His skin was extremely thin and blue veins were easily seen through it. His fingers were highly extensible, but there were no parchment or onionskin scars.

Laboratory tests were normal except that there was an unusual abundance of dibasic amino acids in the urine. In a biopsy of the skin, 21 percent of the total skin collagen content of a biopsy specimen was soluble in dilute salt. (Normal is less than 5 percent). An unusual molecule, rich in dibasic amino acids and apparently capable of acting as a substrate to lysyl oxidase, was associated with the skin collagen.

COMMENT   This patient has a heretofore unnamed condition which precludes surgical repair of his hernia. It is probably inherited. We have seen several other similar patients. Not all recurrent hernias are cured merely by being rerepaired by a different surgeon.

Subsequently, a similarly afflicted younger brother (dislocations, disc degeneration, thin skin) had an upper GI hemorrhage. We operated and closed his incision with large wire sutures. He neither dehisced nor herniated.

Case Report No. 6

A 60-year-old man asked to have his recurrent ventral hernia repaired. He had had a gastrectomy for ulcer done one and one-half years before. A wound infection occurred and a hernia was noted at about four months. The hernia was repaired at four months with implanted polyethylene mesh. Infection again occurred and a worse hernia was present in a maze of draining sinuses a few months later. The plastic mesh was removed to control infection. Despite the hernia repair done at that time, the hernia recurred. All these operations were done in the space of a year. The net result was a large ventral hernia.

The patient was about 30 percent overweight but had no abnormalities of skin or joints. He had no varicose veins and no family history of poor repair.

He was given a strict diet and was told that we would not repair his hernia until one year after the last clinical sign of infection was seen *and* until he reduced to normal weight.

At one year past the last sign of infection he had lost only 10 percent of his weight. We relented and scheduled a repair. He was given full supplementary vitamins and minerals (specifically 0.5 g vitamin C, 25,000 units vitamin A, 220 mg zinc sulphate, and other vitamins and minerals in ordinary doses). He was given specific antibiotic therapy for the most recent organisms found in his wound. The hernia was repaired with polyethylene mesh. Oxygen was supplemented and blood volume was closely supported postoperatively. Blood pressure and urine output were kept at normal levels for him; mucous membranes were kept moist; capillary return over the forehead was kept at less than 1 second; and he could stand from a recumbent position without significant change in blood pressure or pulse.

He healed without infection. One and one-half years later a small recurrence of the hernia was noted at the lower edge of the plastic mesh. He was told he could expect more of these if he did not lose weight. He lost weight. At reoperation, a small recurrence at the edge of the martex was noted, but now the hernia could be repaired without the mesh. The mesh was removed and the entire hernia was replaced with unscarred tissue. Again, the same antibiotics were given starting a day before the operation. Again, hyperoxygenation was used and

158

blood volume was supported with fluids—not blood in his case—though hematocrit fell to 30%. Repair was successful and no recurrence has been found in over three years.

COMMENT The major errors in this case were to use a light closure in an obese man and to reoperate in the infected tissue too soon. Remember that collagen turnover is rapid for at least six months in any case and is even more rapid for a longer time after infection. Sutures simply cut through the rapidly turning-over tissue.

Old infected wounds tend to become reinfected with the same organisms when reopened. This is the reason for the choice of antibiotics in this patient. Though we have seen delayed wound infections arise in apparently healed wounds as long as 28 years after the original operation, the tendency to reinfection seems to decrease with time. The arbitrary figure of 1 year's delay was used here. This is a commonly accepted delay period, but there is little hard evidence to support it. Certainly, the four- and six-month waiting periods used before the first few repairs were too short.

Obesity encourages recurrences. We should have been more stringent the first time. Probably, the low weight should be maintained for at least six months to a year after the operation in order to get best results.

Case Report No. 7

A 60-year-old alcoholic woman sustained a third degree burn of the shoulder and neck. About 10 percent of her body surface was involved. She did not seek help for four days. She arrived at the hospital with severe erythema around the burn. She was toxic and her temperature was 40C. Gram stain of a smear of a biopsy of eschar showed gram-negative bacilli and gram-positive cocci in chains. She was given intravenous penicillin and kanamycin, the last an arbitrary choice. A complete surgical debridement was done as soon as her temperature could be controlled. The wound was not grafted due to the invasive infection.

To avoid contracture, the patient was placed in yoke head traction. Nutritional deficiencies were corrected. Serum vitamin A was very low, as it is in most seriously burned patients; 25,000 units of vitamin A were given daily, in addition to the usual vitamins, minerals, proteins, and calories. About a week after the debridement, a thick split-thickness isograft (0.020 in) was placed. The patient breathed 40 percent oxygen for the first week after the graft was placed. Take was about 95 percent.

When coverage was complete, a plastic neck collar was tailored so that a strategically placed rubber sponge exerted pressure on the healing area. This was worn during waking hours for four months. At the end of this time, head position was normal, but hyperextension of the neck was limited by thin bands of contractured subcutaneous tissue. When extension was passively forced, these contractures stood out as "bow strings" under the grafts. Each of these "strings" was injected with 50 percent Xylocaine and 50 percent Kenalog-40 using a Dermoject pressure injector. Physical therapy was begun. After 3 injections given monthly, she regained full extension.

COMMENT As shown in Figure 2.17, neck burns commonly cause contractures. A combination of pressure, traction, and local steroids was used to conquer this problem. A massive infection was treated with aggressive debridement and specific antibiotics.

Case Report No. 8

A 55-year-old male asked to have two hernias repaired. One was in a small, midline incision through which a perforated ulcer had been closed. The other was a second recurrence of an inguinal hernia. He complained of pain in both. Both had appeared more than six months after the operation.

The patient was slim, had very lax and thin skin, and had onionskin scars on his knees. His fingers and toes were hyperextensible (Ehlers-Danlos Type II or III).

Skin biopsy showed normal soluble collagen, and all other tests were negative. Roentgenograms of his hands showed bony changes consistent with Ehlers-Danlos syndrome.

His hernias were repaired in separate operations. Heavy nonabsorbable sutures were used in the epigastric hernia. In a so-called Halsted repair, a polyethylene mesh was used to reinforce the repair of the inguinal hernia which paralleled the spermatic cord through its exit.

COMMENT   Although it may require special techniques, successful herniorrhaphy is often possible in patients with Ehlers-Danlos syndrome. The author "went to school" with this patient. He did not believe herniorrhaphy could be done and operated under some duress.

Case Report No. 9

A 40-year-old woman, after total colectomy for ulcerative colitis, developed multiple small intestinal fistulae. During the prolonged nasogastric intubation that was required for treatment of the fistulae, she developed a severe lower esophageal stenosis just above a hiatus hernia. In the succeeding six months, two operations designed to relieve the esophageal stenosis failed. The first failed to stop the fibro-contractive process, and, in the second operation, the surgeon was unable to reach the lower esophagus because of the severe inflammation and scarring. The situation seemed surgically insoluble. The patient was able to swallow her saliva only at the cost of weekly dilatations. After a number of months of dilatations without significant progress, steroids were added to the management. After the next dilatation, she was given a large dose of prednisone that was then tapered over the next few days to a maintenance dose. This was repeated the next week. Thereafter, the need for dilatation slowly diminished until she was discharged from the hospital having needed no dilatation in four months and able to eat regular food.

In this case, the steroids were given immediately after dilatation-stretching of the wound. Presumably, it impaired the inflammatory reaction to the dilatation injury. The patient apparently was able to reepithelize the injury without contracting it. The risks of antiinflammatory adrenal steroids, perforation and infection, seemed to be minimal because of the severe fibrous reaction encasing the esophagus.

Based on recent evidence showing that colchicine inhibits wound contraction, this drug may replace steroids in the future for this purpose.

REFERENCES

General

Cline MJ: The White Cell. Cambridge, Harvard University Press, 1975. Note: Superbly illustrated and annotated. A key to the literature.

Dunphy JE, Van Winkle W Jr.: Repair and Regeneration. New York, McGraw-Hill, 1968. Note: A general reference wedding basic science and surgery. Though it is old, it remains an excellent source book.

Gibson T, Van der Meulen (eds): Wound Healing, International Symposium on Wound Healing, Rotterdam, 1974. Montreux, Switzerland, Foundation for International Cooperation in the Medical Sciences, 1975

Kulonen E, Pikkarainen J (eds): Biology of Fibroblasts. New York, Academic Press, 1973. Note: A general and extremely useful source book for many of the above topics.

Mathews MB: The molecular evolution of cartilage. Clin Orthop 48:267, 1966

Montandon D (ed): Symposium on wound healing. Clin Plast Surg 4(3):1–475, 1977

Peacock EE, Jr, Van Winkle W Jr: Surgery and Biology of Wound Repair. Philadelphia, Saunders, 1976. Note: Written by and for surgeons.

The Injury

Bains JW, Crawford DT, Ketcham AS: Effect of chronic anaemia on wound tensile strength: Correlation with blood volume, total red blood cell volume and proteins. Ann Surg 164:243, 1966

Heppenstall R, Littooy FN, Fuchs R, Sheldon GF, Hunt TK: Gas tensions in healing tissues of traumatized patients. Surgery 75:874, 1974

Heughan C, Zederfeldt BH, Grislis G, Hunt TK: Effect of dextran solutions on oxygen transport in wound tissue. Acta Chir Scand 138:639, 1972. Note: A comprehensive view of hemodynamic factors in repair.

Irvin TT, Hunt TK: Pathogenesis and prevention of disruption of colonic anastomosis in traumatized rats. Br J Surg 61:437, 1974

Order SE, Moncrief, JA: The Burn Wound. Springfield, Ill., Thomas, 1965. Note: One of the classic descriptions of the evolution of the burn wound.

Zederfeldt B: Studies on wound healing and trauma, with special reference to intravascular aggregation of erythrocytes. Acta Chir Scand Suppl 224, 1957

Coagulation and Hemostasis

Chen LB, Buchanan JM: Mitogenic activity of blood components. I. Thrombined prothrombin. Proc Nat Acad Sci USA 72:131, 1975

Krizek TJ, Davis JH: The role of the red cell in subcutaneous infection. J Trauma, 5:85, 1965

Richardson DL, Pepper DS, Kay, AB: Chemotaxis for human monocytes by fibrinogen-derived peptides. Br J Haematol 32:507, 1976

162

Arumugam S, Nimmannit S, Enquist IF: The effect of immunosuppression on wound healing. Surg Gynecol Obstet 133:72, 1971

Clark RA, Stone RD, Leung DYK, et al.: Role of macrophages in wound healing. Surg Forum 27:16, 1976

Cline MJ, Lehrer RI, Territo MC, Golde DW: Monocytes and macrophages: Functions and diseases. Ann Intern Med, 88:78, 1978

Cohen BE, Cohen IK: Vitamin A: Adjuvant and steroid antagonist in the immune response. J Immunol III:1376, 1973

Cohen SC, Gabelnick HL, Johnson RK, Goldin A: Effects of antineoplastic agents or wound healing in mice. Surgery 78:238, 1975

Ehrlich HP, Tarver H, Hunt TK: The effects of vitamin A and glucocorticoids upon repair and collagen synthesis. Ann Surg 177:22, 1973

Goldman LI, Lowe S, Al-Saleem T: Effect of fluorouracil on intestinal anastomoses in the rat. Arch Surg 98:303, 1969

Gospodarowicz D, Moran JS: Stimulation of division of sparse and confluent 3T3 cell populations by a fibroblast growth factor, dexamethasone, and insulin. Proc Nat Acad Sci 71:4584, 1974

Grillo HC, Potsaid MS: Studies in wound healing. IV. Retardation of contraction by local X-irradiation and observations relating to the origin of fibroblasts in repair. Ann Surg 154:741, 1961

Hunt TK, Ehrlich HP, Garcia JA, Dunphy JE: Effect of vitamin A on reversing the inhibitory effect of cortisone on healing of open wounds in animals and man. Ann Surg 170:633, 1969

Lee KH: Studies on the mechanism of salicylates. III: Effect of Vitamin A on the wound healing retardation action of aspirin. J Pharm Sci 57:1238, 1968

Leibovich SJ, Ross R: The role of macrophages in wound repair. A study with hydrocortisone and antimacrophage serum. Am J Pathol 78:71, 1975

Newcombe JF: Effect of intra-arterial nitrogen mustard infusion on wound healing in rabbits: Formation of granulation tissue and wound contraction. Ann Surg 163:319, 1966. Note: A good general reference and key to the literature.

Richardson KT: Pharmacology and pathophysiology of inflammation. Arch Ophthalmol 86:706, 1971

Rutherford RB, Ross R: Platelet factors stimulate fibroblasts and smooth muscle cells quiescent in plasma serum to proliferate. J Cell Biol 69:196, 1976

Sandberg N: Time relationship between administration of cortisone and wound healing in rats. Acta Chir Scand 127:446, 1964

Schorlemmer HU, Bitter-Suermann D, Allison AC: Complement activation by the alternative pathway and macrophage enzyme secretion in the pathogenesis of chronic inflammation. Immunology 32:929, 1977

Spector WG, Heesom N, Stevens JE: Factors influencing chronicity in inflammation of rat skin. J Pathol 96:203, 1968

Unanue ER: Secretory function of mononuclear phagocytes: A review. Am J Pathol 83:396, 1976

Velasco M, Guaitero E: A comparative study of some anti-inflammatory drugs in wound healing of the rat. Experientia 29(10):1250, 1973

Werb Z, Gordon S: Elastase secretion by stimulated macrophages. J Exp Med 142:361, 1975

Phagocyte Function

Babior BM: Oxygen-dependent microbial killing by phagocytes (First of two parts). New Engl J Med 298:659, 1978

Babior BM: Oxygen-dependent microbial killing by phagocytes (Second of two parts). New Engl J Med 298:721, 1978

Brunius V: Wound healing impairment from sutures. Acta Chir Scand Suppl 395, 1968

Conolly WB, Hunt TK, Zederfeldt B, Cafferata HT, Dunphy JE: Clinical comparison of surgical wounds closed by suture and adhesive tapes. Am J Surg 117:318, 1969

Edlich RF, Panek PH, Rodeheaver GT, et al.: Physical and chemical configuration of sutures in the development of surgical infection. Ann Surg 177:679, 1973

Hohn DC: Leukocyte phagocytic function and dysfunction. Surg Gynecol Obstet 144:99, 1977

Hohn DC: Hunt TK: Oxidative metabolism and microbicidal activity of rabbit phagocytes: Cells from wounds and from peripheral blood. Surg Forum 26:86, 1975

Hohn DC, McKay RD, Halliday B, Hunt TK: The effect of oxygen tension on the microbicidal function of leukocytes in wounds and in vitro. Surg Forum 27:18, 1976

Howard RJ, Simmons RL: Acquired immunologic deficiencies after trauma and surgical procedures. Surg Gynecol Obstet 139:771, 1974

Hunt TK, Linsey M, Grislis G, Sonne M, Jawetz E: The effect of differing ambient oxygen tensions on wound infection. Ann Surg 181:35, 1975

MacLean LD, Meakins JL, Taguchi K, et al.: Host resistance in sepsis and trauma. Ann Surg 182:207, 1975

Mandell GL: Bactericidal activity of aerobic and anaerobic polymorphonuclear neutrophils. Infect Immun 9:337, 1974

Myers MB, Cherry G: Functional and angiographic vasculature in healing wounds. Am Surgeon 36:750, 1970

Van Winkle W, Hastings H: Considerations in the choice of suture material for suture material for various tissues. Collective Review. Surg Gynecol Obstet 135:113, 1972

Neovascularization

Karppinen V, Myllärniemi H: Vascular reactions in the healing laparotomy wound under cytostatic treatment. Acta Chir Scand 136:675, 1970

The Fibroblast and Collagen Synthesis

Grant ME, Prockop DJ: The biosynthesis of collagen. New Engl J Med 286:194, 1972. Note: This is part of a three-part exhaustive review article.

164

Niinikoski J: Oxygen and wound healing. Clin Plast Surg 4:361, 1977

Nimni ME: Collagen: Its structure and function in normal and pathological connective tissues. Semin Arthritis Rheum 4(2):95, 1974. Note: An exhaustive review with some discussion of pharmacology.

Pharmacologic Inhibitors of Collagen Synthesis and Fiber Formation

Donoff RB: The effect of diphenylhydantoin on open wound healing in guinea pigs. J Surg Res 24:41, 1978

Nyman S: Studies on the influence of estradiol and progesterone on granulation tissue. J Periodont Res Suppl 7, 1971

Wiznitzer T, Orda R, Bawnik JB, et al.: Mitomycin and the healing of intestinal anastomosis. Arch Surg 106:314, 1973

Diseases Resulting in Poor Collagen Accumulation

Bagdade JD, Root RK, Bulger RJ: Impaired leukocyte function in patients with poorly controlled diabetes. Diabetes 23:9, 1974

Bagdade JD, Root RK, Bulger RJ: Impaired leukocyte function in patients with poorly controlled diabetes. Diabetes 23:9, 1974

Bayer, I, Ellis H: Jaundice and wound healing: An experimental study. Br J Surg 63:392, 1976

Bluemle LW Jr, Webster CD Jr, Elkinton JR: Acute tubular necrosis. Arch Intern Med 104:180, 1959

Esmann V: The diabetic leukocyte. Enzyme 13:32, 1972

Ludwig H, Eibl M, Schernthaner G, Erd W, Mayr WR: Humoral immunodeficiency to bacterial antigens in patients with juvenile onset diabetes mellitus. Diabetologia 12:259, 1976

Meyer, EJ, Lorenzi M, Bohannon HV, et al.: Diabetic management by insulin infusion during major surgery. Am J Surg (in press)

McDermott FT: The effect of 10% human uremic serum upon human fibroblastic cell cultures. J Surg Res 11:119, 1971

McDermott FT, Nayman J, deBoer WGRM: The effect of acute renal failure upon wound healing: Histological and autoradiographic studies in the mouse. Ann Surg 168:142, 1968

Nayman J: Effect of renal failure on wound healing: An experimental study. Ann Surg 164:227, 1966

Nayman J, McDermott FT, deBoer WGRM: Effect of acute renal failure upon wound healing in the mouse. Rev Surg 23:453, 1966

Shaw SN, Amos H: Insulin stimulation of glucose entry in chick fibroblasts and hela cells. Biochem Biophys Res Commun 53:357, 1973

Stern AA, Wiersum J: The role of renal dysfunction in abdominal wound dehiscence. J Urol 82:271, 1959

Than T, McGee JO'D, Sokhi GS, Patrick RS, Blumgart LH: Skin prolyl hydroxylase in patients with obstructive jaundice. Lancet II: 807, 1974

165

Disorders of the Balance of Collagen Synthesis and Lysis

Boucek RJ, Alvarez TR: 5-hydroxytryptamine: A cytospecific growth stimulator of cultured fibroblasts. Science 167:898, 1970

Boucek RJ: Serotonin and collagen metabolism. In Essmann WB: Serotonin in Health and Disease vol 4. New York: Spectrum Publications, 1977, pp 1–39

Eltringham WK, Espiner HJ, Windsor CWO, et al.: Sclerosing peritonitis due to practolol: A report on 9 cases and their surgical management. Br J Surg 64:229, 1977

Harker L, Ross R, Slichter S, Scott C: Homocystine-induced arteriosclerosis: The role of endothelial cell injury and platelet response in its genesis. J Clin Invest 1976

Hawley PR, Faulk WP, Hunt TK, Dunphy JE: Collagenase activity in the gastro-intestinal tract. Br J Surg 57:896, 1970

Hunt TK, Hawley PR: Surgical judgment and colonic anastomoses. Dis Colon Rectum 12:167, 1969

Ketchum LD, Cohen IK, Masters FW: Hypertrophic scars and keloids: a collective review. Plast Reconstr Surg 53:140, 1974

Disorders of the Balance of Collagen Synthesis and Lysis

Larson DL, Baur P, Linares HA, et al.: Mechanisms of hypertrophic scar and contracture formation in burns. Burns 1:119, 1975

McKusik VA: Heritable Disorders of Connective Tissue, 4th ed., St. Louis, Mosby, 1972

Morton D, Steinbronn K, Lato M, Chvapil M, Peacock EE: Effect of colchicine on wound healing in rats. Surg Forum 25:47, 1974

Nyman S: Studies on the influence of estradiol and progesterone on granulation tissue. J Peridont Res Suppl 7, 1971

Ross JC, Goldsmith HJ: The combined surgical and medical treatment of retroperitoneal fibrosis. Br J Surg 58:422, 1971

Rudolph R, Woodward M: Spatial orientation of microtubules in contractile fibroblasts in vivo. Anat Rec, in press

Disorders of the Collagen Fiber

Beighton P, Horan FT: Surgical aspects of the Ehlers–Danlos syndrome. Br J Surg 56:255, 1969

Beighton PH, Murdoch JL, Votteler T: Gastrointestinal complications of the Ehlers-Danlos syndrome. Gut 10:1004, 1969

Beighton P, Price A, Lord J, Dickson E: Variants of the Ehlers-Danlos syndrome: Clinical, biochemical, haematological, and chromosomal features of 100 patients. Ann Rheum Dis 28:228, 1969

Gorlin RJ, Sedano H: Cutis laxa syndrome (generalized elastolysis). Mod Med 124:1971

Kang AH, Trelstad RL: A collagen defect in homocystinuria. J Clin Invest 52:2571, 1973

166

Lapiere ChM: Biosynthesis of fibrous proteins. In Gibson T, vander Meulen JC: Wound Healing. International Symposium on Wound Healing. Rotterdam Foundation on International Cooperation in the Medical Sciences. 1974, p. 45

McEntyre RL, Raffensperger JG: Surgical complications of Ehlers-Danlos syndrome in children. J Ped Surg 12(4):531, 1977

McFarland W, Fuller DE: Mortality in Ehlers-Danlos syndrome due to spontaneous rupture of large arteries. New Engl J Med 271:1309, 1964

McKusick VA: Heritable Disorders of Connective Tissue, 4th ed. St. Louis, Mosby, 1972

McKusick VA: Multiple forms of the E-D syndrome. Arch Surg 109:475, 1974

Maxwell E, Esterly NB: Cutis laxa. Am J Dis Child 117:479, 1969

Rowe DW, Starman BJ, Fugimoto WY, Williams RH: Abnormalities in proliferation and protein synthesis in skin fibroblast cultures from patients with diabetes mellitus. Diabetes 26:284, 1977

Epithelization

Maibach HI, Rovee DT (eds).: Epidermal Wound Healing. Chicago, Year Book Medical Publishers, 1972. Note: The best single reference to all topics under this title.

Wound Complications

Ellis H: Intraperitoneal adhesions. Br J Hosp Med 2:401, 1974

Faddis D, Daniel D, Boyer J: Tissue toxicity of antiseptic solutions: A study of rabbit articular and periarticular tissues. J Trauma, 17:895, 1977

Goldsmith HS: The treatment of postsurgical lymphedema. Surg Clin North Am 49:407, 1969

Goligher JC, Irvin TT, Johnston D, et al.: A controlled clinical trial of three methods of closure of laparotomy wounds. Br J Surg 62:823, 1975

Irvin TT, Hunt TK: Pathogenesis and prevention of disruption of colonic anastomosis in traumatized rats. Br J Surg 61:437, 1974

Jacobs E, Blaisdell FW, Hall AD: Use of knitted marlex mesh in the repair of ventral hernias. Am J Surg 110:897, 1965

Lindstedt E, Sandblom P: Wound healing in man: Tensile strength of healing wounds in some patient groups. Ann Surg 181:842, 1975

Maguire T, Young D: Repair of epigastric incisional hernia. Br J Surg 63:125, 1976

May J, Chalmers JP, Loewenthal J, Rountree PM: Factors in the patient contributing to surgical sepsis. Surg Gynecol Obstet 122:28, 1966

McCallum GT, Link RF: The effect of closure techniques on abdominal disruption. Surg Gynec Obstet 119:75, 1964

Novick M, Gard DA, Hardy SB, Melvin S: Burn scar carcinoma: A review and analysis of 46 cases. J Trauma 17:809, 1977

Parerira MD, Serkes KD: Prediction of wound disruption by use of the healing ridge. Surg Gynecol Obstet 115:72, 1962

167

Postlethwait RW, Willigan A, Ulin AW: Human tissue reaction to sutures. Ann Surg 181:144, 1975

Winn HR, Jane JA, Rodeheaver G, Edgerton MT, Edlich RF: Influence of subcuticular sutures on scar formation. Am J Surg 133:257, 1977

The Nonhealing Wound

Enis JE, Sarmiento A: The pathophysiology and management of pressure sores. Orthop Rev 11:25, 1973

Novick M, Gard DA, Hardy SB, Spira M: Burn scar carcinoma: a review and analysis of 46 cases. J Trauma 17:809, 1977

168

3
INFECTION
John F. Burke

In the first two chapters we have traced the reparative response of tissue, from injury to scar, noting in "Disorders of Repair" the points in the sequence at which the process can go amiss.

In the next two chapters, we turn to resistance to infection, a normal property of a normally healing wound. We will show that the same cells that debride injured tissue and guide the reparative cells also seek out, ingest, and kill microorganisms. A healthy wound in a healthy host can clear itself of an extraordinary number of bacteria. As every surgeon knows, however, this remarkable defense system has its limits.

Several hundred years ago, surgeons first recognized that badly damaged tissue resisted infection poorly and, conversely, that gentle handling of wounds rendered them more resistant to invasive infection. About a century ago Pasteur and Koch described the infective properites of bacteria. Acting on this information, Lister and Semmelweis demonstrated that measures designed to reduce the number of bacteria reaching a wound could also reduce the number of invasive and lethal infections.

Up to that time, infection had followed most surgical procedures, and these scientists and others, in developing the principles of antisepsis and asepsis, were opening a new era in surgical practice. The opportunities offered by their discoveries have yet to be fully exploited.

Antibiotics became generally available about 30 years ago and received an overenthusiastic welcome from surgeons. Wounds were dusted and irrigated with antibiotics; patients of all kinds were given antibiotics with all sorts of operations. Undoubtedly, a few patients benefited, but probably just as many suffered. Toxic reactions were common and hospitals became breeding grounds for antibiotic-resistant organisms. It gradually became clear that aseptic precautions and thoughtful, gentle surgical techniques were as important as ever. Experience also showed that antibiotics could help only a particular group of patients, and then only during a short, critical period in their management.

The next chapters deal with the means by which the surgeon can avoid infections and treat those that arise. They emphasize the preservation and augmentation of host defenses. They describe appropriate surgical techniques and develop a rational policy for use of antibiotics in the perioperative period.

In preparing this volume, we discussed whether we should include standards for "acceptable" rates of infection. Obviously, the only acceptable goal is none. Surely the incidence in the case of wounds made in the course of clean, uncontaminated, elective operations should approach zero—less than one percent is a current and probably achievable goal. Some infections, however, are still inevitable, given today's conditions. Some operations inevitably will leave heavily contaminated wounds. But one can never rest with the assumption that infection is inevitable. The past 15 years have seen a gradual decrease of infections in many hospitals. Where this trend will stop, no one knows, but with understanding and diligence we should be able to continue it.

Until recently, measures taken to prevent postoperative infection were aimed almost exclusively at eliminating bacteria from the surgical environment or from the wound itself. Asepsis, which was an outgrowth of antisepsis (once called "Listerism"), has made it possible for surgery to progress as a therapeutic arm of medicine.

Now the important role host resistance can play in the prevention of infection has been recognized, and methods of wound management have been designed to take advantage of these natural defenses. The risk of bacterial infection can be further reduced by improving our techniques for supplementing host resistance.

The history of efforts to control wound infection reflects two general and, in some respects, conflicting trends. The first has been marked by an increasing ability to control the bacterial population in the wound environment. The second has been the extension of surgical therapy to a number of patients who once would have been regarded as prohibitive risks, individuals highly susceptible to bacterial complications. Thus, while the numbers of bacteria presented to the surgical patient have steadily decreased, the number of poor risk patients with low resistance to these organisms has increased.

Statistics on mortality following severe trauma underscore the contradictory nature of these trends: Although there has been a dramatic reduction in deaths due to shock following trauma, this improvement has been offset by an increase in deaths related to infection in the posttrauma weeks. In solving one set of problems, surgeons have uncovered a new set. Due to improved techniques for the management of severe trauma and massive blood loss, patients now live long enough to develop sepsis.

Improved infection control must depend on a twofold campaign: (1) further efforts to eliminate bacteria from the operating environment, and (2) continuing studies of the mechanisms by which the patient defends himself against invasive organisms.

MEASURES TO REDUCE OPERATIVE BACTERIAL CONTAMINATION

Elaborate precautions are taken on the modern surgical service to protect the patient from contamination. They range from chemotherapy to radiation, from steam sterilization to air filtration, and they even include the very architectural design of the operating room itself. These measures are the result of enormous effort, careful experimentation, and accumulated clinical observations, and they provide the surgical patient today with an environment as bacteria-free as possible.

Sources of Bacterial Contamination

Although the ultimate success of any program of asepsis is judged by the postoperative wound infection rate and not by the number of bacteria that reach the wound, a reduction in the number of bacteria contaminating the wound during the surgical procedure must in some way be related to the overall infection rate. The major sources of bacteria, therefore, must be singled out and studied for their possible contribution to wound infections if they are to be eliminated or reduced.

Every surgical wound is contaminated by at least a few bacteria and, in most cases, these organisms are pathogenic. Broadly speaking, they can stem from three leaks in the aseptic environment: the scrubbed surgical team, the patient, or the general operative environment, including the air in the operating room (Fig. 3.1).

In the first instance, the source might be the nose, throat,

174

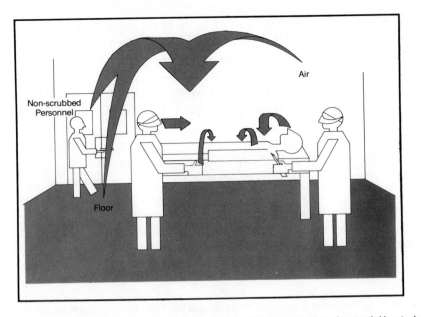

Figure 3.1 Schematic drawing demonstrating the broad categories of potential bacterial contamination of the surgical wound and the relative proportion of each.

skin, or hands of any member of the scrubbed team. Enormous efforts have been directed at improving surgical gloves, surgical masks, and degerming procedures for surgeons' hands. At the present time, the scrubbed team represents a relatively minor source of infective organisms *unless human error introduces a significant break in technique.*

Currently, a more important contributor of bacteria to the wound is the patient. The sources from which patient-borne bacteria emerge start with the skin. Skin cleaning should begin a day or two before the operation with showers or baths using antibacterial soap. Iodine, alcohol, and chlorhexidene are effective for final operative preparation. One percent tincture of iodine is the least expensive and the easiest skin preparation to use, provided that care is taken to wash off excess amounts and to avoid spilling into the patient's eyes or skin creases. Shaving the skin is not a proved means of prophylaxis. If it is necessary, it should be done no more than a few minutes before surgery. Shaving the day before is often harmful because razor nicks actually incubate skin organisms, thus increasing rather than decreasing contamination.

175

The patient's nose and throat have been given less attention, unfortunately, than the incision site. This seeming oversight may be due to the complexities of modern anesthesia. Masking of the patient, at any rate, has never become a widely accepted practice, even though the main areas from which the patient could contaminate his own wound certainly include his nose and throat.

Obviously, the opening of heavily contaminated spaces within the patient constitutes a major infection threat.

The greatest source of contamination in the basically clean operation is the operative environment, a term that covers every other element in the operating room from the nonscrubbed personnel to the air over the surgical wound. This indirect provider of bacteria also supplies the greatest number of individual strains to the wound site (Fig. 3.2).

Figure 3.2 Percent of wounds receiving typable staphylococci from each source (*After Burke JF:* Ann Surg 158: 898, 1963).

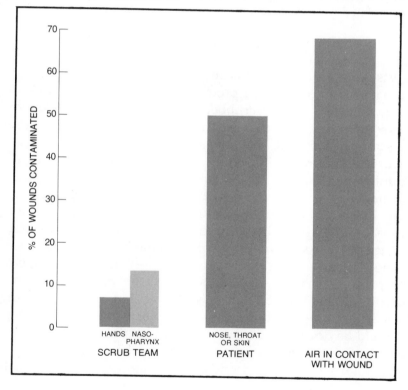

Efforts to clean up the operating environment have largely concentrated on the air-handling system and the physical design of the operating room. Unfortunately, technical improvements in these areas have tended to deemphasize the need to control the behavior of nonscrubbed people in the operating room.

Although vast sums have been spent on elaborate operating rooms and so-called laminar-flow ventilation systems, no one has produced a design that cannot be neutralized by human behavior. In general, the more elaborate systems have added little to the basic principles of asepsis. There is ample evidence, though, that modern operating room designs permit only an occasional colony-forming unit of bacteria to enter by way of the ventilation system. Studies of operating rooms during periods of inactivity indicate that although the walls and floors may contain considerable numbers of bacteria, these organisms do not enter the air of the room. Bacteria do not become airborne unless they are pushed into the air by blasts of air or mechanical brushing.

Thus, human activity accounts for most of the organisms in the air of an operating room. Movement or talking by the nonscrubbed staff leads directly or indirectly to the dissemination of the major portion of bacteria-containing particles in the air. Members of the scrubbed team, so long as they are relatively motionless, contribute little to this contamination.

The rules of behavior in the operating environment come down to simple common sense and a strict "surgical conscience." Movement should be restricted to those functions necessary to conduct the operation. Talking should be minimal. Any break in aseptic procedure should be reported and corrected immediately, *no matter who does the reporting and no matter who has to correct it!*

Sterilizing Techniques

Sterilization of surgical equipment plays a major part in preventing surgical infection. In the autoclaving of instruments and operating room supplies, it is generally agreed that a 30-minute exposure to saturated steam at a pressure of 15 to 17 pounds per square inch and at a temperature of 250 to 254 F provides dependable sterilization. "Flash" autoclaving, which is applicable only to naked unhinged instruments, involves a higher temperature (270 F) and shorter time (three minutes). Each sterilization run must be carefully handled, and the articles to be sterilized must be packaged in holed steel containers and arranged within the autoclave so that the steam will come into direct contact with them.

Most autoclaves used today depend on gravity to help the steam displace air from the chamber and the articles inside it. Disregarding proper packaging procedures and poor positioning of the autoclave contents can, therefore, thwart sterilization efforts even though the required pressures and temperatures are reached for the prescribed time. Autoclaving must be conducted by responsible individuals who understand the principles involved, and spot checks should be made of packages that have been put through the sterilization cycle.

Visual indicators are generally used to demonstrate that autoclave contents have been exposed to heat. These range from adhesive paper (that shows diagonal black strips when it comes into contact with moist heat) to bacterial spores and chemical solutions or solids enclosed in glass tubes. However, while heat-sensitive techniques are useful in indicating that an article has been in the autoclave, *in no way do they prove that the article is sterile.*

A number of materials or substances pose particular problems in sterilization. These include rubber or latex gloves, petrolatum or other greases or oils, powders, certain delicately constructed instruments, and instruments made of plastics. Steam is destructive to these items, so they must be exposed to newer methods of cold chemical or ethylene oxide gas sterilization, or even electron beam irradiation—methods involving sometimes complex and even controversial technologies. We know, however, that the older, simpler methods of quaternary ammonia soaks and boiling water are ineffective and have no place in modern sterilization procedures (Table 3.1).

Aseptic or Sterile Technique

In the past 100 years we have seen the development of complex and perhaps at times even mystical codes of operating room

Table 3.1 Some Acceptable Methods of Sterilization and Disinfection Commonly Used in Operating Room

Basic Principle: Initial cleanliness, adequate contact, sufficient time, and the use of an efficacious agent are the controlling factors in effective sterilization and disinfection.

Method	*Typical Uses*
Autoclave (pressurized wet heat) Normal sterilization cycle 121 C 30 min 15 lb/sq in Flash sterilization cycle 134 C 3 min 29.4 lb/sq in	Sterilization of drapes, gowns, sheets, towels, surgical instruments, lap pads, surgical needles, and other items not damaged by intense heat. For unwrapped, open instruments only, with no linen in tray.
Ethylene Oxide Gas Chemical sterilization under carefully controlled time, temperature, and humidity conditions. Items corporating rubber, plastic, and other nonmetallic materials must be aerated for up to 24 hr after sterilization to dissipate toxic residual gas ("gas aerator" can reduce aeration time).	Sterilization of lensed instruments, ampules, catheters, anesthesia face masks and tubing, pacemakers, and other heat-labile items. (For implantable items up to 72 hr of aeration may be required depending on composition of plastic materials.)
Activated Gluteraldehyde Cold chemical solution effective against vegetative organisms (5 min), T.B. bacilli (10 min), and spores (10 hr.) Items must be rinsed in sterile water before contact with human tissue.	Disinfection of lensed instruments, anesthesia face masks and tubing, and other heat-labile nonporous items.
Povidone-Iodine Kills vegetative organisms (10 min) and T.B. bacilli (20 min) but is not sporicidal.	Patient skin preparation and preoperative hand scrubbing.
70% Ethyl Alcohol Kills vegetative organisms and T.B. bacilli in 5 min. Not sporicidal. Dissolves cement in lensed instruments.	Disinfection of polyethylene tubing, other plastic items, and electrical cords.
Phenolics Kill vegetative organisms and T.B. bacilli when properly applied in effective concentrations for sufficient time.	Cleaning and disinfection of environmental surfaces such as floors, walls, and furniture.

dress and behavior. In Lister's day, "sterile" technique consisted mostly of the liberal use of carbol solution, both as a spray and as a soak. Then, in the last two decades of the 19th century, there was a vigorous argument between the proponents of aseptic and antiseptic surgery.

The surgeons who embraced antiseptics felt that problems of wound infection could be solved by the efficient use of such germicides as carbolic acid. They reasoned that all microorganisms that might come in contact with the wound during the surgical period would be killed by the germicide before the wound was closed. They also believed that the air was by far the most important source of infective bacteria.

On the other hand, the aseptic surgeons held that all objects used in the operating room should be free of bacteria, i.e., sterile, when they were brought into the room. Advocates of this school of thought were the first to insist on scrupulous cleanliness in the operating room and began to wonder about the sterility of hands, the use of coats stained with the blood of previous patients, and the microorganisms that might be exhaled by the surgeon and his assistants. As early as 1866, Ernst von Bergmann of Berlin introduced steam sterilization of all bandages, ligatures, and instruments and thus providing the first major step along the road to modern aseptic surgery. Special gloves, masks, gowns, and the surgical scrub ritual are products of this line of thought.

Years of experience and conclusive experiments have amply vindicated the views of the early aseptic surgeons, although some antiseptic techniques have survived. The elaborate precautions that evolved over the years have accomplished their purpose to a large extent. However, attempts to deal with Lister's original concern, airborne organisms, have not achieved anything like the successes recorded in the area of instrument sterilization for instance, and even the most advanced aseptic techniques have not yet produced a complete absence of bacteria from the operative environment.

Nevertheless, attention to aseptic technique is of utmost importance in minimizing the risk of wound infection in all elective or emergency surgical procedures. In the emergency setting, of course, the use of aseptic technique is complicated by the fact that many injured patients require immediate attention to life-threatening physiologic abnormalities. The need for prompt measures to deal with massive hemorrhage, respiratory insufficiency, or cardiovascular collapse will frequently take precedence over the details of sterile technique and concerns about cross-infection, but this is no excuse for omitting them when they can be used.

The wound is not the only route by which bacteria can invade the traumatically injured patient. The respiratory and urinary tracts and bloodstream may become infected by organisms carried on instruments or equipment used in the rush of an emergency situation. When used for emergency resuscitation without proper precautions, intravenous catheters, tracheostomy tubes, Foley catheters, and dressing sponges can become conduits for cross-infection.

This problem is underscored by the fact that the bacterial species that most frequently cause serious sepsis following trauma are not those likely to contaminate a wound at the time of injury. They are most often gram-negative strains that are probably resistant to antibiotics commonly used in the hospital. The lesson to be drawn is that in both planned operative procedures and general surgical care strict attention must be paid to the details of aseptic technique. *In the emergency situation, the strictness of this attention ultimately is reduced to a matter of personal and team discipline.*

METHODS THAT SUPPORT NATURAL HOST RESISTANCE TO BACTERIAL INFECTION

Research in the past few years has clearly demonstrated the effectiveness of the body's immune mechanisms in preventing bacterial invasion in the person with normal health. The consequences of immunity impairment or suppression are disastrous. Thus, the management of the surgical patient must include operative techniques that minimize injury to the tissue and preserve normal *local physiology* and resistance. It must also include the use of preventive antibiotics, and it must be complemented by overall support of the patient's natural defense mechanism through maintenance of normal systemic physiology. A description of this immunity and its disorders is in the next chapter.

Physiologic Measures Important in Preventing Infection

Meticulous Surgical Technique   There is now agreement, both in
the clinic and the laboratory, that meticulous surgical technique
is crucial to the prevention of postoperative wound sepsis. Although there is ample evidence that the number of bacteria
involved is a major factor in the development of infection (Fig.
3.3), there is equally impressive evidence that trauma and
hypoxia are also critically important.

The exact number of bacteria needed to create a suppurative
lesion varies according to the physiologic state of the tissue in

Figure 3.3   Percent of incisions infected following inoculations with various doses of
bacteria *(After Morris PJ, Barnes BA, Burke JF:* Arch Surg 92: 368, 1966 copyright 1966,
American Medical Association).

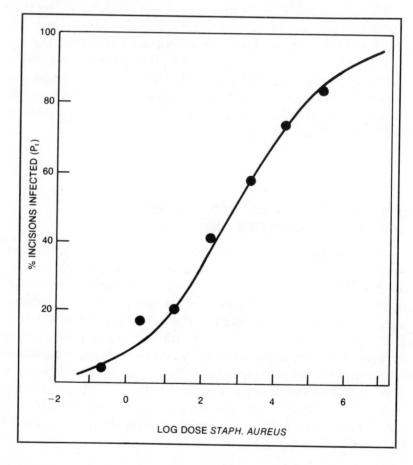

which the bacteria find themselves. Therefore, as noted before, incomplete hemostasis, retained blood clots, and necrotic or traumatized tissue can convert a wound that ordinarily would resist millions of contaminating organisms into one that is susceptible to hundreds.

Thus, surgical techniques must aim at avoidance of tissue damage caused by mechanical trauma or ischemia. Necrotic tissue or foreign substances must be removed. Complete hemostasis is indispensable since it can reduce the chance of hematoma formation and minimize tissue damage. Other essential measures include gentle manipulation of tissue, the use of noncrushing clamps and instruments, the avoidance of rough or prolonged retraction, and judicious use of electrocautery.

Thoughtful selection of sutures on the basis of the task at hand, rather than for the convenience or prejudice of the surgeon, is another important way to reduce tissue damage and the quantity of foreign material left in a wound. Sutures should be used to approximate tissue accurately without causing strangulation. The right number of sutures is the least number required to do the job.

If meticulously adhered to, these principles of surgical technique will help provide a surgical incision whose resistance to bacterial invasion will be at its best.

Accurate anatomic reconstruction of the wound is essential to the success of primary closure. This is as true in the abdominal wall as it is in the reconstruction of a nerve, tendon, or loop of bowel. If repair of the incision restores proper anatomic relationships and does not create spaces for the collection of blood or serum, healing should proceed at an optimal rate and the risk of infection should be minimal.

Any factor that delays wound healing increases the risk of sepsis. In postoperative management, therefore, local dressings, immobilization (especially after debridement and closure of a traumatic wound on an extremity), and the prevention of venous or lymphatic congestion, by elevation of the extremity are as important in preventing infection as is proper shielding of the wound from environmental bacteria.

Maintenance or Reestablishment of Normal Physiology The maintenance or reestablishment of normal physiology is the foundation upon which all other antisepsis measures rest. Maximum control of infection requires maintenance of active host resistance, as bacteria cannot yet be totally eliminated from the operative environment. Without normal perfusion and natural nonspecific immunity, outside means of controlling infection will accomplish little. One must emphasize careful and gentle surgery. A tissue injury resulting from rough or inaccurate surgical technique undermines local host defenses and makes that tissue an easy target for bacterial invasion.

Preservation of local resistance is, however, not the surgeon's only goal. Systemic resistance must also be kept up through the maintenance or reestablishment of normal physiology. Low cardiac output and systemic hypoperfusion will compromise the functioning of the brain, kidneys, and heart, and will seriously weaken the patient's local and systemic antibacterial mechanisms. This loss of host resistance is particularly detrimental in the contaminated wound. Prevention or immediate correction of local or systemic circulatory failure is essential to the prevention of wound sepsis. No antibiotic can penetrate if the injured area is vasoconstricted due to hypovolemia.

Normal respiratory function and adequate gas exchange also must be maintained as must acid–base equilibrium, electrolyte balance, and overall hydration, if the white cells are to function normally. These cells are hampered in hyperosmolar environments, for example, and their mobility is reduced by low intracellular potassium concentrations.

Preexisting disease states, such as diabetes, which alter host resistance, must be controlled as well. Excess exogenous or endogenous steroids inhibit probably all aspects of the immune systems; antiinflammatory steroids should be reduced or, better yet, replaced with cortisol if at all possible. Hyperglycemia should be minimized since it inhibits leukocyte migration, yet adequate supplies of glucose and insulin are necessary to provide energy for phagocytosis, protein synthesis (and thus antibody formation), as well as to ensure normal cardiopulmonary energy resources.

CIRCULATION Nothing in the total management of the surgical patient at risk of sepsis is more important than the rapid and effective use of measures to return circulation to normal. The most meticulous debridement, the most timely and accurate repair of vascular occlusion and the most extensive use of antibiotics will all accomplish little without the simultaneous resumption of normal tissue perfusion. It is obvious that immediate correction of circulatory failure is essential to prevent death. But it is not widely recognized that it is also essential to the prevention of wound sepsis.

The effects of hypotension on the body's ability to defend itself against bacterial invasion have been well documented (Fig. 3.4). Unfortunately, adequate circulation is often thought to have been achieved when urine flow resumes or normal arterial pressure returns. Actually, the peripheral muscle mass and skin may remain seriously underperfused in such cases. This circulatory defect in a wound can allow bacteria to proliferate, at least in part, because the local leukocytes are not being adequately oxygenated and circulating antibodies are not being

Figure 3.4 Increase in lesion size of bacterial infection caused by dehydration shock, and insusceptibility to increases in lesion size of infection when bacterial injection is made two hours following shock (*After Miles:* Br J Exp Path 38: 79–96, 1958).

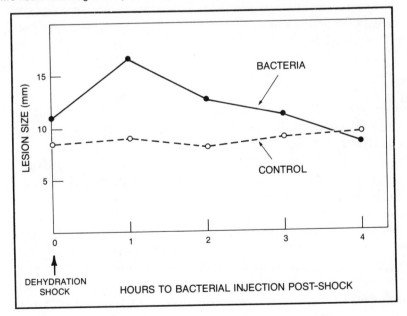

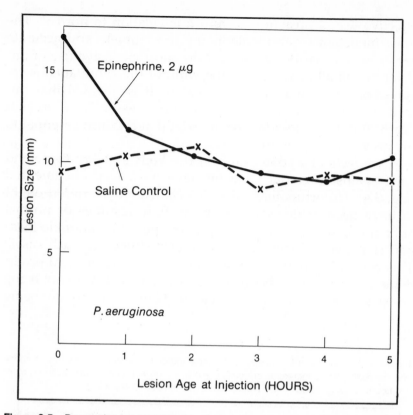

Figure 3.5 Decreasing susceptibility to enhancement of lesion as lesion age increases at time of 2 μg epinephrine injection.

delivered. In this context, the peripheral hypoperfusion produced by vasoconstrictive agents provides a further reason to avoid their use (Fig. 3.5).

Here, clinical examination of the patient is extraordinarily useful. The degree to which the wound is perfused is usually visible. Warm, dry skin (especially at the areas that can be most easily constricted, such as the knees and face), good capillary return in the face or near the wound, lack of postural hypotension, moist tongue, lack of thirst and good eye turgor, all attest to good skin and subcutaneous blood flow, thus assuring maximum resistance to the inevitable contamination. Patients who cannot pass these tests are likely to have poor wound perfusion and are at extra risk of infection. (See Chap. 2).

NUTRITION Malnutrition, particularly protein depletion, seriously hampers the patient's ability to mount a substantial antibacterial effort. Lymphocyte deficiencies, lymphopenia, and immunoprotein deficiencies occur early in acute starvation, but restoration of nutrition can rapidly bolster the patient's immune competence. On the other hand, sepsis increases the patient's nutritional needs and further decreases resistance to bacteria, thus creating a vicious cycle that can be interrupted only by combating both the sepsis and the defect in the host resistance.

Vitamin deficiencies can have a similar effect; vitamins A and C, in particular, are associated with natural immunity. In some mysterious way, vitamin A is both a component of a complete inflammatory reaction and an adjuvant in the development of specific antibody. Vitamin C is probably important to superoxide formation in the oxidative killing mechanism of white cells. For their part, the B vitamins are required for energy production, even in the white cells. Although their role in the immune system has not been established, it is probably important. (Appropriate vitamin dosages will be discussed in a subsequent chapter.)

All this indicates how important a patient's preoperative nutritional state is to infection prevention. Preoperatively, protein starvation, for example, potentiates sepsis more than postoperatively. A complete work-up for surgical candidates must include more than a simple evaluation of hematocrit, a white blood cell count, and a nonprotein nitrogen determination. The patient should be checked for vitamin deficiencies and questioned about weight loss and hair growth. Serum albumin and other indicators of malnutrition should be assessed by appropriate laboratory tests.

CONGENITAL AND ACQUIRED DISEASE Agammaglobulinemia or defects in the complement system can create gaping holes in a patient's defenses, as can hormonal imbalances. Adrenal corticosteroids retard the inflammatory reaction, and in large doses they weaken host resistance. Then, too, there are a number of specific conditions that will sap the antibacterial defenses, among them are Cushing's disease, Addison's disease, diabetes mellitus, the various leukemias, obesity, and liver disease (Table 3.2).

187

Table 3.2 Congenital or acquired conditions that reduce natural or specific immunity to wound infection.*

Congenital Defects
    Agammaglobulinemia
    Chronic granulomatous disease
    White cell disorders

Acquired Defects
    Diabetes mellitus, especially diabetic hyperosmolarity and acidosis
    Cushing's syndrome (endogenous or exogenous)
    Addison's disease
    Leukemias and aplastic anemias
    Severe hemolytic anemia
    Hypersplenism syndromes
    Obesity
    Liver failure
    Heart failure
    Radiation sickness
    Severe trauma
    Active sepsis
    Coagulation disorders
    Malnutrition
        Long-standing bowel obstruction
        Malabsorption and short bowel disorders
    Active tuberculosis, leprosy, fungal disease

Local Defects
    Rheumatic heart valve defects
    Congenital heart and great-vessel disease
    Chronic pulmonary disease
    Radiation tissue damage
    Poor local blood flow
    Regional ischemia
    Neuropathies

*Their presence implies the need to bolster perioperative resistance.

Severe trauma inhibits host resistance; some of the effect is mediated through catecholamine release, hypovolemia, and inadequate oxygenation of leukocytes. However, there are also humoral and specific cell-mediated immune responses that are suppressed by trauma. Burned patients in particular are severely affected: even homograft rejection is suppressed in severely burned patients. At the moment, the only known means of supporting the immune mechanisms in these patients lies in nutrition, support of blood volume, minimization of catecholamine release, and control of existing infection. This is discussed in more detail in Chapter 4.

Supplementing Weakened Host Resistance

Host resistance is the prime factor in preventing sepsis, and its loss cannot be offset by antibiotic therapy. Antibiotics are dependent upon a response from the patient. Normal, intact tissue is usually resistant to bacterial infections (Fig. 3.6). But since the level of natural resistance varies from tissue to tissue, resistance to infection depends on the patient's overall physiologic state. It is imperative that periods of weakened host resistance be quickly recognized, and that the defenses be immediately repaired or supplemented. For example, surgical and anesthetic procedures and various diseases cause marked aberrations in host resistance. In these instances, a small contamination may be large enough to overwhelm the weakened natural resistance, in which case prompt supplementation may tip the balance back in the host's favor.

Understanding Host Resistance   With an increasing number of high-risk patients undergoing operation with low resistance to infection, it is urgent that efforts to understand the basic principles of host defense be expanded. It is increasingly clear that the future of surgery will largely rest on the surgeon's ability to restore his patient to a state of normal resistance to bacteria. An ultimate solution to the sepsis problem in operations to implant prostheses, for example, will involve the following combination: measures to quickly reestablish host resistance, new means of bolstering that resistance, and the already established practices of aseptic technique, meticulous surgery, and control of infection.

The patient's defense system operates on two levels: specific (or acquired) and nonspecific (or natural) immunity. Specific resistance is marked by "learned" activity directed against a particular microorganism, one the host has encountered before. It is characterized by such elements as specific humoral antibody, opsonins, delayed hypersensitivity reactions, and specific cellular immunities mediated through the lymphocyte and macrophage systems. Although it is extremely important in the overall scheme of antibacterial defenses, acquired immunity plays a secondary role in preventing postoperative surgical infection.

Natural, or nonspecific, immunity, on the other hand, is of primary importance in preventing postoperative bacterial problems. It does not depend on the previous experience of the host; the terms "natural" or "nonspecific" refer to innate antimicrobial mechanisms such as phagocytosis, intracellular killing by enzyme systems, and by such extracellular substances as properdin, complement, myeloperoxidase, and lysozyme. Although the systems are different, they do overlap at certain points and complement each other to a great extent.

Studies have shown that an enormous inoculum of viable staphylococci must be injected into the dermis of a normal person before a lesion will develop. The number of bacteria needed to overwhelm normal host defenses runs into the millions. Any lesser number is effectively dealt with, indicating

Figure 3.6 Variations in host resistance and extent to which antibiotics can increase the natural level.

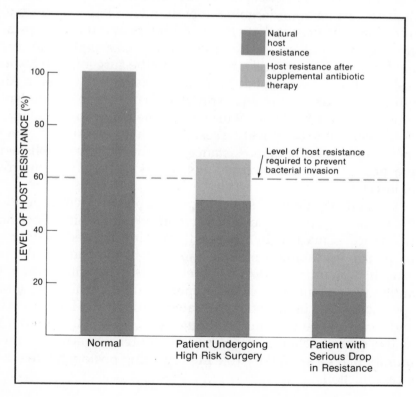

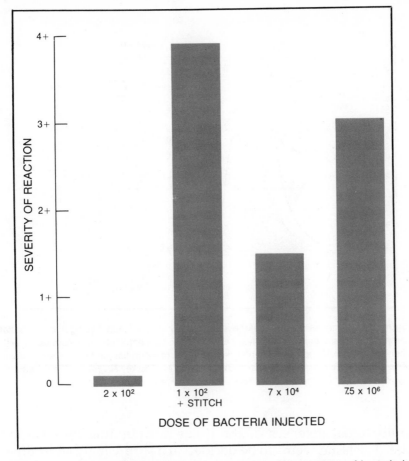

Figure 3.7 Severity of staphylococcal infection as related to numbers of bacteria injected and presence or absence of foreign body in the form of a single silk suture *(After Elek SD:* Ann NY Acad Sci 65: 86, 1956).

the efficiency of intact tissue resistance. However, a foreign body in the form of a single stitch containing approximately 100 viable staphylococci, when put in the dermis, will produce a lesion comparable to that created by an injection of millions of organisms (Fig. 3.7). Obviously, then, the host's defensive forces can easily be confounded by a porous foreign body.

There is a point at which the infecting microorganisms must make their initial lodgement in the tissue. The fate of this "beachhead"—its elimination or its persistence as a staging area for further invasion—depends largely on the state of the

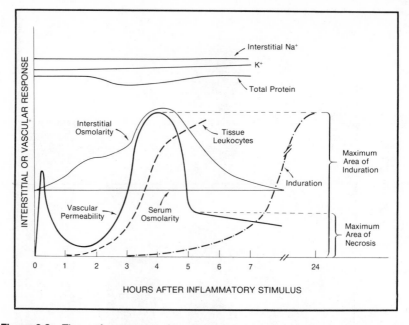

Figure 3.8 Times of occurrence of events in early inflammation. Changes in interstitial composition (osmolarity, electrolyte, and protein concentration) are compared with changes in vascular permeability and development of induration and tissue leukocytosis *(After Leak LV, Burke JF. In Zweifach BW, Grant L, McCluskey RR (eds): The Inflammatory Process, Vol III, 2nd ed. New York, Academic Press, 1974, p 201).*

antibacterial defenses of the tissue surrounding this landing site. The issue seems to be decided in a surprisingly short time, usually in about 3 or 4 hours. Early inflammation (i.e., early inflammatory phase after injury) is a critical period in this intense battle, which is marked by a number of physiologic and biochemical reactions to the contamination (Fig. 3.8). This time has been called the "decisive period in the defense against bacterial invasion."

In a series of animal studies, investigators have examined the effect of blocking various recognized components of early bacterial inflammation on the final size of the bacterial lesion. This type of experiment has confirmed the importance of the individual components of the defense system to the host's overall ability to control bacterial invasion, as evidenced by the eventual lesion size. It has also indicated at about what point during the development of the lesion each of the studied components acts (Fig. 3.9). The mature lesion was chosen as an end

192

point because there is a firm relationship between its diameter and the log number of invading bacteria. It is the number of bacteria that survives the rapid initial killing in the tissue that determines the size of the final mature lesion.

Figure 3.9 The period of active tissue antibacterial activity (decisive period) compared with the arrival of leukocytes in the tissue, the beginning of induration, and the phases of vascular permeability *(After Leak LV, Burke JF. In Zweifach BW, Grant L, McCluskey RR (eds): The Inflammatory Process, Vol III, 2nd ed. New York, Academic Press, 1974, p. 207).*

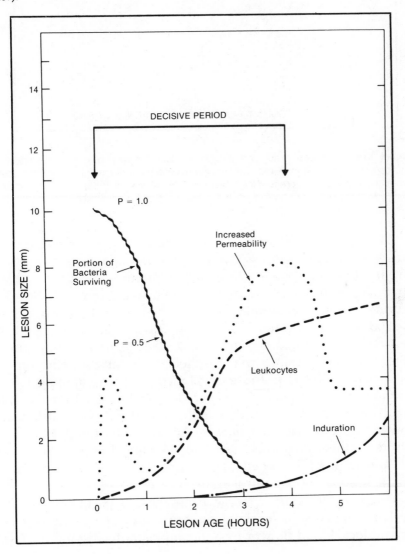

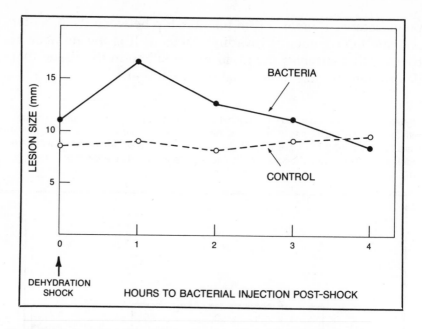

Figure 3.10 Increase in lesion size of bacterial infection caused by dehydration shock, and insusceptibility to increases in lesion size of infection when bacterial injection is made two hours following shock (*After Miles:* Br J Exp Path 38: 79–96, 1958).

An important discovery in the first experiments was that the host's efforts to suppress a developing lesion are greatest during the first few hours following contamination. In three distinct situations—when bacteria were injected into the dermis during a time the animal was in shock (Fig. 3.10), during a period of epinephrine ischemia (Fig. 3.11), or soon after an injection of an anticomplement and anticoagulant compound (Fig. 3.12)—the lesions that resulted were substantially larger and more severe than those developed in control animals with unmodified resistance. However, lesions caused by bacterial injection four or more hours following the same resistance-lowering events *were not enhanced* in size even though they did not reach their maximum dimensions for an additional 20 hours or more (Fig. 3.13). Indeed, at 24 hours, they were the same size as the lesions in the control animals.

Three major points emerge from these experiments. First, certain antibacterial mechanisms are inhibited by reduced or absent local blood flow or by anticomplement substances. (The

194

relationships here are still unclear, but these factors appear to be associated with leukocyte chemotaxis and oxidative killing, and with opsonization, as discussed in other chapters.) Second, these particular antibacterial mechanisms exert their major preventive effect within the first three hours of tissue contamination. Third, it is during this early period that the ultimate size of the lesion is determined. In their normal state, tissue defenses appear to be most efficient over a very short period of time. If they become inoperative before the contaminating organisms are killed, the bacteria multiply and produce an increased area of tissue damage.

An understanding of the events occurring in this decisive period is most important in determining the means by which

Figure 3.11 The enhancement of *S. aureus* infection in the skin by 2 μg epinephrine. The dose of bacteria is plotted logarithmically, and the horizontal distance between the two response lines, measured at the 10 mm lesion diameter, is twelve-fold *(After Miles AA:* Ann NY Acad Sci 66: 357, 1956).

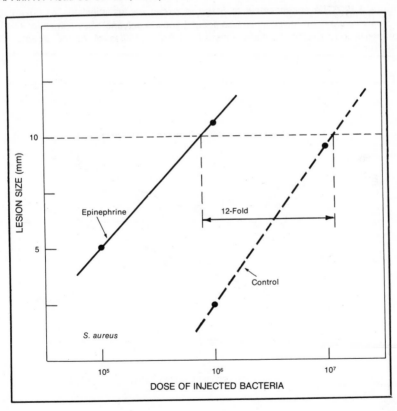

host defenses can be bolstered by exogenous substances such as antibiotics. The crucial nature of this decisive period was underlined by the experimental finding that maximum inhibition of the tissue defenses immediately before, or simultaneously with, initial contamination resulted in the greatest lesion size. Susceptibility to lesion enhancement thereafter declined to the end of the decisive period and then disappeared.

These results suggest that there may be particular value in enhancing host defenses during the critical period. Theoretically, antibiotic substances could augment the natural resistance in the invaded tissue. The bactericidal or bacteriostatic activity of these agents does not perceptibly interfere with natural host mechanisms but affects bacteria directly. The two forces, natural host resistance and antibiotics, should be additive or perhaps even synergistic. Experimental and clinical studies have shown this to be the case.

Figure 3.12 The enhancement of *Staphylococcus aureus* infections by 50 µg anticomplementary and anticoagulant compound sodium polyanetholesulphonate. The increased lesion size of the treated lesions is 240-fold (*After Miles AA:* Ann NY Acad Sci 66: 358, 1956).

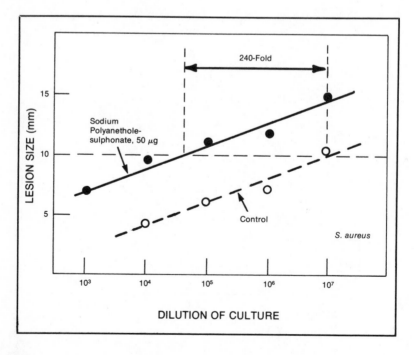

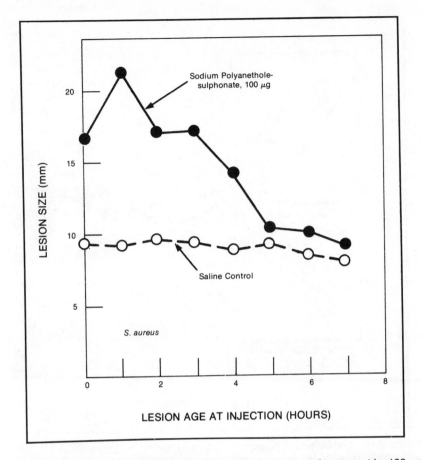

Figure 3.13 Decreasing susceptibility of *S. aureus* lesions to enhancement by 100 µg anticomplementary and anticoagulant compound sodium polyanetholesulphonate with increasing age of the infection. Decisive period 5 hours (*After Miles AA:* Ann NY Acad Sci 66: 359, 1956).

There is a short *effective period,* therefore, during which it is possible to augment the host's antibacterial mechanisms with an antibiotic. In Figure 3.14, *the decisive period,* demonstrated by epinephrine ischemia, is compared with the effective period, demonstrated by the effect of penicillin on an experimental staphylococcal lesion. Studies have shown that if penicillin is given at the same time the wound is contaminated with an organism susceptible to penicillin, the resulting lesion will be similar to one produced by an autoclaved (i.e., killed) bacterial suspension (Fig. 3.15). If, on the other hand, tissue is contaminated and penicillin is not administered until three hours after

197

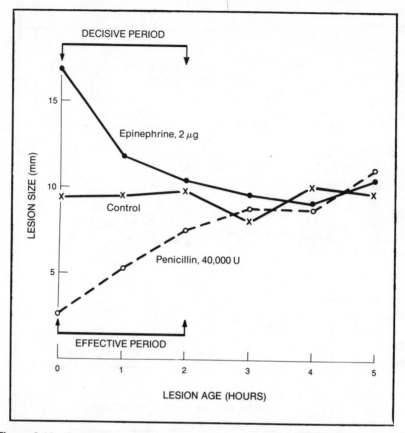

Figure 3.14 Comparison of decisive period as demonstrated by enhancement using epinephrine ischemia with effective period of systemic penicillin, demonstrating that both effects occur during the period of early inflammation depending on whether the natural host defense mechanisms are depressed or supplemented.

the invasion, the lesion will be similar to the one seen in an infected animal given no penicillin at all. That this is a general effect of antibiotics and not peculiar to penicillin is shown in Figure 3.16.

Antibiotics do, in fact, reach the wound after it has been made. Figure 3.17 shows time sequences and concentrations that are typical of cephalosporins. The major point is that the entry of antibiotics is slowed from a few minutes before wounding to over an hour after the wound is made.

Here again, three major conclusions can be drawn. First,

198

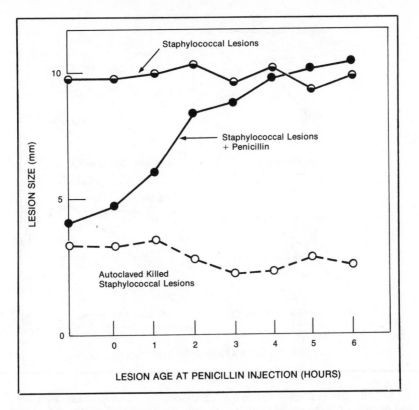

Figure 3.15 Decreasing effect of penicillin on lesion diameter as lesion age at penicillin injection increases. *(From Burke JF:* Surgery 50:1, 161, 1961).

nonspecific host resistance against bacterial invasion is a composite of distinct factors, some of which operate locally. Second, the interaction between the host forces and bacteria begins the moment the invaders arrive in the tissue; there is no "grace period." Third, those defensive forces that have been studied have shown a definitive period of intense, effective activity beginning at the moment of contamination and exerting major detectable effects within a few hours, although the lesion itself continues to develop for another 20 hours or more. Futher, this host activity can be supplemented or undercut by the actions of the surgeon. It is easy to give antibiotics at the proper time and place. It is just as easy to be careless for a moment and leave a hypovolemic or vasoconstricted patient in

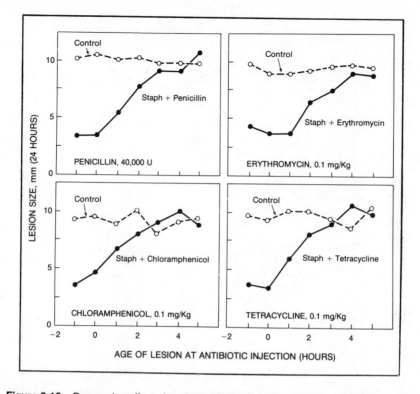

Figure 3.16 Decreasing effect of penicillin, erythromycin, chloramphenicol, and tetracycline on lesion size as age of lesion at antibiotic injection increases. *(From Burke JF: Surgery 50: 1, 161, 1961.)*

the recovery room; and neither antibiotics nor oxygen will be conveyed through constricted local vasculature.

Preventive Antibiotics This use of antibiotics has recently become not only a matter of great importance but frequently of great controversy. Indiscriminate use of antibiotics serves no useful purpose and can often be harmful. At the same time, it is clear that in certain circumstances antibiotics do reduce the risk of postoperative infection.

Experience has shown that in most clean surgical operations the patient's antibacterial mechanisms, even though compromised by the wound, are sufficient to deal with the usual minor bacterial contamination. In these procedures, preventive

200

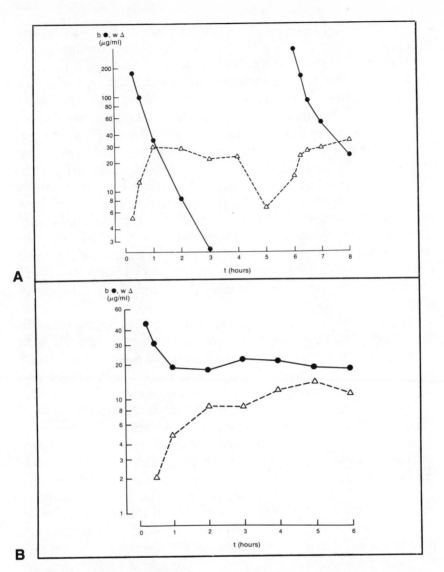

Figure 3.17 **A.** Blood (solid line) and wound fluid (dotted line) cephaloridine concentrations after two intravenous bolus doses of about 50 mg/kg each. Note that equilibrium was not reached until one hour after injection. Concentrations in the wound are well up in the therapeutic range after this high systemic dose. **B.** Blood and wound fluid concentrations of cephaloridine during a constant intravenous infusion (after a small "loading dose"). Note that equilibration occurs only after 5 or 6 hours, and then at a relatively low level.

antibiotics should not be given. However, when the operation involves a physiologic alteration or bacterial contamination large enough to present a serious risk of infection, the surgeon should consider supplementing the host's natural resistance with antibiotics. This supplementation effort must be made within a few hours of bacterial contamination, preferably in anticipation of possible infection. *A preventive antibiotic drug is clearly most effective if it is waiting in the tissue when the bacteria arrive* (Fig. 3.18 and Fig. 3.19).

Unfortunately, of course, antibiotics affect patients in ways other than simply augmenting natural defenses. They can produce allergic or toxic reactions, alterations in the normal bacterial flora, and, in the long-term, resistant strains. Clearly, antibiotics should be administered only when the risk of infection is high. If the patient's own defensive mechanisms are up to the job, there is no need for such a potentially harmful supplement.

The surgical patient represents a somewhat special case in the development of infection. The incision breaches the skin barrier, allowing bacterial contamination of deep tissue. Anesthesia and surgical trauma disturb the normal physiology and decrease the usual cellular and hormonal resistance to bacterial invasion. However, the exact time that both the mechanical barriers will be broken and the patient's natural resistance reduced is known well in advance and is of only short and predictable duration. The surgeon can predict the moment of initial bacterial invasion, and thus can assist the patient through the immediate period of danger with a systemic antiobiotic to supplement the reduced host resistance at the incision site.

A reasonable approach to the use of antibiotics to prevent postsurgical infection can be stated thus: *Preventive antibiotics are indicated if there is a high probability that a patient's natural resistance to bacterial invasion will not overcome the combined bacterial and physiologic challenge of a surgical procedure.* The application of this principle may present problems, though, because the surgeon cannot predict with certainty the probability of infection, or the magnitude of the expected contamination, or even the extent to which normal host defenses will be weakened. Nonetheless, a number of guidelines, but not hard and fast rules, can be put forward.

202

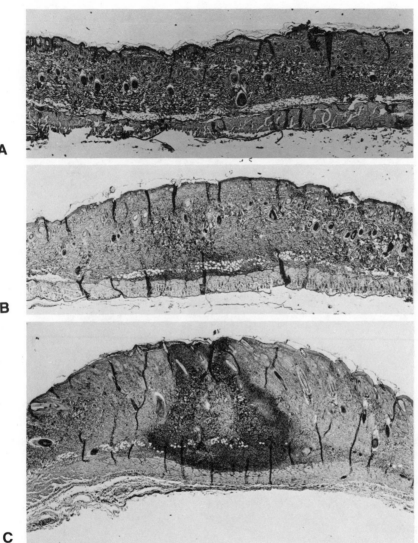

Figure 3.18 Photomicrographs showing histology of control and staphylococcal lesions. Decreasing effect of penicillin is seen as lesion age increases. **A.** Control incision, contaminated with 0.1 ml of saline. **B.** Penicillin, 20,000 units, followed by contamination of the incision with 0.1 ml of live staphylococcal suspension **C.** Incision contaminated with 0.1 ml of live staphylococcal suspension, followed in 3 hours by 40,000 units penicillin (× 39). *(From Burke JF:* Surgery 50: 165, 1961.)

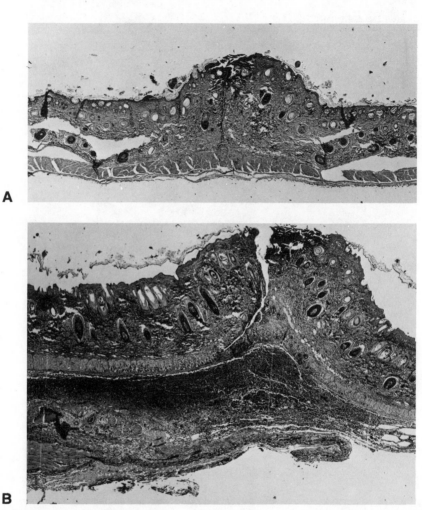

Figure 3.19 A. Control incision, contaminated with sterile normal saline. **B.** Incision contaminated with 0.1 ml of live staphylococcal suspension: no penicillin given.

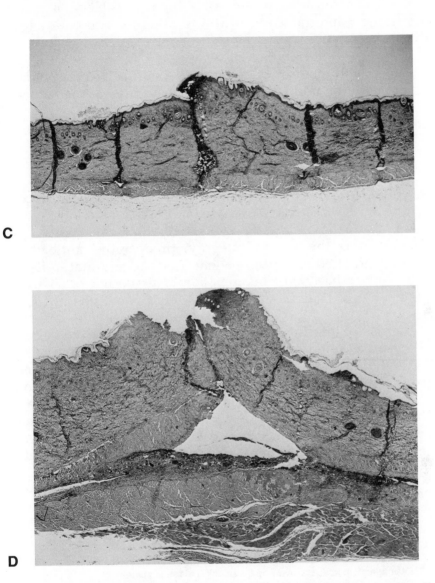

Figure 3.19 **C.** Penicillin, 20,000 units, followed by contamination of the incision with 0.1 ml of staphylococcal suspension. **D.** Incision contaminated with 0.1 ml of staphylococcal suspension, followed in 3 hours by 20,000 units penicillin (× 39). *(From Burke JF: Surgery 50:1 161, 1961.)*

Surgical candidates who have a high probability of post-operative bacterial complications fall into the following categories:

1. Those with diseases or congenital abnormalities that interfere with the normal function of one or more of the natural mechanisms of host resistance.
2. Those in whom the surgical procedure entails a clear hazard of massive bacterial contamination.
3. Those in whom an established local infection would clearly produce disastrous sequelae.
4. Those in whom the extensive nature of the surgical procedure itself threatens to overwhelm host defenses.

Concerning the second category, preoperative antibiotics may be indicated when the patient faces surgery that in itself will produce bacterial contamination of tissue not previously contaminated. Examples of such procedures are listed in Table 3.3.

The risk of infection is obviously proportional to the degree of operative contamination. Table 3.4 summarizes the accepted method of assessing the degree of contamination and the need for antibiotic supplementation. A grey area of difficult decision in so-called clean-contaminated wounds is immediately apparent in the table. The surgeon's dilemma is that despite his preoccupation with infection and his responsibility to prevent sepsis in his patient, he may cause more harm than good with

Table 3.3 Some Surgical Procedures That Will Produce Bacterial Contamination of Tissue Not Previously Contaminated

1. Operation for ruptured appendix
2. Operation for gangrenous cholecystitis
3. Operation for perforated diverticulum or perforated colon carcinoma
4. Drainage of an abscess involving the opening of tissue planes
5. Excision of a localized empyema cavity
6. Decortication in the face of pleural sepsis
7. Excision of a brain abscess
8. Bacterial disease in the watershed of lymph nodes to be excised (this would cover groin dissection at the same time that an ulcerated carcinoma of the foot is excised)
9. Excision of a tuberculous process
10. Debridement of contaminated trauma wounds
11. Excision of a bladder diverticulum in the face of chronic bacterial cystitis
12. Excision of a maxillary sinus tumor complicated by maxillary sinusitis
13. Excision of a bone tumor overlaid by skin ulceration

antibiotics. The complication rate of antibiotics is estimated at about five percent, although not all the problems are serious. However, the harmful results of bacteria being made resistant through antibiotic overuse are incalculable. Many deaths due to such resistant bacteria incubated in surgical wards have been recorded.

The third and fourth categories consist of patients whose operative procedures will seriously compromise their normal physiology. Included are those in whom foreign bodies are to be implanted and those slated for operations in anatomic areas where resistance to bacterial invasion is normally low or where sepsis would result in death or extensive morbidity. The procedures in this classification include a number of neurosurgical, cardiac, orthopedic, and vascular operations.

Although antibiotic schedules have to be individually developed for each patient in each of these categories, the period that is crucial in preventing postoperative sepsis lies clearly between the onset of surgery and the return of normal physiology. The regimen must ensure an adequate level of antibiotic substance in the tissue throughout the entire period of decreased host resistance and probable bacterial contamination. Both experimental and clinical evidence indicate that the antibiotic is most effective if it is already circulating in the interstitial space when the contaminating bacteria arrive.

In the usual operation, bacteria are seeded during the period when the wound is open. The risk of contamination under ordinary circumstances ends with wound closure. There is little evidence to support the use of antibiotics as a preventive measure after the operation; their effective period is limited to the first three hours following bacterial contamination of tissue. (If the rationale for their employment is other than preventive, other considerations would prevail, of course.) Restricting the preventive use of antibiotics to this effective period should minimize the risk of adverse reactions, alterations in bacterial flora, and the creation of resistant strains.

Because host defense mechanisms are most effectively supplemented when a high level of antibiotic is present in the tissue at the time it comes under bacterial attack, the route and time of antibiotic administration are critically important. If delivered intramuscularly, the agent should be given one hour before anesthesia is begun. If delivered intravenously, it may be given following the establishment of the intravenous line

Table 3.4 Operative Wound Classification According to Contamination-Infection Risk

Clean

Nontraumatic

No inflammation encountered

No break in technique

Respiratory, alimentary, genitourinary tracts not entered

Reported infection rates are usually 1 to 4 percent.

In general, no antibiotics are needed unless the host defenses are suppressed or unless the consequences of infection are catastrophic—heart valve replacement, etc.

Drains are not used unless blood or fluid must be evacuated and should be left in no longer than the period of accumulation (usually 24 hours).

Clean-Contaminated

Gastrointestinal or respiratory tracts entered without significant spillage

Appendectomy—not perforated—no cloudy peritoneal exudate

Prepared oropharynx entered

Prepared vagina entered

Genitourinary or biliary tract entered in absence of infected urine or bile

Minor break in technique

Reported infection rates are 5 to 15 percent.

Here the surgeon must use his judgment about using preventive antibiotics.

It will probably not be necessary to use antibiotics in most cases of biliary or small intestinal surgery, unless the operation is to be carried out in the face of invasive bacterial infection or *unless* host defenses are suppressed.

Cases where the consequences of infection are trivial (e.g., minor mouth procedures) do not require antibiotics.

Delayed primary closure may be considered in cases with pre-existing sepsis.

Contaminated

Major break in technique

Gross spillage from gastrointestinal tract

Traumatic wound, fresh

Entrance of genitourinary or biliary tracts in presence of infected urine or bile

Reported infection rates are about 16 to 25 percent, although many centers are reporting lesser rates.

In this category, most patients will need supplementation unless the operation is trivial, as in oral surgery.

Delayed primary or secondary closure techniques should be used frequently.

and prior to the onset of anesthesia in the operating room. In either mode, these administrations should be repeated in three hours, should the operation last that long, and be discontinued at the end of the period of increased risk, with the final injection or infusion given as the patient leaves the operating room (Table 3.5).

208

Table 3.4 *(continued)*

Dirty and Infected	*Infection rates mean little here, but are often over 25 percent.*
Acute bacterial inflammation encountered, without pus	Here, either preventive antibiotics or delayed closure or both should be used.
Transection of "clean" tissue for the purpose of surgical access to a collection of pus	Antibiotics are *not* usually necessary for drainage of a small abscess.
Perforated viscus encountered	
Traumatic wound with retained devitalized tissue, foreign bodies, fecal contamination and/or delayed treatment, or from dirty source	

No benefit is gained by initiating preventive antibiotics earlier than discussed above. Administration started 24 hours before the operative procedure, for instance, adds nothing to the preventive activity and poses the risk of selecting resistant bacterial strains through the prolonged exposure. It also increases the chance of toxic reactions, venous thrombosis, and so on. Nor is there any advantage whatever in continuing antibiotic delivery past the period of bacterial contamination and return of normal physiology. In most surgical patients, therefore, preventive antibiotics should be discontinued after wound closure and the stabilization of postanesthesia cardiorespiratory function.

The question always arises: What antibiotics do you use? Few rules can be given. The predominant wound infections vary with hospitals and circumstances. Hospital "antibiograms" should be consulted. Obviously, preventive antibiotics should be associated with a low frequency of toxic reactions and should match the expected contaminations. For example, if a decortication is being performed for empyema, the surgeon should know in advance which bacterium he will encounter and give an antibiotic known, by test, to be specifically effective

Table 3.5 Timetable for Preventive Antibiotic Therapy

	Intramuscular	*Intravenous*
Begin treatment	1 hr before surgery	When IV line is established
Repeat	Every 3 hr	Every 3 hr
End treatment	In recovery room	In recovery room

against that organism. In some cases, he may select an agent on the basis of a Gram's stain of pus released at surgery. When an incision that was once infected is reopened, the surgeon should order antibiotics effective against the old infecting organism, since bacteria may persist in tissue for many years.

The importance one should place on prevention of anaerobic invasion is still controversial, except in the case of clostridial infection where it has been convincingly proved that debridement of nonviable tissue, particularly muscle, is effective in prevention of clostridial myositis.

Recently, studies have shown that povidone iodine, particularly when used in the aerosolized, dry powder form, has reduced the postoperative wound infection rate to a level comparable with that seen with preventive antibiotics. The timing of delivery of this chemical preventive agent is similar to that demonstrated to be effective in preventive antibiotic management in that the povidone iodine spray was used locally during wound closure. Although studies have not been carried out to demonstrate an effective period for chemical preventive agents similar to that seen with antibiotics, the importance of coordinating the preventive measure with the arrival of bacteria and the uselessness of prolonged treatment after the period of bacterial contamination has ended (as seen with preventive antibiotics) will probably also be true for chemical agents. Experience with dry povidone iodine powder is not extensive enough to clearly assess possible deleterious affects of the agent on wound healing itself so that further studies will be needed. The advantage of avoiding the problem of developing resistant strains of bacteria may be, however, a considerable advantage.

Definitions

A *clean wound* is a nontraumatic, uninfected operative wound in which neither the respiratory, alimentary, or genitourinary tracts nor the oropharyngeal cavities are entered. Clean wounds are made under aseptic conditions. They are usually primarily closed without drains.

Clean-contaminated wounds are operative wounds in which the respiratory, alimentary, or genitourinary tract is entered without unusual contamination.

Contaminated wounds include open, fresh traumatic wounds, operations with a major break in sterile technique (e.g., open cardiac massage) and incisions encountering acute, nonpurulent inflammation such as in cholecystitis or cystitis, or wounds made in or near contaminated or inflamed skin. Unless the procedure is very clean, wounds made for access to the lumen of the colon, belong in this category.

Dirty and infected wounds include old traumatic wounds and those involving clinical infection of perforated viscera. The definition of this classification suggests that the organisms causing postoperative infection are present in the operative field before operation or that pus contaminates the wound.

Assessment of Risk

The risk of wound infection is the sum of the interactions of the following quantities: (1) the degree of bacterial contamination, (2) cracks in the armour of systemic host resistance, and (3) the degree to which the environment of the wound supports the bacterial inoculum. With this conception in mind (it will be developed more fully in the next chapter), the risk of infection in any given operation can be assessed. The major elements governing the magnitude of bacterial contamination are given in Tables 3.3 and 3.4. Host resistance factors are best summarized in Table 3.2. The favorability of the environment is the sum of the trauma the surgeon has inflicted plus the degree to which the circulating system and tissue metabolism has been impaired by tissue damage, blood loss, trauma, anesthesia, and preexisting diseases.

As one might expect, therefore, certain major risk factors can be identified. The major factors dealing with contamination that have been statistically associated with wound infection are the category of contamination (clean, clean-contaminated, and so on), length of operation, the number of blood transfusions given, preoperative shaving, presence of drains and sutures, or other foreign bodies connecting the wound with the outside environment. Those associated with wound environment are obesity, drains, use of the electrosurgical knife, duration of operation, presence of shock, and hypovolemia. Those factors associated with host resistance are the degree of trauma, number of transfusions, diabetes, obesity, malnutrition, administration of antiinflammatory steroids, age, and associated illnesses.

Examples of the degree to which these factors affect infection rates are given in Table 3.6. This does not imply, for instance, that one should never use drains or razors, but it does imply what the price is for using them routinely.

Table 3.6 Factors Increasing the Risk of Surgical Wound Infection

	Approximate Increase
Age over 60 years	3 ×
Malnutrition	3 ×
Active infection elsewhere	2–3 ×
Obesity	2 ×
Steroid therapy	2 ×
Diabetes	2–3 ×
Prolonged preoperative hospitalization:	
over 2 wk	4 ×
1–2 wk	2 ×
Night-time or emergency operation	2–3 ×
Duration of operation over 3 hr	2–3 ×
Preoperative shaving operative site	2 ×
Use of electrosurgical knife	2 ×
Penrose wound drain	2 ×

Data in this table excerpted from two large multifactorial studies each encompassing over 15,000 operated patients (Ann Surg. 160 (Suppl.): 1–192, 1964; Arch Surg 107: 206–211, 1973.)

TREATMENT OF CONTAMINATED AND SPECIAL WOUNDS

Not all of the wounds the surgeon has to deal with are created under aseptic conditions. Traumatic wounds are often contaminated and thus are under bacterial attack from the start. Similarly, the site of a surgical incision made to approach a deep-lying collection of pus is contaminated shortly after it is created. In either case, it is obvious that the bacterial count in the wound is such that infection is almost sure to follow if the wound is closed primarily, despite the most rigorous aseptic

212

precautions and meticulous surgical technique at the time of closure.

Clinical experience has produced two principles for treating wounds that depart from the concepts of tissue preservation and primary wound closure to obtain healing by first intention. Rapid healing and the promise of a return to normal in the shortest period of time may be sacrificed in these cases to avoid the potentially devastating effects of sepsis.

The first of these is to remove bacteria and poorly perfused tissue by excision of the contaminated wound surface. This, in the modern sense of the word, is called "debridement." The second principle is to provide adequate drainage for any possible locus of bacterial inflammation remaining in the wound. Closure is thus delayed to allow the antibacterial forces at the edges of the wound to eliminate the remaining bacteria and to begin repair, with devitalized exudate being removed promptly. Anatomic reconstruction is postponed until the wound edges can be placed together without danger of infection.

Debridement (Fig. 3.20) can convert a heavily contaminated and often poorly perfused wound into a sterile one, so that primary closure, with its obvious advantages, can be em-

Figure 3.20 Area of debridement.

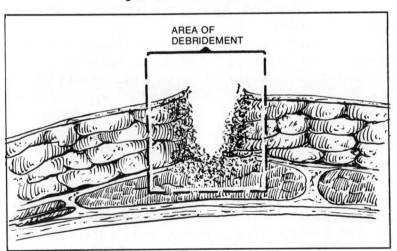

ployed. This approach is most frequently indicated for patients who can be treated less than eight hours following injury, those who have not been in shock and those whose wounds are not massively contaminated. In such cases, debridement and a successful primary closure can decrease postoperative disability and restore function in a relatively short time. However, considerable experience and judgment must be exercised in selecting the cases in which this approach will be successful. Primary closure following debridement should only be tried if all contaminated and devitalized tissue can be removed and if the patient is under the constant scrutiny of trained personnel. Only under these conditions can developing sepsis be detected and attended to immediately. Obviously, debridement is always useful, but primary closure may be hazardous in treatment of mass casualties.

Debridement of all dead and poorly perfused tissue without unnecessary harm often requires extremely precise surgical judgment, especially in areas such as the hand, forearm or face, where removal of potentially viable tissue could create a serious loss of function. Delayed closure gives the surgeon some time to weigh the risk of sepsis against the risk of functional impairment. Where viability is in question, injured tissue can be left in place for careful observation over the postdebridement period and removed if infection develops or continues. Delayed closure also affords reliable drainage of the entire wound, as well as the opportunity for easy and repeated inspection and further debridement if necessary.

A useful and acceptable technique of delayed primary closure is used in cases of borderline contamination when the need for further debridement appears unlikely. In this technique, the edges of the debrided wound are separated by a thin layer of mesh gauze or skin allograft (Fig. 3.21), which allows effective drainage without danger of pocketing. The wound is then covered by an occlusive dressing to prevent further contamination. If exudate, local pain, cellulitis, or a systemic reaction occurs, the wound can be examined without difficulty and further debridement carried out as necessary. If, however, no such indications for inspection arise, it can be left undisturbed for four or five days. Then, if there is no sign of suppuration or further devitalized tissue, it can be closed by direct apposition of all layers of the tissue, including the skin (Fig. 3.21). Several

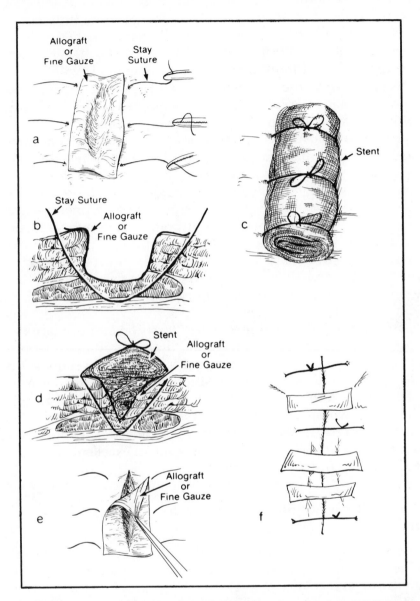

Figure 3.21 Steps in technique of delayed primary closure using allograft or fine gauze wound cover: a) allograft or gauze placed as the usual split thickness skin graft; b) relation of debrided area to allografted surface and stay suture tract; c) and d) stent holding allograft in place on debrided surface; e) removal of allograft or gauze at time of definitive closure; and f) appearance of wound following definitive closure.

studies have shown statistically that closure without infection can be achieved most successfully on the fourth or fifth day.

Delayed primary closure is a time-honored method used to particular advantage by military surgeons. However, if the technique is used indiscriminately, many wounds will become infected despite the delayed closure. The surgeon must develop the skills to recognize which wounds can be closed and which are too contaminated to withstand closure.

Secondary closure is reserved for those wounds that manifest obvious superficial or invasive infection when they are first encountered or for wounds that develop sepsis during the sequence leading to delayed primary closure. In these wounds, closure is delayed until granulation tissue has formed, generally after 10 days or more. At that point, a secondary closure may take two forms, the first being simple joining of the two granulating surfaces. The second method, which usually gives the best functional result, involves the excision of both the granulating tissue and the indurated scar tissue, followed by a joining of the two surfaces.

This technique, sometimes called "excision and primary closure," might be used following the drainage of a perinephric abscess. When the perirenal process no longer floods the wound with purulent material, secondary closure may be used to decrease morbidity. In this case, the granulating wall around the flank wound would be excised and the contaminated granulation tissue and indurated scar removed. Closure of the fresh tissue would then give the wound an excellent chance to heal without further infection.

Burns: Techniques of Primary Excision and Prompt Wound Closure

The most effective treatment of the burn wound, as with any other wound, is prompt excision of all devitalized tissue followed by immediate closure.

Evidence accumulated over recent years indicates that the high mortality rate associated with postburn infections reflects a combination of bacterial invasion and serious defects in the victim's resistance, due to the many consequences of having a large wound open for a prolonged time. Topical or systemic antibiotics serve only as adjuncts in burn therapy; they do not deal directly with the problems created by a large open wound and associated protein and calorie starvation. A solution to the problem of extensive skin loss secondary to burns appears to lie in rapid excision of devitalized skin followed immediately by closure of the wound.

Two techniques can be used to excise the devitalized tissue. The first, *direct excision to the fascia*, is reserved for large areas of unequivocal, full-thickness burn injury. The second, *sequential eschar excision*, includes areas of deep dermal injury as well as full-thickness burns and is appropriate, obviously, in cases of mixed deep dermal and full-thickness injuries and in burns where the exact depth of various areas of the injury cannot be determined unequivocally. In this technique, sequential slices of necrotic tissue are removed (with a knife having a guard to govern the thickness of slices) until viable tissue is reached. In either type of primary excision, the resulting wound is promptly closed by skin grafting.

Topical therapy can provide a high degree of bacterial control on the wound itself. Surface application of an antibacterial agent can reduce the number of organisms in the burn area to levels that will help avoid invasive infection, once the chief cause of death in burn patients. Silver nitrate, silver sulfadiazine, povidone-iodine, and Sulfamylon are among the most frequently used topical agents. Silver nitrate has proved to be the most effective adjunctive agent when primary excision and grafting are employed because it can be easily used to protect freshly grafted areas and donor sites, as well as unexcised burn eschar.

Puncture Wounds

Puncture wounds pose particular infection problems because their depth and narrow entry at the surface prevent efficient cleaning at the time of injury. Such foreign bodies as dirt, rust, or even bits of clothing may be present but undetected and are difficult to remove. Also, purulent exudate from an inflamed puncture wound tends to hide itself in pockets of infection after the wound is sealed by a protein coagulum. For this reason, if there is evidence of deep contamination, such wounds should be opened widely in the emergency room to insure adequate cleaning, debridement, and drainage. If no contamination is found, the wound edges can be allowed to fall together, and, in most cases, such wounds heal uneventfully.

Tetanus prophylaxis must always be considered. Most puncture wounds are infection prone; and depending on their appearance and circumstances, toxoid, antitetanus globulin, and/or penicillin should usually be given.

GENERAL TREATMENT OF ESTABLISHED INFECTIONS

Treatment of an established infection is completely different from prevention of one. The general principles of drainage, elevation, heat, and rest are the cornerstones of management in this setting, with antibiotic therapy now having been added to these classic control measures. Although antibiotics are important in treating localized bacterial infection, their role is often overstated. In a therapeutic mode, as in prevention, antibiotics are simply adjuncts to host resistance and surgical excision or drainage; they do not replace them.

To be an effective supplement in established infection, the antibiotic must be active against the infecting organism and must be used in a concentration that is bactericidal or bacteriostatic. Moreover, it must be given over a period of days, rather than the few hours required for sepsis prevention. Effective antibiotic use in established infection places great stress on the need to restore the patient's normal physiology, nutrition, and anatomy. Selection of longer term therapeutic antibiotics must be made carefully, and their doses precisely adjusted to minimize possible allergic and toxic reactions.

The contaminating organism therefore must be isolated and identified by Gram-stained smear and culture. Its sensitivity pattern must be determined and then matched to a careful, thorough patient history before an appropriate antibiotic is selected. In urgent clinical situations where antibiotic treatment has to be instituted before an exact bacterial diagnosis can be established, a Gram-stained smear of pus may provide vital information until the results of cultures indicate the adjustments that should be made for maximum antibacterial effect.

The methods used to obtain culture material are very important. Tissue biopsy is better than surface smear because it pinpoints the pathogen and not the superficial contaminant. It is far more likely to yield an anaerobe than is a swab. Swabs dry out and often yield no information. Pus usually yields the pathogen, and *pus withdrawn in an airless syringe or placed immediately in anaerobic media is*the only source from which anaerobes are likely to be isolated. Carelessness in obtaining biologic material is far more often the source of inadequate information on the infecting organism than are technical faults in the laboratory.*

The effectiveness of antibiotic treatment has obscured, to an extent, the essential role of host resistance in controlling infection and, unfortunately, has led some surgeons to rely far less on surgical drainage or repair. Thus, it is common to find patients with localized abscesses assigned to a prolonged course of antibiotics where simple drainage could solve the problem with less morbidity and in far less time. Similarly, patients with sepsis due to biliary tract obstruction, for example, may be treated repeatedly with antibiotics when surgical restoration of normal anatomic function would be more likely to produce a permanent cure.

Antibiotics must always be regarded as an adjunct to host resistance and often as an adjunct to an operative procedure such as excision (e.g., in suppurative cholecystitis or acute appendicitis) or drainage of a closed space to allow the effective functioning of host resistance and healing of the wound. Such surgical measures play a major role in the treatment of certain bacterial infections.

Clinical Manifestations of Bacterial Infection

Bacterial infection of tissue usually presents clinically either as *cellulitis* or *abscess*. Cellulitis is a spreading bacterial infection in the tissue planes, causing an intense inflammatory reaction. An abscess, on the other hand, is a localized infection marked by a circumscribed area of necrotic tissue and pus. Bacterial invasion of the vascular spaces, with subsequent dissemination via the blood, is called bacteremia and is a life-threatening condition. Septicemia denotes multiplication of bacteria within the bloodstream as a progression of bacteremia. In lymphangitis, bacteria spread through the lymphatics. Septic phlebitis

219

("pylephlebitis" in the case of the portal vein) occurs when there is infection within the lumen of a vein. Often, thrombus breaks down to produce septic emboli.

Cellulitis   Although all bacterial infections that originate in tissues rather than in the bloodstream begin as cellulitis, most usually remain localized and form abscesses if not eliminated. Only certain bacterial species (β-hemolytic *streptococcus* and some staphylococci) usually spread through tissue as extending cellulitis—defined as a spreading infectious inflammation of connective tissue without suppuration.

The local manifestations of cellulitis are pain and local tenderness, swelling, redness, and local heat.

Rest is an important element in the treatment of cellulitis, for it reduces the possibility that muscle contractures will force the bacteria into lymphatics or veins. Cellulitis of the limbs can usually be ameliorated by elevating the limbs. This procedure aids host resistance with a normal blood supply and frees it of the impediment of dependent edema.

Because in cellulitis there are no localized areas of pus formation, drainage is indicated only to relieve any pressure that may cause ischemia. However, local abscesses may sometimes be surrounded by areas of cellulitis, and here drainage of the abscess, as well as treatment with antibiotics, are essential therapeutic measures.

The bacterial organism most likely to produce the classic picture of cellulitis is the hemolytic streptococcus; here, penicillin therapy is specific. For other bacterial species the choice of antibiotic is not as clear-cut, and identification of the organism and its antibiotic sensitivity is required for effective therapy.

Abscess   Abscess formation is marked by the local collection of necrotic tissue, bacteria, and white cells, commonly called pus. Superficial abscesses can be detected by their localized nature, tendency to develop point tenderness, and fluctuation on palpation. All abscesses should be drained or excised for they present a considerable hazard of further bacterial spread. Because of the enzymatic processes that go on in the abscess, there is increased osmotic pressure within the cavity itself through the splitting of large molecules into fragments. Water migrating into the area under the generated osmotic force produces considerable pressure, and this raises the risk of bacterial spread along tissue planes or by way of blood or lymphatic vessels. Open drainage not only can relieve this pressure but will reduce bacteria number, and thus toxin production, and will permit white cells to operate efficiently. The cavity must be kept open until it is obliterated by natural healing; for, if it is allowed to seal, another closed space and increased pressure will again be created. Incision and prolonged drainage with a drain kept free of coagulation by a wet and frequently changed dressing is often effective when combined with rest, heat, and elevation.

Surgical abscesses are most frequently produced by *S. aureus*. Treatment may require antibiotic therapy in addition to drainage or excision, particularly if there are systemic signs of infection (fever, chills, malaise) or surrounding cellulitis. Staphylococcal strains are no longer commonly sensitive to penicillin, so a penicillinase-resistant drug should be used even if such an infection has been acquired outside the hospital.

Abscesses are easily recognized in the skin or subcutaneous tissue, and also when they begin deeper but point, or migrate, toward the surface of the skin. There are, however, deep-lying abscesses that present far more complex problems of diagnosis and therapy. The ones that develop deep within the body or lie hidden by major anatomic features are difficult to locate and treat. For instance, a brain abscess under the motor cortex cannot be handled by simple incision and drainage. Instead, careful excision of the abscess and its wall may be the best approach. Although excision generally involves a more complicated procedure than incision—and also poses a greater risk of bacterial spread as a result of surgical manipulation—there are clinical problems for which it is the procedure of choice, as in the foregoing situation. As a preventive measure, the control of bacterial spread through the judicious use of antibiotics begun before the operation is extremely important. Here the choice of a preventive antibiotic is often dependent on clinical judgment, for the exact infecting organism may not be known.

Blood and Lymphatic Infections Bacterial infections of the lymphatic or blood systems are usually extensions of localized areas of cellulitis or abscess formation. The rapid dissemination of pathogens through these pathways demand that bacteremia or lymphangitis must always be immediately and vigorously treated with appropriate antibiotics. Local therapy should be directed at the original lesion, with surgical drainage in the case of an abscess.

Bacterial Infections Requiring Surgical Treatment   Besides the infections that result from contamination of tissues, there are a number of bacterial conditions caused by abnormalities of organ function, and these usually produce disease through the development of an obstruction. This may take the form of a stricture, as in the lower urinary tract, or a foreign body, such as biliary and urinary tract stones. The obstruction may also result from the loss or distortion of normal anatomic structure, as in the case of inflammation of a colonic diverticulum. Congenital abnormalities such as those that produce ureteral valve malfunction will also lead to infection. These diseases often present added problems regarding wound infection and must be included in an overall view of surgical infections. Here, as in the treatment of abscesses, recovery from sepsis depends on surgical removal of the obstruction or correction of the anatomic abnormality, not on antibiotics alone.

TREATMENT OF INFECTIONS
ACCORDING TO CAUSATIVE ORGANISM
β-Hemolytic Streptococcal Infections

β-hemolytic streptococci produce a rapidly invasive, spreading infection tending to cause extensive cellulitis with a marked systemic response. One example is erysipelas, which may begin hours after the traumatic contamination of a wound and proceed to fatal septicemia in a matter of days. The infection is accompanied by chills, high fever, rapid pulse, and severe toxemia. Purulent material, if present, is thin and watery, and invasion of the blood and lymphatic streams is frequent and early.

The β-hemolytic streptococcus is highly sensitive to penicillin therapy and, due to an inability to develop resistance, is easily controlled by the use of preventive antibiotics. If an infection does develop, early use of therapeutic antibiotics (penicillin) is effective. Such treatment plus rest, heat, and elevation of the infected area provide early control of the invasive process.

The danger of this infection lies in its ability to produce a rapidly evolving systemic infection increasing the possibility of extensive bacterial invasion before diagnosis and treatment can be implemented. A point to consider is the fact that in mixed bacterial populations such as is often seen in the pharynx or a wound, a penicillinase-producing bacteria, such as a resistant staphylococcus, will protect the β-streptococci from penicillin by destroying the antibiotic. Here, the use of an effective antibiotic which is not subject to penicillinase should be used.

Gram-Negative Organisms

Gram-negative sepsis has increased over the past decade and now accounts for more than half the infections reported following trauma or surgery. *Escherichia coli, Pseudomonas aeruginosa,* and strains of *Proteus* and *Klebsiella* have become frequent adversaries. An explanation of this trend lies not so much in changes of endogenous flora due to the use of antibiotics but, more importantly, because seriously ill patients with weakened natural defenses are now being operated on with reasonable surgical safety. Debilitated individuals, or those in whom debridement of dead tissue has been incomplete, are especially prone to invasion by these low-virulence strains which often result in serious infection, or even death.

The treatment of infections produced by gram-negative bacteria includes surgical incision and drainage of any abscesses, excision of necrotic tissue, and appropriate antibiotic therapy. Most important, though, it demands extensive physiologic and nutritional support. Since these organisms are usually of relatively low virulence, their ability to invade may indicate serious physiologic and/or nutritional abnormalities in the patient.

Tetanus

Tetanus is caused by a toxin produced by *Clostridium tetani,* a spore-forming, strictly anaerobic, gram-positive bacillus widely distributed in nature. It is commonly found in the gastrointestinal tract of domestic animals and in soil. Unlike the usual infective bacteria, which produce their effects by direct invasion, the tetanus bacillus causes disease simply by elaborating toxin, which diffuses throughout the tissue. Severe or even lethal tetanus can thus result from a limited growth of this organism in the most minor of wounds with little inflammation.

Natural tissue resistance to the tetanus bacillus is high; contamination of tissue by this bacillus or its spores ordinarily does not result in bacterial growth or invasion. However, devitalized tissue and/or foreign bodies remaining in a wound, accompanied by poor perfusion, can produce anaerobic conditions under which a tetanus infection can take hold.

Because of prophylactic measures, clinical tetanus is rarely encountered today. It is generally prevented in the normal population by three subcutaneous 0.5 ml doses of absorbed tetanus toxoid. The second injection is given 4 to 6 weeks after the first, and the third is given 6 to 12 months after the second. The immunization afforded by this regimen lasts for at least a year, and a booster shot of 0.5 ml tetanus toxoid within the following 10 years produces a rapid rise in antitoxin titer. This response to the booster dose may last as long as 25 years after active immunization, and in many patients it provides lifetime protection.

For minor injuries in a patient who has undergone tetanus immunization within the previous five years, a booster dose is all that is required. In the immunized patient who has had a booster within the year, no specific antitetanus treatment is indicated. However, when there are extensive destruction of tissue and contamination, passive immunization and penicillin or tetracycline should be given. In the unimmunized patient, passive immunity can be established by an intramuscular injection of human antitetanus globulin. The usual recommended dose is 250 units, although larger amounts have been proposed. Besides the administration of antibody for passive immunity, inoculations to assure active immunity should be started immediately, according to the aforementioned schedule, and should be given in a different limb with a different syringe.

Tetanus may be suspected in a patient who shows insomnia, irritability, tremor, spasms, and rigidity of the muscles adjacent to a wound. The incubation period varies from 4 to 21 days, but is usually between 7 and 10 days. The severity of the clinical disease and the risk of mortality, it should be noted, are *in-*

versely proportional to the length of incubation; the shorter the incubation, the more serious the condition.

The major objectives in treating tetanus are to remove the sources of toxin production and neutralize the toxin already circulating. The first goal is accomplished by thoroughly debriding any traumatic wound by wide excision. Anaerobic conditions must be prevented at all costs, and the wound, therefore, is usually left open following debridement.

Any tetanus toxin subsequently entering the circulation is destroyed by administering 500 units of immune human globulin daily for about 10 days. Antibiotics—usually penicillin, cephalosporin, or tetracycline—are given to prevent further growth of the tetanus bacillus. Because the victim's main symptoms are muscle spasms, it is essential that he or she be sedated and kept in a quiet, dark environment. In severely ill patients with pharyngeal spasm, a nasotracheal tube should be installed or a tracheostomy performed, with muscle relaxants and mechanical respiration being used as necessary adjuncts to ensure adequate respiration. Nutrition can be maintained through a nasogastric tube in such patients who require constant nursing care.

Patients being treated for tetanus should undergo a program of active immunization; the clinical disease does not uniformly confer immunity.

Clostridial Myositis (Gas Gangrene)

Clostridial organisms can produce a spectrum of problems ranging from simple contamination to abscess, from superficial cellulitis to a life-threatening gangrenous infection of muscle. An invasive gangrene—rapidly progressive and causing extensive systemic as well as local lesions—usually arises after injuries associated with devitalized muscle and an acute depression of oxygen tension and oxidation-induction potential.

Pain is an early symptom, usually appearing within 24 hours of the injury. Crepitus may be present in the tissue at this time, but extensive edema can occur in clostridial myositis without gas formation. The patient develops rapidly progressing systemic and local signs: pain, a striking facial pallor, weakness, apathy, profuse sweating, prostration, and shortness of breath.

The pulse is rapid and feeble, but the patient's fever is seldom over 101F. The wound discharge is thin, watery-brown, and foul-smelling, and it usually contains many bacteria and red blood cells but few white cells.

Soluble toxins diffusing into the circulation from the involved tissue can produce a severe hemolytic anemia and renal, cardiac, and liver damage, as well as septic shock, which, without vigorous intervention, may lead to death. Laboratory data include a severe anemia and a relatively low white count, seldom exceeding 15,000 cells per cubic millimeter.

Gas gangrene must be diagnosed early in its course if treatment is to be successful. This can be difficult at times because other infections following treatment of a severe injury may obscure the early signs of a clostridial infection. However, continued pain at the injury site and a rapid and faint pulse with minimal fever, combined with a rapidly spreading toxemia, demand immediate surgical exploration of the wound. Other important signs include a thin, watery-brown and foul-smelling exudate, dusky or bronze-appearing skin overlying the wound (with vesicles filled with dark red fluid), crepitus and herniation of discolored dark red muscle.

Treatment calls for immediate surgical exploration of the wound, with a wide incision and debridement of involved muscle. Intensive antibiotic therapy should be employed—usually penicillin given intravenously.

Supportive therapy is crucial to maintaining fluid and electrolyte balance, as well as to correcting the severe anemia and decreased circulatory volume produced by the infection. Hyperbaric oxygen treatment of gas gangrene may preserve tissue, and perhaps even life, but it should be regarded as a measure adjunctive to surgery.

EPILOGUE

1. Throughout surgical history, control of infection has been the single most important prerequisite to the major advances, and the limits of control have yet to be reached.
2. Surgeons tend to accept the standards of their own practice and time. Undoubtedly, many readers will feel that the battle has been won, that we have reached the irreducible

minimum of infection. Remember, however, that Paré was vilified for suggesting that he could do better than his contemporaries. As it turned out, he was right. For similar reasons, the entreaties of Lister and Semmelweis went unheeded for years.

3. It is unlikely that we will soon see another event as important as the promulgation of aseptic technique. In the absence of such obvious turning points, the rest of the way to zero infection rates will be traveled in slow, probably agonizingly small steps. The development of techniques for restoration and enhancing of natural and acquired immunity is the most logical approach to this objective. With the current knowledge of host defenses dissected and exposed, the reader may find more ways to combat and prevent infection than first seem apparent.

It is therefore logical that the next chapter should examine in more detail the subject of systemic and local host resistance and the management of its disorders.

APPENDIX A
Protocol for Prophylaxis

Cardiac Valvular Disease

50,000 units of procaine penicillin one or two hours prior to operation is considered sufficient. Obviously, intravenous penicillin could be used as well.

Tuberculosis

INH for six weeks prior to operation. Ideally, cultures should be negative.

Summary of Prospective Randomized Studies in Preventive Antibiotic Use

Investigators	Operations	Agents and Dosage	Administration Schedule
Bernard, Cole: Surgery, 56:151, 1964	Gastrointestinal and pancreaticobiliary operations	Penicillin G 600,000 U Methicillin 1 g Chloramphenicol 200 mg	IM 1-2h preop IV intraop IV 4h postop
Campbell: Lancet, 2:805, 1965	General and thoracic surgery operations	Penicillin G 10,000,000 U	IV 15 min. preop Intraop + or − None, postop
Karl, Mertz, Veith, Dineen: N Engl J Med., 275:305, 1966	General surgery operations	Methicillin 2 g Chloramphenicol 500 mg	IM 2h preop IV intraop IV 2h postop
Feltis, Hamit: Am J Surg, 114:867, 1967	Gastrointestinal operations including appendectomy	Penicillin G 300,000 U Methicillin 1 g Chloramphenicol 500 mg	IV preop intraop and postop
Goodman, Schaffner, Collins, Battersby, Koenig: N Engl J Med, 278:117, 1968	Cardiac operations	Penicillin G 1,500,000 U Streptomycin 250 mg	IM on call to OR IM q6h for 3d
Fekety, Cluff, Sabiston, Seidl, Smith, Thoburn: J Thorac Cardiovasc Surg., 57:757, 1969	Cardiac operations without cardiopulmonary bypass	Oxacillin 1 g Penicillin G 500,000 U‡ Penicillin G 1,000,000 U‡ Penicillin G 500,000 U‡ Methicillin 1 g‡ Methicillin 2 g‡ Methicillin 1 g‡	IM 8 and 12h preop IM on arrival in OR IM q6h 6d postop IM 8 and 12h preop IM on arrival in OR IM q6h 6d postop
Polk, Lopez-Mayor: Surgery, 66:97, 1969	Gastrointestinal operations	Cephaloridine 1 g	IM on call to OR IM 5h postop IM 10h postop
Fogelberg, Zitzmann, Stinchfield: J Bone Joint Surg, 52A: 95, 1970	Mold arthroplasty Spine fusion	Penicillin G 600,000 U Penicillin G 5,000,000 U Penicillin G 600,000 U	IM preop IV intraop IM postop 5d

Controls				
(No Antibiotic)		(Antibiotic)		
Number	Wound Infection (%)*	Number	Wound Infection (%)*	P
63	25.3	55	5.4	<0.01
78	16.6	67	8.9	=0.18
70	12.9	65	18.5	
336	11.0	189	1.5	<0.001
15	13.3†	30	6.6†	
		27	11.0†	
		37	2.7§	
22	13.6§			>0.1
		36	2.8§	
98	29.5¶	101	5.9¶	<0.001
112	8.9	120	1.7	>0.025

(continued on pp. 230-1)

Summary of Prospective Randomized
Studies in Preventive Antibiotic Use

Investigators	Operations	Agents and Dosage	Administration Schedule
Ledger, Sweet, Headington: Am J Obstet Gynecol 115:766, 1973	Vaginal hysterectomy	Cephaloridine 1 g	On call to OR Twice postop Route not stated
Boyd, Burke, Colton: J Bone Joint Surg, 55A: 1251, 1973	Hip fracture operations	Nafcillin 500 mg	IM on call to OR IM q6h for 48h
Pavel, Smith, Ballard, Larsen: J Bone Joint Surg, 56A:777, 1974	Clean orthopaedic operations	Cephaloridine 1 g	IM 1h preop IV intraop and postop for 4h

From Altemeier, et al.: Manual on Control of Infection in Surgical Patients, Philadelphia, Lippincott 1976.

*Except where noted, these were wound infections.

†Endocarditis or septicemia.

‡Proportionate doses for children.

§Includes some lung infections.

| Controls | | | | |
| (No Antibiotic) | | (Antibiotic) | | |
Number	Wound Infection (%)*	Number	Wound Infection (%)*	P
50	8.0#	50	8.0#	<0.005
145	4.8**	135	0.8**	=0.041
740	5.0	887	2.8	=0.025

¶Includes intracavitary infections.

#Pelvic infections.

**If infected hematomata are included, the rates are controls, 7.5%; nafcillin group, 5.1%.

††This table contains no cases of trauma, no retrospective analyses and only those studies done between the years 1964–1974.

APPENDIX C
Incidence of Infection
in Relation to Wound Classification

	5 Hospitals (1964)	Foothills Hospital (1973)	Univ. Calif. Hospitals (1975)
Distribution of operations (no. and %)			
Total number	15,613	23,649	7,570
Clean (%)	74.8	76.4	64.6
Clean-contaminated (%)	16.5	17.5	22.3
Contaminated (%)	4.3	3.2	7.9
Dirty (%)	3.7	2.9	5.2
Incidence of wound infection (%)			
Total	7.4	4.8	2.1
Clean	5.0	1.8	1.4
Clean-contaminated	10.8	8.9	3.6
Contaminated	16.3	21.5	4.3
Dirty	28.5	38.3	—

(From Cruse JPE, Foord, R: Arch Surg, 107:206, 1973; and Howard JM, et al.: Ann Surg 160 (Suppl): 1–192, 1964; University of California data given courtesy of A. Giuliano, M.D., and T.K. Hunt, M.D.)

Note: These are examples of infection rates in the four-category classification system. The rates in the five hospitals categories are based on 1964 data. General rates are thought to be only slightly lower today. However, the Foothills Hospital and University of California Hospitals data support our belief that infection rates can and should be considerably lower today. The infection rates for "dirty" cases in the University of California study are not given because liberal use of secondary and delayed primary closure make the figure meaningless. This is also part of the reason why the heavily contaminated category rate is so low. But delayed primary closure does not affect the statistic for clean contaminated cases.

APPENDIX D
Organisms Most Likely to Be Associated with Selected Infections

Infection	Probable Organism
Erysipelas	Streptococcus
Acute necrotizing fasciitis	Polymicrobic
Acute lymphangitis	Streptococcus
Meleney's synergistic gangrene	Streptococcus and Staphylococcus
Breast abscess	Staphylococcus, but often polymicrobic
Subcutaneous abscess (not hospital-acquired)	Staphylococcus
Human bite (infected)	Polymicrobic, spirochetes
Abscess of hand	Staphylococcus
Abdominal wound	
Gastrointestinal or genitourinary tract entered	Polymicrobic, Bacteroides important
Gastrointestinal or genitourinary tracts not entered	Staphylococcus
Peritonitis following appendicitis or injury to intestine	Polymicrobic
Perirectal, appendiceal, intra-abdominal, retroperitoneal, or subphrenic abscess	Polymicrobic; anaerobes
Cholecystic abscess and cholangitis	Polymicrobic; Clostridia
Crepitant myositis	Clostridia
Enterocolitis following antibiotic bowel preparation	Staphylococcus
Septicemia following burn injury	Polymicrobic
Septicemia following genitourinary instrumentation	E. coli
Septicemia from contaminated intravenous solutions or associated with indwelling intravenous catheters	Enteric bacteria, often Pseudomonas, Serratia, or Mimeae
Septicemia from superinfections during antibiotic therapy	Gram-negative pathogens or Candida
Primary pneumonia	Pneumonococcus
Pneumonia complicating respirator treatment or intubation	Gram-negative pathogen, often Pseudomonas

Modified from Altemeier WA, Alexander JW. In Sabiston DC Jr (ed): Textbook of Surgery. Philadelphia, Saunders, 1972

APPENDIX E
A Guide to Prophylaxis against Tetanus in Wound Management

General Principles

I. The attending physician must determine for each patient with a wound, individually, what is required for adequate prophylaxis against tetanus.

II. Regardless of the active immunization status of the patient, meticulous surgical care, including removal of all devitalized tissue and foreign bodies, should be provided immediately for all wounds. Such care is essential as part of the prophylaxis against tetanus.

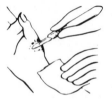

III. Each patient with a wound should receive adsorbed tetanus toxoid* intramuscularly at the time of injury, either as an initial immunizing dose, or as a booster for previous immunization, unless he has received a booster or has completed his initial immunization series within

This guide from the Committee on Trauma of the American College of Surgeons is the work of the ad hoc subcommittee on prophylaxis against tetanus: Roger T. Sherman, MD, FACS, Tampa, Florida, Chairman; Wesley Furste, MD, FACS, Columbus, Ohio; Paul A. Skudder, MD, FACS, New York; and Oscar P. Hampton, Jr., MD, FACS, St. Louis.

*The Public Health Service Advisory Committee on Immunization Practices in 1972 recommended DTP (diphtheria and tetanus toxoids combined with pertussis vaccine) for basic immunization in infants and children from two months through the sixth year of age, and Td (combined tetanus and diphtheria toxoids: adult type) for basic immunization of those over six years of age. For the latter group, Td toxoid was recommended for routine or wound boosters; but, if there is any reason to suspect hypersensitivity to the diphtheria component, tetanus toxoid (T) should be substituted for Td.

(*Morbidity and Mortality Weekly Report*, Vol. 21, No. 25, National Communicable Disease Center)

234

the past five years. As the antigen concentration varies in different products, specific information on the volume of a single dose is provided on the label of the package.

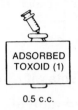

0.5 c.c.

IV. Whether or not to provide passive immunization with tetanus immune globulin (human) must be decided individually for each patient. The characteristics of the wound, conditions under which it was incurred, its treatment, its age, and the previous active immunization status of the patient must be considered.

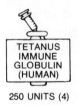

250 UNITS (4)

V. To every wounded patient, give a written record of the immunization provided, instructing him to carry the record at all times, and, if indicated, to complete active immunization. For precise tetanus prophylaxis, an accurate and immediately available history regarding previous active immunization against tetanus is required.

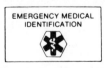

VI. Basic immunization with adsorbed tetanus toxoid requires three injections. A booster of adsorbed tetanus toxoid is indicated ten years after the third injection or ten years after an *intervening* wound booster. All individuals, including pregnant women, should have basic immunization and indicated booster injections.

235

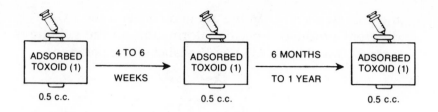

ADSORBED TOXOID (1) — 0.5 c.c. → 4 TO 6 WEEKS → ADSORBED TOXOID (1) — 0.5 c.c. → 6 MONTHS TO 1 YEAR → ADSORBED TOXOID (1) — 0.5 c.c.

Specific Measures for Patients with Wounds

I. **Previously immunized individuals**
   A. When the patient has been actively immunized within the past 10 years:
      1. To the great majority, give 0.5 cc of adsorbed tetanus toxoid* as a booster unless it is certain that the patient has received a booster within the previous five years.
      2. To those with severe, neglected, or old (more than 24 hours) tetanus-prone wounds, give 0.5 cc of adsorbed tetanus toxoid* unless it is certain that the patient has received a booster within the previous year.
   B. When the patient has been actively immunized more than 10 years previously:
      1. To the great majority, give 0.5 ml of adsorbed tetanus toxoid*.
      2. To those with severe, neglected, or old (more than 24 hours) tetanus-prone wounds:
         a) Give 0.5 cc of adsorbed tetanus toxoid*‡
         b) Give 250 units§ of tetanus immune globulin (human)
         c) Consider providing oxytetracycline or penicillin.

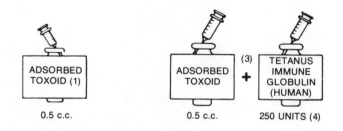

ADSORBED TOXOID (1) — 0.5 c.c.   ADSORBED TOXOID — 0.5 c.c. + (3) TETANUS IMMUNE GLOBULIN (HUMAN) — 250 UNITS (4)

II. Individuals NOT previously immunized

A. With clean minor wounds in which tetanus is most unlikely, give 0.5 cc of adsorbed tetanus toxoid* (initial immunizing dose).

B. With all other wounds:
1. Give 0.5 cc of adsorbed tetanus toxoid* (initial immunizing dose)‡
2. Give 250 units§ of tetanus immune globulin (human)‡
3. Consider providing oxytetracycline or penicillin.

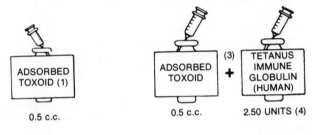

‡Use different syringes, needles, and sites of injection.

§In severe, neglected, or old (more than 24 hours) tetanus-prone wounds, 500 units of tetanus immune globulin (human) are advisable.

PRECAUTIONS regarding passive immunization with tetanus antitoxin (equine):

If the patient is not sensitive to tetanus antitoxin (equine), and if the decision is made to administer it for passive immunization, give at least 3,000 units.

Do not administer tetanus antitoxin (equine) except when tetanus immune globulin (human) is not available within 24 hours, and only if the possibility of tetanus outweighs the danger of reaction to heterologous tetanus antitoxin.

Before using tetanus antitoxin (equine), question the patient for a history of allergy and test for sensitivity. If the patient is sensitive to tetanus antitoxin (equine), do not use it, as the danger of anaphylaxis probably outweighs the danger of tetanus; rely on penicillin or oxytetracycline. Do not attempt desensitization, as it is not worthwhile.

NOTE: With different preparations of toxoid, the volume of a single booster dose should be modified as stated on the package label.

REFERENCES

Altemeier WA, Burke JF, Pruitt BA, Sandusky WR: Manual on Control of Infection in Surgical Patients. American College of Surgeons. Philadelphia, Lippincott, 1976. Basic text on surgical infection control.

Ballinger WF, Collins JA, Drucker WR, Dudrich SJ, Zeppa R: Manual of Surgical Nutrition. American College of Surgeons. Philadelphia, Saunders, 1975. Basic text on surgical nutrition.

Cave EF, Burke JF, Boyd RJ: (eds): Trauma Management. Chicago, Year Book Medical Publishers, 1974. General reference to the problems of general trauma.

Dunphy JE, Way LW (eds): Current Surgical Diagnosis and Treatment, 3rd ed. Los Atlos, California, Lange, 1977. Excellent text on surgical problems.

Florey Lord (ed): General Pathology, 4th ed. Philadelphia, Saunders, 1970. Best general work on pathology of inflammation.

Hendren WH III, (ed): Surgical Clinics of North America: Symposium on Pediatric Surgery. Philadelphia, Saunders, 1976. General reference to modern burn surgery.

Nardi GL, Zuidema GD (eds): Surgery: A Concise Guide to Clinical Practice, 3rd ed. Boston, Little, Brown, 1972. Excellent text on inflammation infection in surgery.

Zweifach BW, Grant L, McClusky RR (eds): The Inflammatory Process, vol III, 2nd ed. New York, Academic Press, 1974. Outstanding reference: key to the literature.

BIBLIOGRAPHY

Epidemiology of Surgical Infection

Burke JF: Identification of the sources of staphylococcus contaminating the surgical wound during operation. Ann Surg 158:898, 1963

Cruse PJE, Foord R: A five-year prospective study of 23,649 surgical wounds. Arch Surg 107:206, 1973

Hunt TK, Linsey M, Grislis G, Sonne M, Jawetz E: The effect of differing ambient oxygen tensions on wound infection. Ann Surg 181:35–39, 1975

Host Defense (specific)

Howard RJ, Simmons RL: Acquired immunologic deficiencies after trauma and surgical procedures (collective review). Surg Gynecol Obstet 139:771, 1974

Law DK, Dudrick SJ, Abdou NI: Immunocompetency of patients with protein-calorie malnutrition. The effects of nutritional repletion. Ann Intern Med 79:545, 1973

MacLean LD, Meakins JL, Taguchi K, et al.: Host resistance in sepsis and trauma. Ann Surg 182:207, 1975

Host Defense (nonspecific)

Elek SD: Experimental staphylococcal infections in the skin of man. Ann NY Acad Sci 65:85, 1956

Hohn DC: Leukocyte phagocytic function and dysfunction. Surg Gynecol Obstet 144:99, 1977

Hohn DC, Hunt TK: Oxidative metabolism and microbicidal activity of rabbit phagocytes: Cells from wounds and from peripheral blood. Surg Forum 26:86, 1975

Hohn DC, Ponce B, Burton RW, Hunt TK: Antimicrobial systems of the surgical wound. I. A comparison of oxidative metabolism and microbicidal capacity of phagocytes from wounds and from peripheral blood. Am J Surg 133:597, 1977

Hohn DC, Granelli SG, Burton RW, Hunt TK: Antimicrobial systems of the surgical wound. II. Detection of antimicrobial protein in cell-free wound fluid. Am J Surg 133:601, 1977

Hohn DC, MacKay RD, Hunt TK: The effect of O_2 tension on the microbicidal function of leukocytes in wounds and in vitro. Surg Forum 27:18, 1976

Leak LV, Burke JF: Early events of tissue injury and the role of the lymphatic system in early inflammation. In Zweifach BW, Grant L, McCluskey RR (eds): The Inflammatory Process; Vol III, 2nd ed. New York, Academic Press, 1974

Miles AA: Nonspecific defense reactions in bacterial infections. Ann NY Acad Sci 66:356, 1956

Miles AA, Miles EM, Burke JF: The value and duration of defense reactions of the skin to the primary lodgement of bacteria. Br J Exp Pathol 38:79, 1957

Weinberg ED: Iron and susceptibility to infectious disease. Science 184:952, 1974

Pharmacology of Antibiotics

Alexander JW, Alexander NS: The influence of route of administration on wound fluid concentration of prophylactic antibiotics. J Trauma 16(6):488, 1976

Ehrlich HP, Licko V, Hunt TK: Kinetics of cephaloridine in experimental wounds. Am J Med Sci 265:33, 1973

Preventive Antibiotics

Alexander JW: Emerging concepts in the control of surgical infections. Surgery 75(6):934, 1974

Burke JF: The effective period of preventive antibiotic action in experimental incisions and dermal lesions. Surgery 50:1, 161, 1961

Hunt TK, Alexander JW, Burke JF, MacLean LD: Antibiotics in surgery. Arch Surg 110:148, 1975

Rodeheaver G, Marsh D, Edgerton MT, Edlich RF: Proteolytic enzymes as adjuncts to antimicrobial prophylaxis of contaminated wounds. Am J Surg 130:341, 1975

Surgical Infection

Bierens de Haan B, Ellis H, Wilks M: The role of infection on wound healing. Surg Gynecol Obstet 138:693, 1974

Conolly WB, Hunt TK, Sonne M, Dunphy JE: Influence of distant trauma on local wound infection. Surg Gynecol Obstet 128:713, 1969

Edlich RF, Waid R, Kasper G, et al.: Studies in the management of the contaminated wound. Am J Surg 117:323, 1969

Morris PJ, Barnes BA, Burke JF: The nature of the "irreducible minimum" rate of incisional sepsis. Arch Surg 92:367, 1966

Postoperative wound infections. Ann Surg (Supplement) 160:2,23, 1964

Robson MC, Duke WF, Kirzek TJ: Rapid bacterial screening in the treatment of civilian wounds. J Surg Res 14:426, 1973

Robson MC, Shaw RC, Heggers JP: Reclosure of postoperative incisional abscesses based on bacterial quantification of wound. Ann Surg 171:279, 1970

Wound Healing

Conolly WB, Hunt TK, Zederfeldt B, Cafferata HT, Dunphy JE: Clinical comparison of surgical wounds closed by suture and adhesive tapes. Am J Surg 117:318, 1969

Egerton MT, Edlich RF: Potentiation of wound infection by surgical drains. Am J Surg 131:547, 1976

240

4

HOST DEFENSE MECHANISMS, WOUND HEALING, AND INFECTION

Jonathan L. Meakins

The work reported herein is the result of research performed by many in the Department of Surgery of the Royal Victoria Hospital with the guidance and direction of Dr. Lloyd D. MacLean. The body composition measurements were performed by Dr. Harry M. Shizgal. Many data cited in this chapter are from studies that were supported in part by The Medical Research Council of Canada.

From the era of the barber surgeon to the midportion of the 20th century, surgeons were considered applied anatomists; and the principles of surgical practice were learned in the dissecting room. However, during the past few decades, surgeons have become much more than functional anatomists. They are, in fact, also practical physiologists. The clearest example of the practical application of physiology is found in the surgical approaches to the management of the wound healing process. It is too simple to think of wound healing as simply the process that allows surgeons to remove stitches from a wound. As described in earlier chapters, it is an exceedingly complex process that requires not only deposition of collagen to weld tissue discontinuities together, but also the delivery of the appropriate cellular and humoral constituents to an area of inflammation and potential infection.

The failure of wound healing is commonly a result of infection in one form or another. Whether the injury is caused by an incision made with a cold knife or by the traumatic disruption of tissue planes, the fundamental reparative processes are similar, and the development of infection in either of these settings signifies a failure of wound healing. This chapter examines the host-related factors that are involved in the process of wound healing and, in this context, with the control of infection.

DETERMINANTS OF INFECTION

Every infectious process, regardless of its location, involves (1) the microorganism which causes the infection, (2) the environment (locale) in which the infection takes place, and (3) the host defense mechanisms that are designed to control invasive bacteria in any environment. The interactions and influences of these three determinants are schematically represented in Figure 4.1. In normal homeostasis, these circles intersect at a point, indicating that the probability of sepsis* in that setting is essentially zero. The philosophical basis for the circles is the mathematical theory of sets or the theoretical use of Venn diagrams. The schematic representations of pathologic situations illus-

*As used here, sepsis is defined as "the presence in the blood or other tissues of pathogenic microorganisms or their toxins. The condition associated with such presence." From Dorland's Medical Dictionary, 25th ed. Philadelphia, Saunders, 1974.

244

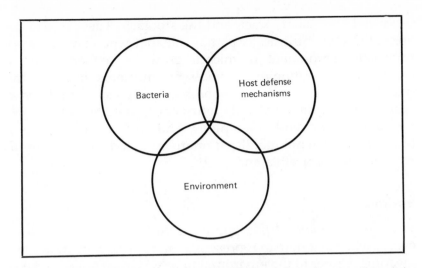

Figure 4.1 In homeostasis, the normal state is shown by the intersection of the circles representing the relationship between the determinants of infectious bacteria, environment, and host defense mechanisms at a point indicating zero probability of sepsis.

trated later in this chapter show the overlapping influences of specific determinants; and the size of the area circumscribed by the intersections indicates the increased probability of an infectious process taking place.

Microorganisms

The *bacteria* generally encountered by surgeons may be classified as exogenous or endogenous. Exogenous bacteria usually become troublesome following trauma where such contaminants as street flora and bacteria residing in the earth are introduced into the tissues through wounds. In the operating room the major sources of exogenous bacteria are the operating team, including surgeons, nurses, and anesthetists, as well as the room itself. Organisms from the operating room environment usually are the ones associated with infection in clean surgical operations such as the inguinal hernia repair. The organisms most commonly seen in this setting are *S. aureus* or *S. epidermidis* and occasionally streptococci.

Endogenous organisms, which now present a much greater threat, reside in or on the patient, in the mouth, the gastrointestinal tract, and, in pathologic situations, the tracheo-

245

bronchial tree, biliary tract, and the stomach. These organisms are not always intrinsically pathogenic, but when given the appropriate environment in which to grow, i.e., either a reduced oxygen concentration or the necessary nutrients, infection frequently results. These infections may manifest themselves as wound infections, wound dehiscence, fistulae, abscesses, peritonitis, empyema, meningitis, and so forth. If host resistance factors are not mobilized or are inhibited, such infections may end in septicemia and death.

Environment

The term *environment* is a popular contemporary word. However, I will use it here to represent a microcosm of its traditional meaning. I refer to the environment in which an infection takes place; the local conditions which, in balance, usually *prevent* the *lodgement* of bacteria at that site. Specifics of these conditions have been discussed in Chapters 1 and 2 and will be further amplified here, in the next chapter, and in Chapter 6.

At the point of contamination, the principle responsibility of tissues and their defenses is to prevent bacteria from establishing themselves as potential pathogens. There are several basic ways in which the body prevents lodgement. The skin and mucous membranes, of course, provide a mechanical barrier. However, there are, in addition, a number of biologic decontamination processes: (1) mechanical decontamination that may be as simple as tears washing bacteria from the eyes or as complicated as the process of ciliary movement in the tracheobronchial tree; (2) chemical decontamination, which relates not only to tears and saliva but also to the fatty acids produced on the skin that have antibacterial properties and help to control pathogenic skin flora; (3) the normal bacterial flora are able to prevent cutaneous establishment of pathogenic bacteria. Normal flora functions in its protective sense in the mouth, oronasopharynx, and throughout the gastrointestinal tract. Most mucous membranes harbor some bacteria, and in certain areas these normal flora are enormously populous. Their functions vary but one is to prevent the establishment of critical masses of pathogenic bacteria that otherwise might establish an infection.

Obviously, environmental factors and host defense mechanisms may interact or even become one and the same in some instances.

Host Defense Mechanisms

The last of the three determinants, the substance of this chapter, is *host defense mechanisms*, or, those local and systemic factors involved with the *containment* of a microorganism resolution of potential infection, which has penetrated the tissues. Traditionally, it is stated that host defense mechanisms are made up of five components: the inflammatory response, humoral factors, phagocytic systems, cell-mediated immunity, and complement. In the context of normal wound healing and its physiologic application to surgery, I think it is more important to organize these components in a series as depicted in Figure 4.2. It is most likely that immunologic damage to organisms initiated via any of the five components will be mediated and finally expressed through a form of the inflammatory response where common factors such as kinin activation, vasoactive peptides, Hageman factor, and prostaglandins all become part of a final process that will, of course, include the leukocyte in most cases. Although different stimuli trigger the response of the various immunologic components, the host response is generally mediated through common pathways. The reason for expressing them as a series is to imply that in many cases a defect in one component of the series may seri-

Figure 4.2 The components of host defense, their interaction, and function.

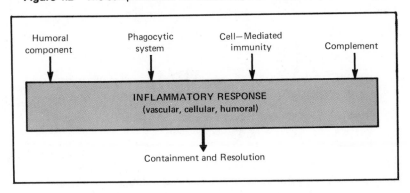

ously impair all steps that follow. For instance, it is of little comfort to a patient that the killing capacity of his leukocytes is normal if he cannot produce opsonins, and, his leukocytes cannot phagocytose bacteria.

Interaction of Determinants

In practice the separation of the three determinants of infection into the Venn diagram may appear artificial; however, conceptually the approach is realistic and provides direction for therapy. The following examples show how alterations of one, two, or three determinants relate to the probability of sepsis.

S. aureus is a primary pathogen that, when it gains access to tissue, often establishes infection. These infections are often controlled locally by systemic defense mechanisms, but they nevertheless produce pustules, boils, furuncles, or abcesses. Alterations in the local environment made, for instance, by silk sutures or other foreign bodies provide the staphylococcus with an opportunity to become established, enhancing its basic pathogenicity, which is its major property. The schema changes to reflect this (Fig. 4.3), and so the probability of infection increases substantially as represented by the central com-

Figure 4.3 Staphylococcal infection: The pathogenicity of S. aureus is represented by the increased size of bacteria circle and presence of the common central area representing increased probability of sepsis.

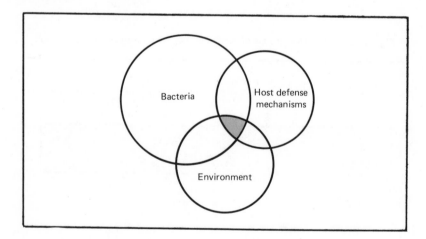

248

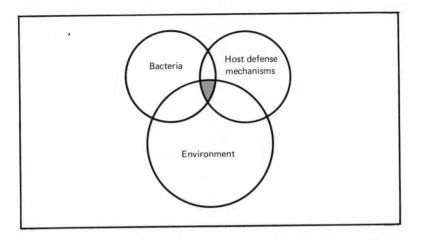

Figure 4.4 Clostridial infection: The presence of Clostridia (slightly increased circle) in an abnormal environment, necrotic muscle (very large circle) indicate the major problems in this infection is local environment.

mon area. Should the local environment change or there be abnormalities of host defense mechanisms, (HDM), the central area representing probability of sepsis would be even larger (i.e. burn wounds and *S. aureus*).

Clostridial infection or gas gangrene continues to threaten the clinician. However, physicians and nurses have a pathologic fear of the organism. The true determinant in clostridial sepsis is not so much the presence of the potentially pathogenic *Clostridium welchii*, but rather the presence of a suitable environment (Fig. 4.4) in which the organism may flourish. This organism requires a very specialized environment in which to grow. The redox potential must be low and tissue therefore anaerobic. For instance, clostridia in the dog's liver live happily without infection unless there is a failure of oxygenation. If a dog's hepatic artery is ligated, gas gangrene results. In humans, the issue of whether clostridia will infect or not is settled by the state of the tissue in which the organism finds itself. Therefore, the infection is most commonly found in traumatized limbs where there has been inadequate debridement, with the presence of necrotic muscle and foreign bodies, or inappropriate primary closure. The most important determinant of this infection is the appropriate environment for bacterial growth.

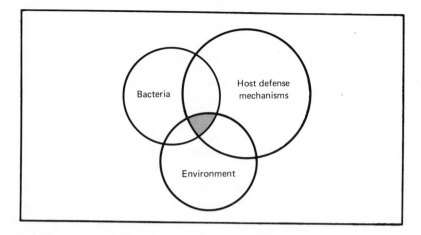

Figure 4.5 Transplant recipient: The increased probability of sepsis is a function of the altered host defenses because of immunosuppressive drugs.

Kidney transplant patients (Fig. 4.5), are uremic and have some alterations in the state of their tissues, but have no peculiarities in their internal environment or the bacteria to which they are exposed. The transplant involves a surgical procedure that, of necessity, alters the retroperitoneal space and invades the bladder. Aside from the surgical insult, there are no intrinsic factors at the local level that change a transplant patient's susceptibility to infection. However, in the peri- and posttransplant period, the use of potent immunosuppressive agents, required to combat allograft rejection, places the recipient at risk of a large variety of major infectious complications involving all varieties of microorganisms including bacteria, viruses, fungi, and protozoa. The immunosuppresive drugs utilized for control of graft rejection exert their primary influence on the cell-mediated immune system. It is therefore not surprising that infections due to intracellular parasites, such as cytomegalic inclusion virus, herpes virus, and a variety of frightening fungal invaders, are common in this population. In recent years, immunosuppression has been more skillfully managed and these infectious complications have become less common, although they are still seen. It is reasonable to say that in the transplant patient decreased host defense is the primary determinant of increased infection.

In the burn injury, two determinants are affected. There is an obvious alteration of the patient's local defenses with substantial environmental changes subsequent to the thermal injury. In addition, there are vast alterations in host defense mechanisms. These alterations as shown in Figure 4.6 indicate that the probability of infection is high. If we had the physiologic tools to dissect the pathophysiology of infection in each burn patient, we would be able to ascribe a mathematical probability to each one of the three determinants and define the cause for each specific infection. Our immunobiologic knowledge has not yet reached that state, but intuitively it seems obvious that these two alterations clearly contribute to the high incidence of sepsis in burn injuries.

The patient in the surgical intensive care unit (SICU) is at risk (Fig. 4.7) by virtue of changes in all three determinants. A hospital environment causes normal flora to alter toward largely hospital-based bacteria, particularly gram-negative rods which, together with *S. aureus,* tend to be resistant to many antibiotics. These patients generally have intravenous and arterial lines, catheters, open wounds, and fistulae, all of which alter the local environment and may become primarily or sec-

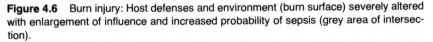

Figure 4.6 Burn injury: Host defenses and environment (burn surface) severely altered with enlargement of influence and increased probability of sepsis (grey area of intersection).

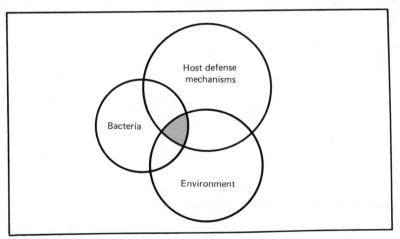

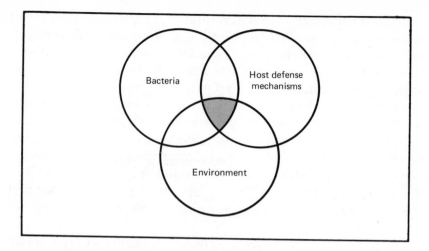

Figure 4.7 Intensive care patient: All three determinants are altered with consequent greatly increased probability of sepsis.

ondarily contaminated or infected by the antibiotic-resistant and pathogenic organisms residing in the intensive care unit. Last, host defense mechanisms in this patient population are altered by their underlying illnesses such as sepsis, cancer, or major trauma as well as by such basic problems as inadequate oxygenation, malnutrition, and altered blood volume. Therefore, because of the increased influence of each determinant, a patient has a greater probability of sepsis simply because he is seriously ill and because he is in an intensive care environment.

NORMAL HOST DEFENSE MECHANISMS

To be effective, host defense requires the integrated and efficient function of a variety of component parts mediated through the inflammatory response. The failure of any component of the system can result in infection, as is apparent in congenital immunologic deficiencies, such as chronic granulomatous disease, that affect single-cell or enzyme systems and frequently result in recurrent, persistent, or lethal sepsis.

Initially the inflammatory response acts as the basic delivery system. The classical signs of inflammation, such as rubor, dolor, tumor, and calor can be explained by examining the vascular, cellular, and molecular components of the inflammatory response.

Vascular Response

The vascular changes in inflammation are largely mediated through vasoactive amines, notably histamine, serotonin, and the kinins. These substances are coordinated to produce the vascular and endothelial changes that then allow delivery of the fluid and cellular components to the focus of inflammation. The precise sequence in which these components act is not completely understood; but basically the vascular response, initially vasoconstriction, occurs within minutes of the initial lesion; and is followed in 10 to 30 minutes by a persistent vasodilation. The overt cutaneous signs comprise the triple response of Lewis.

Vasodilation is accompanied by vessel wall changes and, subsequently by changes in blood flow. Stasis of blood is associated with increased margination and adherence to the endothelial lining by polymorphonuclear leukocytes (PMN).Endothelial changes allow diapedesis of the PMN into the focus of inflammation. The altered vessel wall and elevated capillary pressure increase vascular permeability leading to delivery of plasma proteins, notably immunoglobulins, complement, and fibrinogen. The breakdown of certain large protein molecules and the increased fluidity of the tissue ground substance also contribute to the "tumor" associated with inflammation.

Humoral Response

The humoral opsonic component is composed of complement and immunoglobulins. Complement has many functions, but in the context of bacterial invasion, it facilitates immune adherence, bacterial cytolysis, PMN chemotaxis, and phagocytosis. Immunoglobulins, notably G(IgG) and M(IgM) are, together with complement, involved in PMN bacterial phagocytosis. Complement and immunoglobulin acting in concert can lyse bacteria but this mechanism plays only a small part in the control of invasive bacteria. The crucial role of complement is to attract PMNs to the bacteria and then, with IgG, to opsonize them for effective phagocytosis by PMNs. In the absence of complement or immunoglobulins, phagocytosis is substantially decreased. Fibrin deposition facilitates localization of the infection as seen in abscesses and also supplies a fiber matrix against which neutrophils can phagocytize the bacteria that are not opsonized. Thus, the humoral and cellular components work together to control bacterial growth.

Cellular Response

The development of the cellular exudate parallels the formation of the fluid exudate. Initially, it consists almost exclusively of PMNs. After the first 24 hours, the monocyte tends to replace the neutrophil as the predominant phagocytic cell. When activated by foreign substances the monocyte becomes a more effective phagocyte. However, the macrophage also processes bacterial and other antigens for delivery to the lymphocyte and thus enhances production of specific antibody. As the inflammatory process develops, the lymphatics enlarge, in part secondary to local swelling, and lymphatic flow increases aiding delivery of antigen to the regional lymph nodes.

The similarity between this process and that of the production of granulation tissue during first few days of wound healing is striking. Although the processes seem to be mobilized for different purposes, they are fundamentally identical and differ only in emphasis on certain components. The failure of this response, totally or in part, frequently results in infection as well as in failure of healing. For purposes of this chapter, however, the inflammatory exudate is considered primarily in its role as host defense mechanism.

The Polymorphonuclear Cell

PMN activity constitutes the initial cellular response to a lesion. PMNs are actively phagocytic when delivered by means of diapededis to the inflammatory focus. Even in a wound, they survive the journey through the vascular system, the vessel wall, edema, and extravasated blood to arrive intact and with undiminished antibacterial capacities. Where the bacterium is ingested, it is encased in a membrane lined sac, the phagosome, which becomes a phagolysosome with degranulation of the enzyme-rich contents of PMN lysosomes. The many enzymatic and metabolic processes that result in bacterial killing take place in the lysosomes. PMN's, short-lived cells (half-life in circulation, 6 hours), are constantly being produced by the bone marrow. Of the 2 to 3 billion PMNs in circulation, 50 percent are marginated on vessel walls or in closed capillary loops. Maintained in reserve in the bone marrow are 200 to 300 billion PMNs so that large numbers can be delivered when required. The PMN is the initial bactericidal cell and is essential to the maintenance of intact host defense. Cyclic variations of neutrophil function have been demonstrated in burn and transplant patients, and appear related to the development of sepsis in burn patients. Patients receiving cancer chemotherapy who develop profound neutropenia have a very high incidence of septicemia that may not be controlled until either the bone marrow recovers and neutropenia abates or granulocytes are transfused. The inability of PMNs to contain an infection (even when present in normal number) is a major and critical deficiency that often permits systemic microbial invasion.

Monocyte

The second line of phagocytic response is the monocyte. When a monocyte enters an area of inflammation, it is activated to become a macrophage, an aggressive phagocytic and bactericidal cell with a long half-life. Chemotaxis, bacterial phagocytosis, and intracellular killing by macrophages require antibody and complement just as with PMNs. After ingestion and digestion, the microbial antigen is processed by the macrophage and transported locally or regionally to lymphocytes for production of specific antibody. The cells that take part in this activity may be bursal equivalent (B) lymphocytes or thymus derived (T) lymphocytes. B cells produce specific antibodies; T cells produce specifically sensitized lymphocytes with a major role in protection against intracellular parasites through interaction with macrophages, which, when activated, become the effective microbicidal cells.

The wandering or "resident" macrophage is an effective "mop-up" cell that is able to ingest and dispose of cellular debris, fibrin, and other particulate matter. The PMN is primarily bactericidal and does not have the other extensive functions of the wandering macrophage. There are numerous tissue macrophages, probably also derived from monocytes, that are essential to the microbial host defense. These cells constitute the fixed RES made up of Kupffer cells (liver), littoral cells (spleen), microglial cells (brain), and pulmonary alveolar macrophages. There are macrophages in most other tissues and organ systems, but they are less numerous and are intensely supplemented by circulating cells when required.

The fixed RES is primarily a blood filter, and as such is the clearance mechanism for particulate matter as well as for any microbes that may have entered the circulation. Kupffer cells form the largest mass of the RES and are instrumental in control of systemic as well as transient portal vein bacteremia. The alveolar macrophage is important in controlling pulmonary sepsis and clearing any particulate matter that is not removed by the liver. Therefore, the lung may become a target organ in generalized sepsis and other comparable low-flow states.

Cell-Mediated Immunity

In this discussion, cell-mediated immunity (CMI) will be considered to be limited to intracellular parasites, most notably *Mycobacterium tuberculosis,* salmonella and *Listeria monocytogenes,* and fungal infections. However, CMI is also of importance in viral infections, tumor and transplant immunity, and autoimmune disease. Classically, delayed hypersensitivity is mediated through and often thought to be a reflection of CMI. Failure to respond appropriately can reflect an alteration in any of a number of immune responses that may be nonspecific and not necessarily closely related to CMI. For instance, the end point of an inflammatory response can be deficient and thus an intact CMI cannot be expressed in the usual tests. The antimicrobial action of CMI is mediated through a complex system of cell recognition and activation involving different cells and numerous humoral mediators. In simplified terms, the cell-mediated antimicrobial system is based on recognition of antigen by T lymphocytes and subsequent macrophage attraction and stimulation. If the body has not previously been infected with the specific organism, some time is required before sensitized lymphocytes are produced. In this situation the reaction will work somewhat in reverse; that is, the bacterial antigen will be processed by macrophages and delivered to lymphocytes for production of specifically sensitized T cells, which then will be effective at the site of infection.

When the host has previously been infected with a particular microbe, specific T cells are attracted to the focus of infection, where they are specifically activated to produce lymphokines, a family of soluble humoral mediators, some of which can affect macrophages. The lymphokines of specific interest are migration inhibition factor (MIF) and macrophage activation factor (MAF). MIF attracts macrophages to the infective focus and retains them in the area; MAF converts them into activated cells capable of effective antibacterial function. The mechanisms of intracellular killing are similar to those typical of PMNs. Failure of T cell function, or congenital absence of T cells, results in failure to mount an effective antimicrobial response against intracellular parasites.

Table 4.1 Efficacy of the Three Compartments of Host Defense in Countering Various Infectious Organisms (Greatly Simplified)

Humoral	Cell-Mediated	Phagocytic
Bacteria:	Bacteria:	Bacteria:
Pneumococcus	Mycobacteria	Staphylococcus*
Streptococcus	Listeria	Klebsiella
Hemophilus	Brucella	Aerobacter
Meningococcus	Salmonella	Serratia
Pseudomonas	Staphylococcus*	Proteus
		Probably most other enteric and anaerobic bacteria
Toxins:	Fungi:	Fungi:
Diphtheria	Candida spp*	Candida
Tetanus	Aspergillus	
	Histoplasma	
	Mucor	
Viruses:	Viruses:	
Polio	Vaccinia	
Hepatitis	Cytomegalic inclusion	
Rubella	disease	
Others	Most others	
	Parasites:	
	Pneumocystis carinii	

*Many infectious agents are attacked by two compartments of host defense; selecting the predominant compartment may not be possible.

Each of the three components of host defense—humoral, phagocytic, and cell-mediated immunity— is most effective against certain organisms or classes of organisms (Table 4.1). The host has a complex defense system; often two of the three components are active against invading microbes though one is usually critical. For example, in the absence of specific antibody, the pneumococcus is not phagocytized by PMNs, but once antibody is present, phagocytosis and intracellular killing proceed rapidly. The key to this defense is the specific antibody, although control of the actual infection is a two component effort.

ABNORMALITIES OF HOST DEFENSE

The hallmark of abnormalities of HDM is recurrent infection or an increased incidence of infection. HDM abnormalities were first identified in children with recurrent episodes of infection. Individual defects in cell function, neutrophil, B lymphocyte, T lymphocyte, or defects in production of immunoglobulins or complement could be defined. There are a few congenital defects that affect many components of host defense, but the majority are specific defects in the function of a single HDM component. The technical methodology for evaluation of the patient's immune response therefore was developed.

Much more common, and at present not completely defined, are the secondary, or acquired, defects in host defense. These are, by implication, secondary to some other influence: usually a disease process, an event, or drug therapy. The list of factors that can produce these defects is an impressive and continually growing one. Characteristically these defects do not involve a single component but rather produce a range of abnormalities in several of the components of host defense. These defects may be variable in severity and are only occasionally equivalent to the complete failure of cell function seen in the congenital HDM abnormalities. The clinical factors that may contribute to these acquired defects are common and are to be found on all wards in any general hospital. Marked or continuing stress or a catastrophic event are usual precipating factors. Malnutrition, sepsis, fistulae, trauma, surgery, advanced age, diabetes, shock, burns, advanced cancer, and combinations of these problems may all produce acquired immunodeficiency. When patients on immunosuppressive drugs and other drug regimens that affect the immune system are added to the previous group, the high rates of morbidity and mortality associated with nosocomial infection are not surprising.

The value of identification and definition of the abnormalities of host defense is becoming increasingly apparent. The components of the immune response have been identified and their relative importance in the development of sepsis has been assigned in many cases. Also the methodology for identification and description of these patients with HDM defects has become available. Therefore, it is possible and reasonable to approach these clinical problems from an objective physiologic point of view. In patients with acquired abnormalities, the role of host defenses in development of sepsis may not always be obvious because other medical and surgical problems complicate assessment. In a child with chronic granulomatous disease the recurrent infections are clearly a result of abnormal neutrophil function. However, a burn patient (Fig. 4.6) who develops sepsis has an ideal site (the burn wound) for bacterial growth and subsequent tissue invasion regardless of gross host defense abnormalities. However, the burn patient has acquired abnormalities of host defenses that have been investigated extensively. In fact, the burn patient has become a prototype of the surgical patient with major and significant acquired defects of resistance to infection. The burn patient is easy to identify. The real problem is the identification of patients who appear physiologically normal but have, or are prone to develop, acquired defects of host resistance. There is no doubt that such patients are commonly encountered.

IDENTIFICATION OF THE PATIENT WITH ACQUIRED DEFECTS OF HOST DEFENSE

In clinical practice there are a number of situations where one intuitively suspects an increased incidence of sepsis and therefore a possibility of alterations in the host's ability to handle infection. These include advanced age with significant illness, major surgery, trauma, diabetes, uremia, serious coexistent illness (intensive care patients), pancreatitis, hemorrhagic shock, and sepsis itself to list but a few. Not all of these patients have

259

abnormalities of host defense nor do they all develop sepsis. Identification of those likely to develop sepsis is clearly clinically relevant and defines the population for immunologic study.

Patients with potential for abnormalities of host defense are a large and heterogenous group. Random evaluation of host defenses in surgical patients has been tried but is unrewarding and expensive. A simple and easily performed screening test is required. Our approach to this problem was initiated by the study of a 13-year-old boy referred to our hospital two months after surgery for perforated appendicitis and generalized peritonitis. At that time he had high output intestinal fistulae, intraabdominal abscesses requiring drainage, septicemia, respiratory failure, and malnutrition. Despite repeated drainage of abscesses, parenteral nutrition at the rate of 2,500 to 3,500 calories per day, antibiotics, immunologic support such as transfer factor and others, he died 5 months after admission. Because of his persistent inability to localize and control infection, we examined aspects of his immune response. He was anergic to recall antigens (mumps, purified protein derivative [PPD], trichophyton, varidase, and candida), accepted a skin graft without signs of rejection for 44 days, and had a serum factor which inhibited the mixed lymphocyte culture (MLC) response of his own lymphocytes to allogenic lymphocytes. Other aspects of lymphocyte and neutrophil function were normal and there were normal circulating levels of immunoglobulins. A subsequent pilot study of 50 preoperative patients and 55 seriously ill patients indicated that anergic and relatively anergic patients had a significantly increased incidence of sepsis when compared to those whose skin tests were normal. These data suggested that immune competence could be measured through responses to skin tests with recall antigens, and that abnormalities were related to the incidence of sepsis and its clinical outcome.

Utilizing the recall antigens PPD, mumps, trichophyton, varidase, and candida and defining the skin test results as in Table 4.2, a prospective study of 520 patients was conducted. Neutrophil and lymphocyte studies and the effect of autologous anergic serum on these cell functions were evaluated in anergic patients and normal controls.

The patients were divided into three groups: those studied

Table 4.2 Responses to Recall Antigens

Antigens
  Candida
  Mumps
  PPD
  Trichophyton
  Varidase

Normal response: 5 mm or more of induration at 24 or 48 hours

Anergy (A) = no response (0/5)
Relative Anergy (RA) = single response (1/5)
Normal (N) = two or more responses (2^+/5)

preoperatively, those studied postoperatively and posttrauma, and those who did not require operation. These data are summarized in Table 4.3. The surgical procedures in the preoperative tested group were major biliary tract procedures or operations on the stomach, pancreas, liver, and large and small intestine. [Sepsis, in the subsequent discussion, is defined as a positive blood culture or an abscess found at surgery or autopsy.] In the 322 patients studied preoperatively, those 42 patients with altered responses, either anergy (A) or relative anergy (RA), had a 21.4 percent incidence of sepsis and one-third died. These data show that skin testing identifies a group of patients at risk for increased sepsis and mortality following surgery.

The 115 patients studied in the intensive care unit were all

Table 4.3 Sepsis And Mortality Following Initial Skin Test

Response	Number	Sepsis (%)	Death (%)
Preoperative tests: 322 patients			
Anergy	21	19	33.3
Relative anergy	21	23.8	33.3
Normal	280	4.6	4.3
Postoperative and/or Posttrauma Tests:			
115 patients			
Anergy	71	62	33.8
Relative anergy	25	60	24.0
Normal	19	26.3	5.3
Nonoperative: 83 patients			
Anergy	23	21.7	47.8
Relative anergy	4	25	25
Normal	56	0	1.8

tested following emergency, surgery, trauma (with or without operation), or development of postoperative complications. These patients were very ill, accounting for the high incidence of altered responses (83.5 percent) and remarkable incidence (61.5 percent) of sepsis in patients with altered responses as compared to those with normal cutaneous reactions (26.3 percent). While these are clinically and statistically significant differing rates of sepsis, the major difference was in the mortality rate: 5.3 percent for normal response compared to 31.3 percent of those with altered responses.

In those 83 patients who were not operated upon, 27 had altered responses to skin tests with a 22 percent sepsis rate and 44 percent mortality, compared to no sepsis and one death in normally responsive patients. These patients were admitted with upper and lower gastrointestinal hemmorrhage, bowel obstruction not requiring surgery, pancreatitis, inflammatory bowel disease, and cancer.

Table 4.4 Sequential Testing in 247 Patients

Skin Tests	No.	Sepsis (%)	Death (%)
Anergy: Anergy	41	23 (56.1)	30 (73.2)
Anergy: Rel. anergy	11	4 (36.4)	3 (27.3)
Anergy: Normal	50	21 (42.0)	2 (4.0)
Rel. anergy: Anergy	7	4 (57.1)	7 (100.0)
Rel. anergy: Rel. anergy	6	2 (33.3)	4 (66.7)
Rel. anergy: Normal	44	15 (34.1)	2 (4.5)
Normal: Anergy	5	5 (100.0)	5 (100.0)
Normal: Rel. anergy	0	0 (0.0)	0 (0.0)
Normal: Normal	83	9 (10.8)	1 (1.2)

Sequential skin testing was performed two or more times in 247 patients. Table 4.4 shows how patient outcome is related to the evolution of skin tests. It is clear that patients with either abnormal or normal initial responses whose skin tests become or remain normal have a substantially better prognosis than those whose responses remain abnormal or become abnormal. The development of anergy in a previously normally responsive patient is a grave prognostic sign.

Therefore skin test responses, a classical reflection of CMI, have predictive value in terms of patient sepsis and mortality.

Table 4.5 Organisms in Blood Cultures of 91 Patients

Organisms	Normal	Rel. Anergy	Anergy
Gram-negative rods	17	19	58
Gram-positive cocci	34	18	57
Gram-positive rods	0	0	5
Fungi	0	0	5
Total	51	37	125

Furthermore, they can identify a patient population that is unusually sensitive to major infection. It is of interest that the majority of organisms that caused sepsis were common gram-negative and gram-positive bacteria (Table 4.5). Infections with these organisms are not usually thought to be related to defects in CMI. Individual organisms are not listed. It is of interest that *S. epidermidis* was the organism identified in 49 percent of positive cultures from the normal responders. Of positive cultures from the A and RA groups, 24 percent and 20 percent contained *S. epidermidis*.

We feel that the high incidence of this organism, previously not thought to be a contaminant, is indication of a new pathogen. In normally responsive patients it was usually related to catheter sepsis and parenteral nutrition.

In conjunction with skin testing, numerous other indices of host defense were assessed. Delayed hypersensitivity responses are generally considered a reflection of CMI, so lymphocyte function was examined exhaustively. Mixed lymphocyte culture, lymphocyte response to phytohemagglutinin and pokeweed mitogen, cell-mediated lympholysis, and lymphocyte generation of blastogenic factor were the same in normal patients and nonhospitalized control subjects. In four anergic patients there was a serum inhibitor of their MLC. The only lymphocyte test that was abnormal in the anergic or relatively anergic patients was a reduction in the percentage of rosetting T-lymphocytes and in the total lymphocyte count.

Neutrophil function, particularly neutrophil chemotaxis, was then evaluated using the leading front technique of Zigmond and Hirsch (1973) that gives a migration distance in microns with narrow standard errors as the measure of chemotactic (CTX) response in A and RA patients. CTX is clearly reduced in patients with altered skin test responses and significantly re-

263

Table 4.6 Neutrophil Chemotaxis in Anergic and Relatively Anergic Patients

Skin Test Response	Stimualted Migration (μm)
Anergy (40)	81.7 ± 2,3
Relative anergy (15)	97.2 ± 3.8*
Normal control (19)	117.5 ± 1.6*

*P < 0.001

Table 4.7 Evolution of Chemotaxis Following Restoration of Normal Skin Test Responses

Skin Test Responses	Stimulated Migration (μm)
Anergic patients (14)	78.2 ± 5.4*
Following restoration of cutaneous responses (14)	107.2 ± 4.0
Normal controls	117.5 ± 1.6

*P < 0.01

turns toward normal with recovery of normal responses (Tables 4.6 and 4.7). This evolution of chemotaxis to normal is more clearly seen in the trauma group (see below). The influence of anergic and normal serum upon anergic and normal neutrophils shows that serum from anergic patients inhibits chemotaxis of normal and possibly anergic neutrophils. "Anergic serum" consistently inhibits chemotaxis of normal cells (Table 4.8 and Fig. 4.8). We are in the process of characterizing the inhibitors in anergic serum. In a series of 12 patients, a weak, but statistically significant, correlation between neutrophil chemotaxis and neutrophil phagocytosis and bactericidal killing was established.

The presence of abnormal skin tests identifies patients who are susceptible to sepsis. The same population has abnor-

Table 4.8 Influence of Serum on Neutrophil Chemotaxis

	Stimulated Migration (μm)
Anergic cells: Normal serum	93.0 ± 3.7*
Anergic cells: Anergic serum	86.2 ± 3.5*
Normal cells: Normal serum	121.2 ± 1.6†
Normal cells: Anergic serum	103.6 ± 2.6†

*P < 0.01
†P < 0.001

264

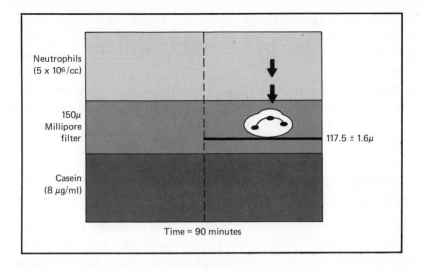

Neutrophils
(5 x 10⁶/cc)

150μ
Millipore
filter

Casein
(8 μg/ml)

117.5 ± 1.6μ

Time = 90 minutes

Figure 4.8 Schematic representation of leading front technique of measuring neutrophil chemotaxis in a Sykes-Moore Chamber. There are two compartments separated by a 150 μ millipore filter with 3 μ sized holes. The cells to be examined are placed in the upper chamber and an attractant, casein, in the lower. The distance the neutrophils migrate into the filter in 90 minutes is the chemotactic response.

malities of some components of host defense which, when found in patients with primary defects (genetic immune abnormalities), are related to recurrent infection. We have concluded that in these numerous and often complicated patients, the failure of delayed hypersensitivity is a nonspecific indicator of altered antibacterial host defenses and is not related to CMI as currently identified.

The results of the preoperative study clearly indicate that anergy present at the time of operation is associated with the subsequent development of sepsis. In other patients it is more

Table 4.9 Clinical Associations in 165 Anergic Patients

	(No.)	(%)
Sepsis	67	41
Multiple factors	51	31
Trauma	22	13
Shock	14	8.5
Malnutrition	6	3.6
Unknown	5	3

difficult to judge whether sepsis is a result, or a cause, of abnormal host defenses. The etiologic factors in Table 4.9 indicate that sepsis itself is a major etiologic factor in the evolution of abnormal skin tests and associated defects in host defense. Malnutrition is a more significant factor than it appears to be in the table, since it was present in most of the patients with multifactorial problems and in many of those with sepsis.

FACTORS ASSOCIATED WITH ACQUIRED DEFECTS OF HOST DEFENSE

The incidence of transiently altered host defense is significant. There are many disease states, events, drugs, and physiologic settings that may contribute to alterations of the host response. Many of these factors overlap, but we will attempt to isolate what is known of HDM alterations in various pathologic situations.

Trauma and the Burn Injury

As an extension of the investigations already outlined, and to ascertain whether anergy and altered host defenses precede sepsis, we studied 53 patients who had sustained blunt trauma. The severity of injury was assessed by assigning one point each to long bone fracture, pelvic fracture, abdominal injury, chest injury, and head injury to a maximum of five. Anergy and relative anergy were found to be a function of the age of the patient and the severity of injury (Fig. 4.9). Patients who became A or RA did so promptly after the injury and had a higher incidence of sepsis than normal responders. The mortality rate was statistically higher, although numbers are small.

Neutrophil chemotaxis was studied in 32 trauma patients and was found reduced in both A and RA patients. Patients with minimal trauma and normal skin tests have normal chemotaxis. However, normal skin tests in the presence of multiple injury, averaging 2.5 points, produced a transient abnormality of neutrophil CTX in all A and RA patients, can be seen in Figure 4.10. The evolution of chemotaxis in four patients of about the same age, but with differing degrees of trauma, is

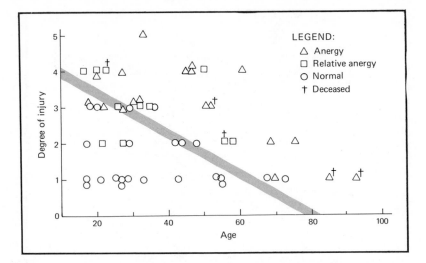

Figure 4.9 Graphic representation of relationship between patient's age, degree of injury, and skin test responses. The shaded area is hypothetical line between advancing age, degree of injury, and development of anergy. Patients who died are indicated. (From Meakins, et al.: J. Trauma 18(4): 240, 1978, Williams & Wilkins Co., Baltimore.)

Figure 4.10 Regression of the two groups of normals and all patients with altered cutaneous responses on days following the injury. **A.** Normal ST: single injury. **B.** Normal ST: multiple injury. **C.** Altered ST: multiple injury. (From Meakins, et al.: J. Trauma (18(4): 243, 1978, Williams & Wilkins Co., Baltimore.)

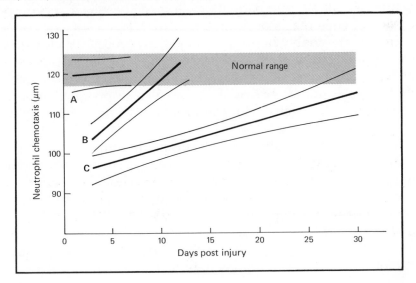

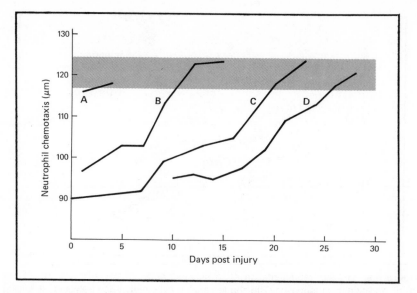

Figure 4.11 Four patients of similar age and different injury and skin text responses showing patterns of abnormality and recovery to normal of neutrophil chemotaxis. **A.** N. 42 F. # sternum, # humerus. **B.** N. 36 M, # pelvis, # skull, # 4 ribs. **C.** RA, 32 M # skull, flail chest, bilateral femoral #'s. **D.** A, 30 M, spinal injury, flail chest, abdominal injury. (From Meakins, et al.: J. Trauma 18(4): 244, 1978, Williams & Wilkins Co., Baltimore)

seen in Figure 4.11. Abnormal chemotaxis was found to be a more accurate predictor of the development of sepsis than skin testing. In all anergic patients examined there is a serum inhibitor of chemotaxis of normal neutrophils.

In this reasonably homogenous patient group it is clear that the injury, and not sepsis, is responsible for development of anergy and abnormal neutrophil function. It is therefore likely that these acquired abnormalities are also responsible, at least in part, for the high incidence of sepsis in the anergic traumatized patient.

The prototype for the study of altered immune responses in trauma patients is the thermal injury. Thermal injury is the most severe injury that can be treated successfully, and it imposes an enormous stress upon the human body and its resources. It is a multiple system injury and one of the systems that is altered is the immune response. All aspects of the immune response are affected by the burn injury. The humoral response to primary antigens is reduced, although the anam-

268

nestic response is normal. Neutrophil function, particularly chemotaxis and bactericidal ability, is severely reduced; and there is evidence to suggest that alterations in neutrophil bactericidal function precedes both the development of invasive burn wound sepsis and changes in qualitative and quantitative microbiology in the burn wound itself. Cell-mediated immunity is also markedly altered as evidenced by altered lymphocyte function, the ability to accept a skin graft without rejection, absence of response to recall antigens, the inability to be sensitized to Dinitrochlorobenzene (DNCB), and abnormal T cell response to Phytohemagglutinin (PHA). Commonly there are alterations in the complement cascade that may, in part, be a result of excessive consumption, but also appear related to inadequate production. With this broad range of immunologic alterations characteristic of the patient with acquired abnormalities of host defense, it is not surprising that the incidence of infections in burn patients is very high. When added to the alterations in the cutaneous surface presenting an appropriate environment for bacterial growth, (Fig. 4.6) it is even more apparent why sepsis is prevalent.

Sepsis

It is ironic that infection itself can alter host defenses. Nevertheless there is a significant amount of data to suggest that this is so. Neutrophil bactericidal function is depressed secondary to sepsis, indicating that abnormal neutrophil function may be a cause, as well as a result, of sepsis. The loss of either immunoglobulins or complement though consumption can be significant and has been termed consumptive opsoninopathy by Alexander (1974). In the group we have skin tested, sepsis contributed in some as yet undefined way to the development of anergy. There have been innumerable patients who, upon development of the septic crisis, i.e., disrupted colonic anastomosis, promptly became anergic. Restoration of skin test responses, together with recovery of neutrophil chemotaxis, has similarly been noted following drainage of a hidden subphrenic abscess or infected common duct, suggesting that resolution of the septic focus can restore host defenses (Fig. 4.12). This reinforces the surgical adage, "never let the sun set on an undrained abscess." It is then apparent that abnormal host de-

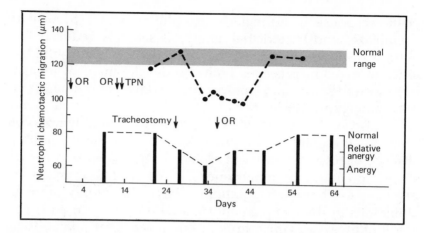

Figure 4.12 The clinical course, skin test reactivity, and neutrophil chemotaxis in 63-year-old male who was admitted with bowel obstruction secondary to gallstone ileus and operated upon promptly. On the ninth hospital day, a second operation for drainage of a small subphrenic abscess was required and followed by institution of total parenteral nutrition. His cutaneous responses remained normal but deteriorated when persistent respiratory failure necessitated tracheostomy and ascending cholangitis required emergency cholecystectomy and common duct exploration. Subsequently, neutrophil chemotaxis and cutaneous responses returned to normal. The hospital course was prolonged but he was discharged on the 86th hospital day.

fenses can not only be a cause but also a result of sepsis thus creating a vicious circle which may become increasingly difficult to break, as host defenses deteriorate.

Shock

Although in this discussion I refer to shock as a state secondary to hemorrhage, other low flow, hypoperfusion or hypovolemic states may have similar effects. We have seen a surprising number of patients with upper gastrointestinal hemorrhage who are anergic upon admission, or who promptly become anergic. Restoration of blood volume and control of hemorrhage with no other therapeutic intervention, can be shown (Fig. 4.13) to promote restoration of normal cutaneous responses. In this context, control of blood volume and red cell mass is a form of immunologic support. This agrees with other observations of the effect of hypoxia and diminished local blood flow on establishment of infection in experimental animals mentioned in Chapter 2 and 3.

Nutrition

It has been stated that as many as a third of the patients on a surgical service are in a state of malnutrition. This does not include obese patients in whom malnutrition is a function of inappropriate eating habits and subsequent alteration of body composition. Most commonly, surgical patients have protein-calorie malnutrition or protein depletion. These two states in their most extensive form are known as marasmus or kwashiorkor (see Chap. 5). The numbers of immunologic abnormalities seen in the setting of malnutrition are strikingly similar to those seen in the burn injury. The development of severe malnutrition in infants and very young children can lead to failure of lymphoid tissue genesis and inability to respond appropriately to antigens. This may affect both B cell function and humoral immunity and T cell function and cell-mediated immunity. Gross changes include thymic atrophy and reduction in the lymphoid mass in the spleen, lymph nodes, Peyer's patches, appendix, and tonsils. Immunoglobulins are often

Figure 4.13   The restoration of skin test responses following control of hemorrhage in a 61-year-old cirrhotic patient, admitted to hospital with hematemesis and melena. Endoscopy revealed bleeding esophageal varices. He continued to bleed on nonoperative management, became hypotensive, and was taken to surgery (OR). A hepatoma was found at laparotomy, the varices were ligated, bleeding was controlled, and blood volume was restored to normal. Skin testing on the first day after operation showed anergy. With maintenance of normal cardiac filling pressure and cardiac output over the subsequent two weeks, the patient converted to relative anergy on the eighth day after operation and to normal reactivity on the twelfth day. The patient's hospital recovery was uneventful.

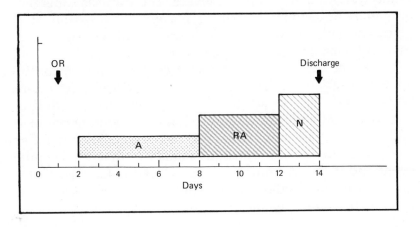

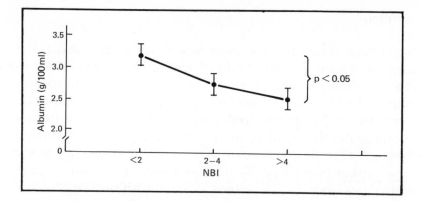

Figure 4.14 Serum albumin and neutrophil bactericidal index (NBI) evaluated in same patients within 24 hours. Neutrophil function is significantly correlated with abnormally low serum albumin.

elevated, usually in response to the chronic or repeated infections to which these children are exposed. Nevertheless, their response to a specific fresh antigen is variable and generally decreased. Cell-mediated immunity and T cell function are abnormal and there are reduced responses to PHA together with altered delayed hypersensitivity reactions and an inability to be sensitized to DNCB. Interestingly, there are alterations in complement activities, specifically including low levels of all components of the classical complement sequence with the exception of C4. Neutrophil function is abnormal, particularly intracellular killing (Fig. 4.14), although chemotaxis may also be reduced when malnutrition is severe. There are also alterations of metabolic activity in leukocytes with depression of the glycolytic pathway activity and reduced NADPH oxidase activity and hence loss of energy for bacterial killing.

It may be argued that, in many respects, the majority of altered host defenses seen on surgical wards relate to trauma, sepsis, shock, or malnutrition. This is particularly true if one considers that all forms of surgical intervention are traumatic, and that surgical complications are exceptionally stressful and may affect the body in a manner similar to that of a traumatic event and therefore stimulate or produce the factor(s) that are involved in the production of cellular and humoral mediated host defense abnormalities.

This view may be slightly simplistic, but it does permit a more functionally directed therapeutic approach which will be discussed. However, there are also a number of other clinical situations in which acquired abnormalities to the immune response are seen. They result from the underlying disease, physiologic alterations imposed by that disease, or by drug manipulations employed in treating the patient's basic illness.

Cancer

Neoplastic disease affects the immune system primarily, and also as a secondary result of its metastases and complications. Patients with malignancies involving lymphoid organs develop immune deficiencies that are usually a function of the extent and type of involvement. Patients with Hodgkin's disease frequently develop abnormalities of T lymphocytes and this may account for the apparently higher rate of infection with intracellular parasites. The leading cause of death in many hematologic malignancies is now sepsis, undoubtedly influenced by complications of chemotherapy.

Cancer patients whose immune response is intact respond better to chemotherapy and live longer. It is not clear whether a true immunologic failure allows the development of a neoplasm. Patients who are subjected to long term immunosuppression have an increased incidence of cancer, particularly those involving hematologic elements. Therefore, in the patient with advanced esophageal carcinoma the carcinoma is clearly a major problem, but it is malnutrition that is probably the major cause of depressed immunity, perhaps encouraging the rapid progression of the cancer. It is not known if cancer per se produces an increased incidence of anergy in patients when compared to other patients who do not have cancer. It does appear, however, that patients with cancer have a markedly increased mortality but less infection following identification of their anergic state when compared to similar patients without cancer. It would therefore appear that those patients with cancer who have altered skin test responses tend not to recover if any complications develop. This may result from the complications of the neoplasm itself, but the alterations that attend far advanced disease may also be responsible. Unfortunately, in malignant disease it is difficult to ascertain whether the alterations in host defense are directly related to the development of the neoplasm, were a cause of the neoplasm, or are secondary to the general effect that extensive neoplastic disease has upon the host.

Drugs

Transplantation   A review of early experience shows infection was a major contributor to morbidity and mortality following renal and other forms of organ transplantation. With a clearer understanding of the effects of immunosuppressive agents (e.g., imuran, prednisone, cyclophosphamide, and/or antilymphocyte globulin), use of these drugs has been modified to produce a much lower complication rate with consequent reduction in sepsis. The alterations in the immune response produced by these agents not only prevents rejection but also suppresses the humoral and CMI response to facultative intracellular parasites (viruses and fungi) together with slight alterations in the ability to respond to specific humoral antigens and decrease in neutrophil function. Bone marrow suppression following exuberant immunosuppression is less common today. As a consequence, the occurrence of neutropenia and the incidence and severity of early bacterial infections have been markedly reduced.

Adrenocortical Steroids   Since their discovery in the 1950s adrenocortical steroids have been known to have immunosuppressive properties. They have been reported to alter neutrophil function in vitro, although the data appear to be somewhat conflicting. Certainly their end result is to delay or prevent the entry of leukocytes into wounds. There is, however, no question that lymphocyte function is altered and that adrenocortical steroids in high doses may, in fact, be lympholytic. They have a pronounced effect on cell-mediated immunity, and this is seen most specifically in the prolongation of transplant survival in experimental animals and humans. In experimental systems, adrenocortical steroids have also been used to increase survival of tumor allografts and xenografts. Although they are used in certain settings as part of cancer chemotherapy, they tend to facilitate development of metastases in

274

experimental animals. When steroids are given prior to stimulation with antigen, antibody responses are reduced although fully differentiated plasma cells will respond normally. Adrenocortical steroids alter cell membranes and have a major antiinflammatory effect. Many of these immunosuppressive features may be mediated not only at the cell surface but also through interference with basic mediating molecules such as the prostaglandins. Further clarification is required, but it is clear now that adrenocortical steroids have a broad effect on the immune response. Their use allows the development not only of common bacterial infections but also facultative intracellular parasites such as tuberculosis, viruses, and sometimes fungi; thus accounting for their tendency to cause a flare up of a long quiescent tuberculous lesion.

Obviously, it is important that when surgery is being performed on patients who are receiving adrenocortical steroids, particular attention be paid to concepts of wound healing and surgical technique, as these are themselves a form of immunotherapy. Good technical surgery supports the host's local response, reduces the probability of an infectious process occurring (as discussed in Chap. 6) and reduces the task which the steroid-retarded wound has to perform in order to heal.

Cancer Chemotherapy　The broad range of drugs used in cancer chemotherapy precludes a detailed discussion of their effects on the immune response. Nevertheless, all who have experience with these agents will testify that the incidence of sepsis is much higher in patients receiving them. They have profound effects on the immune response in terms of neutrophil function, cell-mediated immunity, and the ability to develop a specific antibody response. Many also alter the inflammatory response, which may be a function of interference with the action or production of basic mediating molecules. The effect on the bone marrow is particularly significant and neutropenia associated with chemotherapy is a particularly dangerous situation. The approach to treatment in these settings is usually "an ounce of prevention is worth a pound of cure." However, when neutropenia develops, white cell transfusions as a specific form of therapy appear to be most critical. There are some immunomodulating agents that may be useful in the immunosuppressed patient. These are discussed on page 282.

Diabetic patients exhibit a high incidence of infection related to (1) potential defects in host defense, (2) anatomic changes due to vascular disease, and (3) metabolic alterations, particularly of acid/base balance in the presence of ketoacidosis. The contribution of each of these factors varies from time to time. For instance, the infected foot of the diabetic is more a function of the failed physiology of the peripheral vasculature than of any alteration in cell function, but wound healing and bacterial |killing by leukocytes vary with metabolic control as noted in Chapter 2. Ketoacidosis and severe acid/base disturbance, affects oxygen delivery and peripheral perfusion, both of which affect local factors involved in prevention of infection as well as systemic host defense factors, particularly neutrophil function. Infection is therefore aided by alteration in two determinants of infection, environment and host defenses, as a result of metabolic acidosis.

The uremic patient also develops acquired defects of host resistance that primarily affect the humoral and cell-mediated immune system. These alterations are multifactorial, dependent to some extent upon the state of nutrition, adequacy of dialysis, presence of other diseases, and adherence of the patient to his diet. There is some evidence to suggest that a patient on dialysis for a prolonged period becomes increasingly immunosuppressed, and renal transplantation is accordingly more successful.

These various problems indicate that HDM failure and subsequent infection is multifactorial, but also suggest that there are many aspects of basic care that may correct these abnormalities.

IMMUNOLOGIC SUPPORT
General Measures

The previous discussion has focused on the biology and consequences of defective host defenses. The purpose of describing the biology of the infectious process is to delineate and apply physiologically sound therapeutic approaches. Manipulation of the host's physiology can alter two of the three determinants of infection, the environment and host defenses. Approaches to each of these determinants are similar and reflect sound patient care. Many principles of management that thoughtful physicians have found useful in the past can now be identified with sound biologic principles. Many of these lessons have been learned, forgotten, or ignored, and relearned many times over the years because of the changing fashions in medical and surgical practice.

The technical skills of tissue management have historical roots in the work of the French war surgeon Paré, and more recently in the work of Halsted. The concept that gentle handling of tissues, accurate hemostasis, sharp dissection, abscence of dead space, precise ligating with the smallest possible sutures, have immunobiologic implications could hardly have been known at the time these surgical principles were first described. Nevertheless, in light of the evidence presented elsewhere in this book, these principles clearly do have implications for host defenses. The serum and cellular components of host defense that promote wound healing and contain or resolve any infectious potential, cannot function optimally in an environment of debris, seroma, hematoma, and large bites of dead tissue with big ligatures. Studies have proved conclusively that these surgeon-controlled technical factors directly influence infection rates. (See Chap. 6). Cruse (1973) has demonstrated this indirectly, but firmly, when he showed that wound infection rates could be halved by wide publication of an unacceptably high infection rate. Clearly surgical technique has immunobiologic implications that are directly related to failed wound healing, i.e., infection.

The same philosophy must be applied to management of the multitude of invasive devices in common use on surgical wards and intensive care areas. The management of these devices, i.e. IV, central venous pressure (CVP), and TPN lines, Swan–Ganz catheters, Foley catheters, drains, chest tubes, and tracheostomy tubes can be reduced to scrupulous care and attention to detail.

The maintenance of Bernard's "Milieu Interieure" may not be thought to have implications for host defense in the view of the classical immunologist. Yet if there is potential for infection, such as following traumatic splenectomy, and if the cells and serum components needed to fight infection are unable to get to the site, or if once there they are unable to function because of abnormal systemic physiology, the probability of sepsis is high. This situation is not in the least farfetched. Normal physiology includes adequate blood volume and therefore adequate tissue perfusion, thus ensuring delivery of the components of host defense so critical to the control of infection. Similarly, the environment must be such that the cells can function; thus oxygenation and acid base balance must be near normal.

In summary, good basic care includes:

1. Restoration and maintenance of blood volume
2. Maintenance of good tissue perfusion
3. Adequate arterial Po_2
4. Physiologic acid/base balance

All of these have profound implications for host defenses and, as a consequence, on normal wound healing and prevention of infection. Therefore, when the seemingly empty phrase, "maintain or boost the host resistance" is uttered, there are several very basic and sound concepts of good patient care which can be applied. It is fundamental, however, that these must be applied accurately or the concepts have no meaning.

As noted before, drainage of infection also has profound effects upon the immune response. Sepsis itself has immunosuppressive properties. Sepsis was the major contributing factor to anergy in 41 percent of our anergic patients. While there is no panacea that will eliminate an infectious process, its drainage is crucial. We usually think of drainage as being required only for abscesses or closed spaces, and forget its importance in tracheobronchial, biliary, and urinary tract infections. We have frequently seen host responses promptly return to normal following drainage of a common duct, an abscess or, in the case of multiple abscesses, drainage of the final abscess. In this setting, the persistence of anergy frequently indicates that there is more pus or infection that requires attention.

The synthesis of these points regarding surgical technique and patient care based upon physiologic principles can be visualized in the management of the injured patient and resolution of his trauma. The recovery of skin test responses and associated return to normal of neutrophil CTX are obviously secondary to the issue of patient recovery. They nevertheless serve as objective measures of management and have clear implications for the patient with regard to development of infection and concurrent recovery. Following recovery from the acute phase of injury and early respiratory insufficiency, sepsis is the major cause of death in the trauma patient. It is therefore of considerable significance that all aspects of a patient's physiology be supported with equal enthusiasm starting from the moment the patient enters the emergency room. For instance, apart from meticulous debridement and maintenance of blood volume and tissue perfusion, the active prevention of hypoxia at all times is essential. We have no embarrassment in asking patients to use a mask to keep arterial Po_2 in the high physiologic range.

Specific Approaches

Nutrition   Of the four horsemen of the apocalypse, pestilence and famine have sadly visited more frequently than the others. They have been linked together for eons, and to the modern day scientist in third world areas, it is still not always clear which problem, infection or malnutrition, strikes first. Major infections impose huge caloric and nutritional demands not only as a result of the catabolic effects of the infectious process but secondary to fever, fluid loss, and so on, as well.

It is apparent from earlier discussion and figures that infection and malnutrition can individually depress host defenses. The sum, in turn, appears to aggravate the seriousness of the infectious insult. The single most significant event in surgical management in the past 10 years has been the development of a global approach to nutrition that allows surgeons to give normal or supernormal nutrition via parenteral or enteric routes.

Body composition studies in anergic patients have been of some value in providing data that support the use of total parenteral nutrition (TPN). About one-third of our patients have responded to TPN with restoration of normal host defenses as measured by cutaneous responses (Table 4.10). It is not clear why the others failed to respond similarly. However, because

Table 4.10 Effect of Total Parenteral Nutrition

	Patients	Na_e/K_e Pre-TPN	Post-TPN
Remained anergic	19	1.60 ± 0.16	1.48 ± 0.13
Restored to normal	8	1.62 ± 0.26	1.11 ± 0.10

the population was quite heterogenous, and the illnesses complex, it should not be concluded that TPN did not help the other patients. One can conclude only that proof was lacking one way or the other.

Experimental studies with rats and dogs in various states of protein calorie malnutrition have very nicely shown the value of TPN in restorating components of the immune response in animals. Law has also shown, in an unselected group of patients, that TPN can restore some components of host defense. The data for a patient with carcinoma of the larynx (Figure 4.15) supports this concept clearly. In appropriate situations enteric nutritional support may prove to have greater effect upon the

Figure 4.15 Malnutrition and effect of total parenteral nutrition. Mr. M., a 51-year-old man with cancer of the larynx, was treated previously with radiotherapy before he was admitted to hospital for surgery. He was severely malnourished, with a total exchangeable sodium to total exchangeable potassium ratio (Na_e/K_e) of 3.2 (normal = 0.98, Shizgal). He was anergic and was started on TPN. After three weeks his skin test responses had become normal. He was operated on and recovered uneventfully. The post-operative body composition (Na_e/K_e = 0.98) studies confirmed a return to normal of body composition.

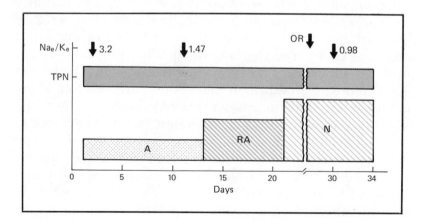

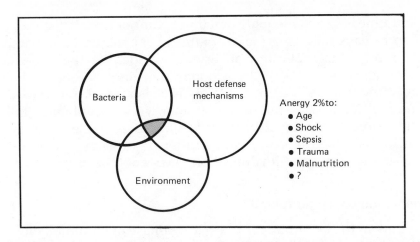

Figure 4.16 In the figure, there are three overlapping circles labeled Bacteria, Host defense mechanisms, and Environment, with a list: Anergy 2%to: Age, Shock, Sepsis, Trauma, Malnutrition, ?

Figure 4.16 Anergy, etiologic features, and resultant alteration in host defenses with resultant known increase in incidence and probability of sepsis.

immune response than TPN. This has proved to be the case in burn patients receiving equivalent amounts of calories orally (or via tube) versus parenterally. All available laboratory data and clinical experience lead us to view nutrition as a form of immunotherapy, which provides the caloric requirements for healing and also for support of the immune system.

A frequently asked question, and one for which there is no single ready answer, is: How should we manage the preoperatively identified anergic patient? At the present time,if the required operation is not an emergency, 7 to 10 days of total parental nutrition is probably a reasonable approach. The patient in Figure 4.15 required three weeks of TPN because he was grossly malnourished. However, relatively few patients are in that severe a state of malnutrition. If there are other potential causes for anergy, (e.g. sepsis, bleeding, etc.) these should be appropriately managed before operation (Fig. 4.16).

In the postoperative period the development of anergy is a grave sign and the basic cause must be identified. However, in this setting we feel that TPN is generally required. The initiating factors for anergy exert a severe catabolic effect, and there is no other direct method of supporting the immune system. In trauma, we have no way of being certain that TPN should be initiated in the anergic injured patient. Our policy at the present time is that if adequate oral intake cannot be anticipated by 7 to 10 days following major trauma, TPN should be initiated promptly. Pragmatically, on Friday we identify the patients who may need TPN. If by Monday morning there is no improvement in their calorie intake, TPN is started. Otherwise, the decision is often put off for another week by hedging while the vicious cycle of malnutrition leading to depressed host defense, increased infection and further depression of host defense and worsening malnutrition takes another turn or two.

Immunomodulating Agents

We are at the beginning of an exciting phase of immunobiology anticipated in 1906 by G. B. Shaw in his spoof on the medical profession, *The Doctor's Dilemma:*

There is at bottom only one genuinely scientific treatment for all diseases, and that is to stimulate the phagocytes. Stimulate the phagocytes. Drugs are a delusion.

While medicine has progressed considerably over the past 70 years, we still do not have effective direct means of stimulating the immune system during an acute surgical situation. While control of polio, tetanus, measles, whooping cough, diphtheria, and rubella has been achieved via specific immunologic stimulation, the methods do not apply to problems faced by surgeons. The most active research in modulation of major segments of the immune response is in cancer therapy where *C. parvum*, Bacille Calmette-Guerin (BCG), Glucan, Levamisole, and a host of other pharmacologic or microbial products are being tested. The effort is directed toward stimulating immune responses, or restoring abnormal immune responses to normal, as a means of controlling or curing cancer.

Surgeons probably can assume that in the not too distant future, we will be able to stimulate and restore immune responses in patients whose acquired defects predispose them to sepsis. We will directly treat immune responses as well as indirectly support them. Nevertheless, the immune responses need their energy, their protein sources, their oxygen, their vitamins. No amount of "stimulation" can change that. As we await the future, we should realize that while we may not now be able to actually *increase* the immune response to much more than its normal potential with our present supportive methods, we can regularly maintain it at a higher level than surgeons have ever experienced before.

BIBLIOGRAPHY

Alexander JW: Emerging concepts in control of clinical infection. Surgery 75:934, 1974

Alexander JW, Good RA: Fundamentals of Clinical Immunology. Philadelphia, Saunders, 1977

Alexander JW, Meakins JL: A physiologic basis for the development of opportunistic infections in man. Ann Surg 176:273, 1972

Bubenik O, Meakins JL: Neutrophil chemotaxis in surgical patients: Effect of cardiopulmonary bypass. Surg Forum 27:267, 1976

Cline MJ: The White Cell. Cambridge, Harvard University Press, 1975

Cruse PJE: Surgical wound sepsis. Can Med Assoc J 102:251, 1970

Cruse PJE: Incidence of wound infection on surgical services. Surg Clin North Am 55:1269, 1975

Cruse PJE, Foord R: A five-year prospective study of 23,649 surgical wounds. Arch Surg 107:206, 1973

Dionigi R, Zonta A, Dominioni L, Gnes F, Ballabio A: The effects of total parenteral nutrition on immunodepression due to malnutrition. Ann Surg 185:467, 1977

Dhillon K, MacLean LD, Meakins JL: Neutrophil function in surgical patients: Correlation of neutrophil bactericidal function, serum albumin and sepsis. Surg Forum 26:27, 1975

Dubos RJ: The micro-environment of inflammation or Metchnikoff revisited. Lancet 2:1, 1955

Eilber FR, Morton DL: Imparied immunologic reactivity and recurrence following cancer. Cancer 25:362, 1970

Good RA: Progress toward a cellular engineering. JAMA 214:1289, 1970

Hirsch JG: Immunity to infectious disease: Review of some concepts of Metchnikoff. Bact Revs 23:48, 1959

Hohn DC: Leukocyte phagocytic function and dysfunction. Surg Gynecol Obstet 144:99, 1977

Howard RJ, Simmons RL: Acquired immunodeficiencies after trauma and surgical procedures. Surg Gynecol Obstet 139:771, 1974

Law DK, Dudrick SJ, Abdou NI: Immunocompetence of patients with protein-calorie malnutrition. The effects of nutritional repletion. Ann Intern Med 79:545, 1973

283

Law DK, Dudrick SJ, Abdou NI: The effect of dietary protein depletion on immunocompetence. The importance of nutritional repletion prior to immunologic induction. Ann Surg 179:168, 1974

Lennard ES, Bjornson AB, Petering HG, et al.: An immunologic and nutritional evaluation of burn neutrophil function. J Surg Res 16:286, 1974

MacLean LD, Meakins JL, Taguchi K, et al.: Host resistance in sepsis and trauma. Ann Surg 132:207, 1975

Majno G: The Healing Hand. Man and Wound in the Ancient World. Cambridge, Harvard University Press, 1975

Meakins JL: Pathophysiologic determinants and prediction of sepsis. Surg Clin North Am 56:847, 1976

Meakins JL: Infection control in the surgical intensive care unit. Can J Surg 28:78, 1978

Meakins JL, Pietsch JB, Bubenik O, et al.: Delayed hypersensitivity: Indicator of acquired failure of host defenses in sepsis and trauma. Ann Surg 186:241, 1977

Meakins JL, MacLean APH, Kelly R, et al.: Delayed hypersensitivity response and neutrophil chemotaxis: Effect of trauma. J Trauma 18:240, 1978

Metchnikoff E: Immunity in Infective Diseases. London, Cambridge University Press, 1907.

Metchnikoff E: Lectures on the comparative pathology of inflammation. London, Kegan Paul, Trench, Truber and Co., 1893. Quoted in Hirsch JG: Phagocytosis. Ann Rev Micro 19:339, 1965

Palmer DL, Reed WP: Delayed hypersensitivity skin testing. I. Response-rates in a hospitalized population. J Infect Dis 130:132, 1974

Palmer DL, Reed WP: Delayed hypersensitivity skin testing. II. Clinical correlates and anergy. J Infect Dis 130:138, 1974

Pietsch JB, Meakins JL, Gotto D, MacLean LD: Delayed hypersensitivity responses: The effect of surgery. J Surg Res 22:228, 1977

Pietsch JB, Meakins JL, MacLean LD: The delayed hypersensitivity response: Application in clinical surgery. Surgery 82:349, 1977

Robson MC, Krizek TJ, Heggers JP: Biology of surgical infection. Curr Probl Surg 3 13:1–62, 1973

Saba TM: Reticuloendothelial system host defense after surgery and traumatic shock. Circ Shock 2:9, 1975

Scrimshaw NS, Taylor CE, Gordon JE (eds): Interactions of Nutrition and Infection. Monograph series, No. 57. Geneva, World Health Organization, 1968

Shizgal HM: Total body composition and nutritional status. Surg Clin North Am 56:1185, 1976

Slade MS, Simmons RL, Yunis EJ, Greenberg LJ: Immunodepression after major surgery in normal patients. Surgery 78:363, 1975

Sokal JE: Measurement of delayed hypersensitivity responses. New Engl J Med 293:501, 1975

Spanier AH, Pietsch J, Meakins JL, MacLean LD, Shizgal HM: The relationship between immune competence and nutrition. Surg Forum 27:332, 1976

Stossel TP: Phagocytosis. New Engl J Med 209:717–723, 774–780, 883–889, 1974

Warden GD, Mason AD, Pruitt BA: Suppression of leukocyte chemotaxis in vitro by chemotherapeutic agents used in the management of thermal injuries. Ann Surg 181:363, 1975

Westwood JCN, Legacé, S, Mitchell MA: Acquired infection: Present and future impact and need for positive action. Can Med Assoc J 110:769, 1974

Zigmond SH, Hirsch JG: Leukocyte locomotion and chemotaxis. J Exp Med 137:387, 1973

5

NUTRITION
Stanley Levenson
Eli Seifter
Walton Van Winkle, Jr.

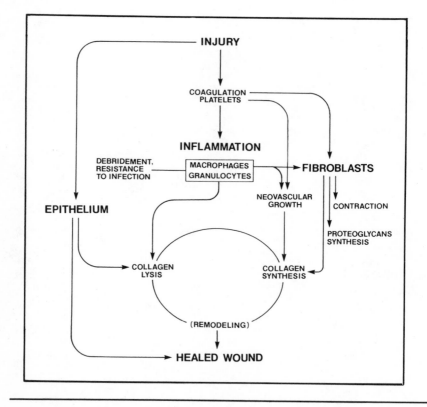

The research reported by two of the authors was supported in part by Grant DADA 17-70-C-009 from the Army Medical Research and Development Command, Grants K 69 M 14,208 (Research Career Award, S. M. Levenson) and 1 R01 GM 19328 from the National Institutes of Health to the Albert Einstein College of Medicine.

Wherefore I say that such constitutions as suffer quickly and strongly from errors in diet are weaker than others that do not; and that a weak person is in a state very nearly approaching to one in disease. . . . And this I know, moreover, that to the human body it makes a great difference whether the bread be fine or coarse, of wheat with or without the hull, whether mixed with much or with little water, strongly wrought or scarcely at all, baked or raw. . . . Whoever pays no attention to these things, or paying attention, does not comprehend them, how can he understand the diseases which befall a man? For by every one of these things, a man is affected and changed this way or that, and the whole of his life is subjected to them, whether in health, convalescence or disease. Nothing else, then, can be more important or more necessary to know than these things.

So stated Hippocrates some 2,300 years ago, sounding a warning to succeeding generations of physicians that has not been entirely heeded. Although we recognize the close link between nutrition and disease (including injury and the healing of wounds), we do not yet fully understand all the component factors—those "things" Hippocrates considered so vital.

As described in the earlier chapters, wound healing is a dynamic process, a spectacular progression of biochemical, physiologic, and morphologic changes. These events are highly integrated and follow an orderly sequence. However, the process is responsive to well-directed aid, and is influenced dramatically by metabolic and nutritional factors.

At no other time are the body's nutritional demands as great as they become following serious injury, especially if complicated by infection. Our understanding of this has led to advances in the surgeon's ability to meet those demands. And because of this progress, along with an expansion of our nutrient-providing resources, patients are surviving operations, injuries, and infections that in former days would have been fatal.

No longer must we, as in Paré's time, simply dress the wound and trust in God to heal it.

METABOLIC REACTIONS TO TRAUMA

What are the specific mechanisms and clinical consequences of the metabolic and nutritional derangements prompted by grave injury or acute illness? A complete series of answers—for the question is complex—will be provided only by further, more extensive research; but we can outline our present state of knowledge.

Müller was among the first to study these problems, having noted in 1884 that typhoid fever patients excreted unusually large amounts of nitrogen in their urine. Some 25 years later, Coleman, Shaffer, and DuBois began their investigations of metabolic changes in patients with a variety of diseases. But another 20 years passed before the first systematic study of the effects of injury on metabolism was conducted by Cuthbertson, who described the accelerated metabolic rate, weight loss, and increased urinary excretion of nitrogen, potassium, and sulfur characteristic of patients and animals with long-bone fractures.

Trauma abruptly alters the metabolic "steady state" of the healthy adult. The postinjury state is marked by increased heat production and gluconeogenesis; negative nitrogen, potassium, sulfur, and phosphorus balances; early hyperglycemia; and modifications in carbohydrate utilization. Other metabolic alterations produce elevated serum concentrations of free fatty acids and a tendency to ketosis; retention of sodium, chloride, and water; an increased need for ascorbic acid, thiamin, riboflavin, nicotinamide, and vitamin A; and possible deficiencies of certain trace metals, particularly zinc, iron, and copper.

These changes are usually accompanied by an involution of lymphoid tissue and of the thymus. Lymphopenia, eosinopenia, leukocytosis, adrenal cortical hypertrophy (with an associated depletion of cholesterol and ascorbic acid), and an increase in the secretion of catecholamines, adrenal glucocorticoids and antidiuretic hormone are also noted in the postinjury state.

An early increase in plasma glucagon is followed by a return to normal levels, while an initial drop in plasma insulin is followed by a rise. Plasma growth hormone levels are often elevated. Thyroid hormone levels do not increase and may decrease. A lessening of adrenal steroid conjugation is one of the indices of alteration in liver function.

Thus, the body's reaction to acute injury or illness appears to involve almost all its metabolic pathways. The response is dynamic, and although the pattern is ever-changing, it is generally predictable.

The pathogenesis of these responses and clarification of cer-

289

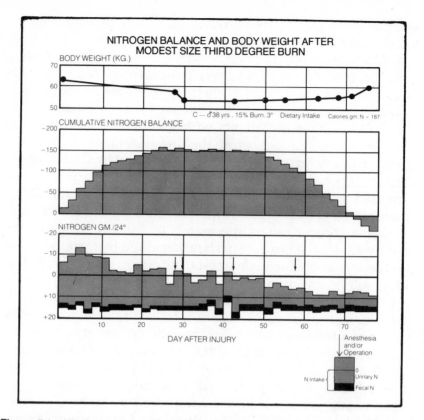

Figure 5.1 Nitrogen balance of previously healthy 38-year-old man with deep burns involving about 15 percent of body surface. In the lower third of the graph, nitrogen intake is plotted from the zero line down, fecal N in solid black going up from the intake line; above is urinary N. The middle section depicts the cumulative N balance. His daily food intake averaged 100 g protein (1½ g/kg body wt.) and 2950 calories (45 cal/kg body wt.). Despite this he was in negative nitrogen balance for 25 days. His weight loss was 9 kg and his cumulative nitrogen loss was 150 g; loss of "muscle" was calculated as 4.8 kg. "Muscle" equivalent calculated as follows: N × 6.25 × 5; N × 6.25 = protein, protein × 5 = muscle (protein = 20 percent muscle. *(Reprinted from Federation Proceedings 18: 1155–1190, 1950.)*

tain critical metabolic events, such as the metabolism of specific amino acids, have yet to be completely elucidated. Many conditioning and modulating factors are involved, including the age, sex, and pretrauma nutritional status of the patient, the severity of the injury, the degree of immobilization following injury, the patient's temperature, and the environmental temperature and humidity. For example, previously healthy young men suf-

290

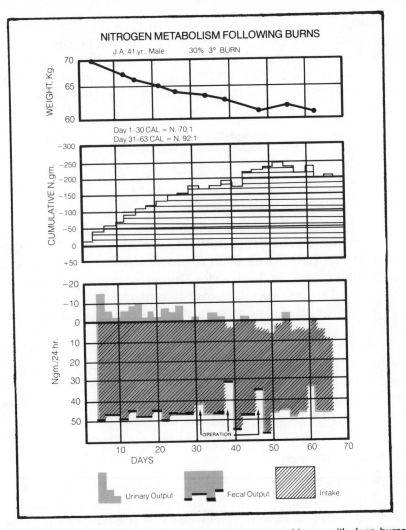

Figure 5.2 Nitrogen balance of previously healthy 41-year-old man with deep burns involving about 35 percent of his body surface. Daily food intake after injury averaged 280 g protein (4 g/kg body wt.) and 45 to 60 cal/kg. Despite this, note the marked negative nitrogen balance during the first seven weeks. Cumulative N loss (food minus urine and fecal N) was −250 g; muscle equivalent 8.1 kg. Surface nitrogen loss was not measured so that the actual negative nitrogen balance was even greater than indicated on the graph.

fering traumatic injury show the greatest metabolic derangements, these being roughly proportional to the severity of the injury (Figs. 5.1, 5.2).

Young women show less severe metabolic derangements, and children and the aged show less metabolic disturbances early than the young adults.

Individuals who have undergone elective operations, even very extensive ones, experience less marked alterations.

Nitrogen "Loss" in a Patient
with Severe Battle Wounds and Renal Failures

10-Day Loss*

Nitrogen	450 g
Tissue equivalent	14.4 kg

As for the mechanisms initiating these metabolic changes, most studies have focused on neuroendocrine responses, such as the role of the cerebral cortex, hypothalamus, pituitary, adrenals, and so on. Recent investigations have emphasized the key role the catecholamines play in the accelerated metabolic rate seen after serious injury.

Although the consequences of disturbances in metabolic pathways have not been fully delineated, it is clear that persistent imbalances can produce serious malnutrition, impair wound repair, and render the patient more susceptible to infection.

Demanding Wounds

Wound repair is influenced by the nutritional disorders (dysnutrition) stemming from the altered metabolic processes associated with severe injury, as well as by the patient's previous nutritional status. Superimposed on these disturbances are other problems posed by contaminating microorganisms, foreign bodies, and compromised blood supply to the injured tissues. Maintenence of the patient in a good state of nutrition must be a high priority, both to sustain healing and avoid infection. This is especially so in patients with large complex wounds—those that involve a number of different tissues and organs. Consider the formidable healing tasks depicted in the photographs of the wounded soldier in Figure 5.3. Shrapnel

*Calculated N and tissue ("muscle") loss of previously healthy young man with massive battle wounds and acute renal failure.

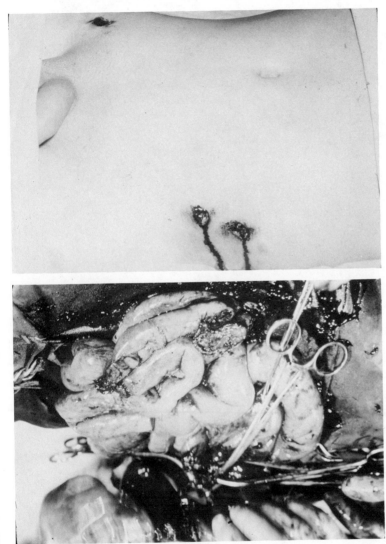

Figure 5.3 Severely wounded soldier. **A.** Abdomen before surgery shows penetrating wounds. **B.** Intraoperatively there is considerable blood in the peritoneal cavity stemming from torn vessels (chiefly mesenteric veins); small and large intestines are perforated in several sites (continued on p. 294).

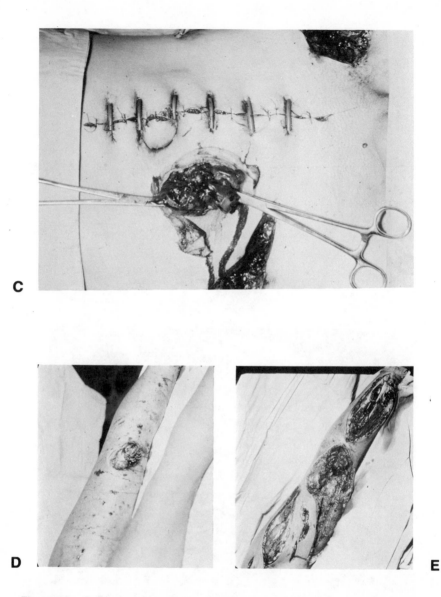

Figure 5.3 **C.** Seen postoperatively, abdominal shrapnel wounds have been debrided and left open, while the laparotomy wound has been sutured. **D.** Leg, preoperatively—innumerable penetrating wounds. **E.** Leg, postoperatively—after debridement; wounds, left open, dressing applied. Secondary closure several days later. *(Courtesy U.S. Army Medical Service, Walter Reed Army Institute of Research.)*

294

caused innumerable leg wounds and also penetrated his abdomen, tearing muscle, fascia, blood vessels, and intestine. Wound healing in this patient became a fight for survival, one in which prevention of nutritional deterioration was vital.

Patients with thermal burns also present varied and special metabolic, nutritional, and healing problems. The author first became interested in the nutritional facets of surgical therapy when treating severely burned victims of Boston's Coconut

Figure 5.4. Appearance of 19-year-old girl **(A)** and **(B,C)** 12 days after injury. Edema of face associated with burns has disappeared. The rounded appearance of her face and breasts is indicative of her normal well-nourished state. She had extensive deep burns, particularly on her back and arms. **D,E,F.** Same patient about 2 months later. Note the obvious weight loss, edematous, friable granulations over hand and forearm (dependent areas), and scanty granulations over her back. *(From Lund CC, Levenson SM. In Cole WH (ed): Operative Technique. New York, Appleton, 1949 pp. 51–84).*

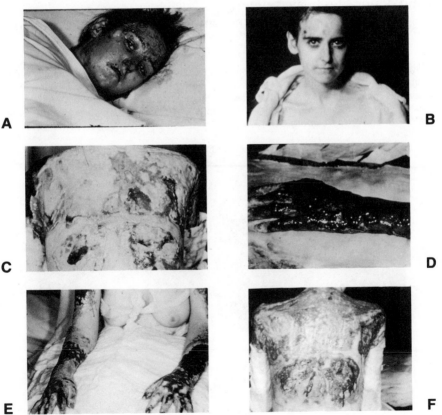

Grove fire in November 1942. On the night of that disaster, which took more than 500 lives, 132 burned patients—most of them of college age and previously healthy and well nourished—were admitted to the Boston City Hospital. The rapid nutritional deterioration observed in some of those extensively burned, such as the 19-year-old girl shown in Figure 5.4 was startling. Accompanying the malnutrition in these patients was weakness, a greater susceptibility to anesthetics and shock, impaired liver and gastrointestinal tract function, slowed wound healing, serious infection, long hospitalization, and death.

Sloughing of the deep third-degree burns proceeded at the rate expected in such patients, but as seen in Figs. 5.4 and 5.5 the underlying granulation tissue was edematous, friable, and often scanty. It proved highly susceptible to infection, and the "take" of skin grafts was poor. Epithelization from the periphery of the burns was delayed or completely inhibited, and donor sites healed slowly.

Since then we have learned much about the metabolic and

Figure 5.5 Appearance of young woman with extensive deep burns two months after injury. The burned skin has sloughed. The patient has lost considerable weight and is severely malnourished. Granulation tissue is soggy and edematous. *(From Margen S, (ed): Progress in Human Nutrition, vol 1, chap. 13, 1971 p.148. Used with permission of AVI, PO Box 831, Westport, Conn. 06880)*

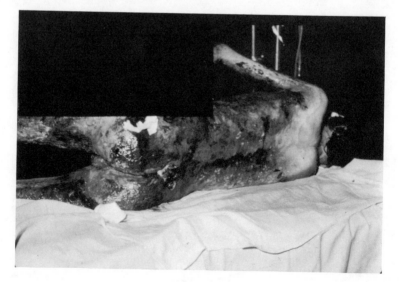

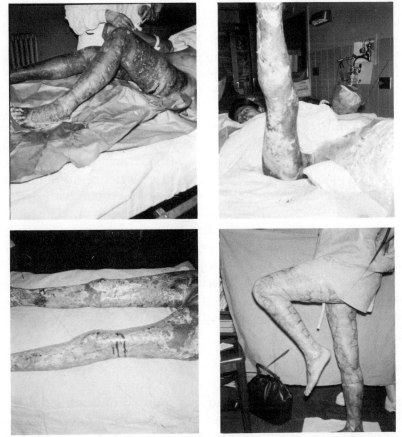

Figure 5.6 **A,B.** Deep flame burns involving both legs of a young woman; appearance one week after injury. **C.** Appearance of patient five weeks later. Most of the slough has separated. Granulation tissue is firm and healthy. Autografts were applied. **D.** Appearance of patient on discharge from hospital. Skin coverage is complete, function is good. Patient remained in a well-nourished state throughout hospitalization. *(From Levenson SM: In Lynch JB, Lewis SR (eds): Symposium on Treatment of Burns. St. Louis, Mosby, 1973 vol. 5, chap. 3, pp. 9–30.)*

physiologic problems involved in such patients. Today, maintenance of severely burned patients in a good nutritional state is a major factor in their recovery, increasing their resistance to infection and inducing granulation tissue that is firm, flat, and red. Grafts can be placed on such tissue with excellent "takes" and rapid healing of the donor sites, as indicated in Figure 5.6. (A more detailed discussion of the healing of burn wounds is presented in Chapter 7.)

Patients undergoing major elective surgery may also present serious metabolic and nutritional derangements. For example, a man with a carcinoma in the lower third of his esophagus is likely to be in a less than optimal nutritional state at the time of surgery. Such a patient requires nutritional support before and after operation if he is to heal the several anastomoses and major incisional wounds. Similar problems are presented by surgical patients with such gastrointestinal disorders as ulcerative colitis, Crohn's disease or a chronically impaired blood supply to the gut, and by those with cirrhosis of the liver or chronic pancreatitis. Others who will experience difficulties in wound healing include patients with severe renal dysfunction, those with endocrine disorders, such as diabetes and Cushing's disease, and those with conditions requiring treatment with certain drugs, such as glucocorticoids (rheumatoid arthritis) or penicillamine (Wilson's disease).

Malignancies can pose special problems; they *may* have a primary systemic effect on reparative processes, and they *do* have secondary effects through associated nutritional disturbances.

Patients undergoing major elective surgery who have no nutritional disturbances prior to operation are not apt to develop wound healing problems secondary to metabolic changes induced by the operation itself unless some complication, such as serious shock, infection, or renal or liver failure develops. This is because the metabolic derangements associated with uncomplicated elective surgery are moderate, and preventive and therapeutic steps can be taken fairly readily, as will be described later.

Clinical experience indicates that wounds in the elderly tend to heal poorly, become infected, and develop other complications. Several studies have found a relationship between age and the incidence of wound dehiscence, one putting it at 1.3 percent among patients under 45 years of age and at 5.4 percent among those over 45. Does this increased incidence reflect the effects of aging per se, or is it due to underlying disorders such as decreased resistance to infection, impaired peripheral circulation, or the poor nutrition frequently encountered in the elderly? Some experiments suggest that aging directly retards key steps in the healing process, for example, fibroblastic proliferation and collagen synthesis. In addition, repair can be im-

298

peded secondarily in the aged by the local and systemic factors already mentioned, including inadequate nutrition.

All the steps involved in wound healing require numerous syntheses and other energy-consuming reactions. The wound itself makes a nutritional demand, and unless that demand is met by dietary sources, the body is forced to turn on itself, catabolizing certain of its own tissues to acquire the metabolites needed for repair, as well as to support the metabolic and physiologic processes going on in the rest of the body. A patient with massive trauma and minimal food intake may lose the equivalent of a kilogram of muscle a day, in addition to considerable body fat.

Cuthbertson has suggested that the rapid breakdown of glycogen fat, and labile protein after injury serves to provide energy and/or amino acids needed for healing—a protective response of a wounded animal whose ability to feed itself has been reduced. He pointed out that a similar view had been expressed in the late 18th century by John Hunter, who wrote: "There is a circumstance attending accidental injury which does not belong to disease—namely, that the injury done has, in all cases, a tendency to produce both the disposition and the means of cure."

This so-called catabolic reaction to injury may be a useful design of nature, but it does not assure optimal wound repair following injury. Moore has noted that most closed incisional wounds heal to "tensile integrity" during the time of negative nitrogen balance, but we do not know whether the wounds are healing at a normal rate. The healing appears to be satisfactory but it may be neither normal nor optimal. Our lack of information on this important matter stems from two interrelated factors: the complexity of the problem and the absence of controlled, definitive, clinical studies.

ROLE OF NUTRIENTS ON WOUND REPAIR

Ideally, one would like to follow the healing process in patients by taking serial biopsies of the wounds—observing histologic and biochemical changes and measuring breaking strengths. But such an extensive assessment of wound repair cannot be readily carried out in humans, although some initial steps have been taken in that direction. For the present, our data in this area come largely from in vitro culture studies and animal experiments that the investigator can control to a degree impossible in clinical studies. However, the problems that arise during the healing of injured patients are far more complex than those observed in the laboratory.

For instance, repair of simple incisions proceeds more slowly in man than in the animals commonly used in experiments. In rats subjected to skin incisions, rapid collagen synthesis begins on about the fifth day after injury; fibrous protein accumulates in the wound rapidly over the first six weeks, then begins a very gradual decline (Fig. 5.7). There is a slight but progressive

Figure 5.7 Histologic appearances of experimental dorsal skin incisions in healthy rats; van Gieson's stain. Postoperative days: **A.** 7; **B.** 14; **C.** 21; **D.** 42. *(From Levenson SM, Geever EF, Crowley LV, et al.: Ann Surg 161:293, 1965.)*

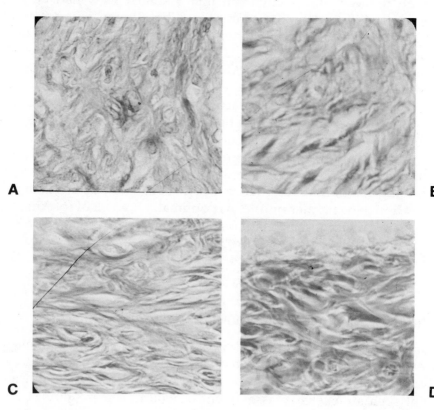

A B C D

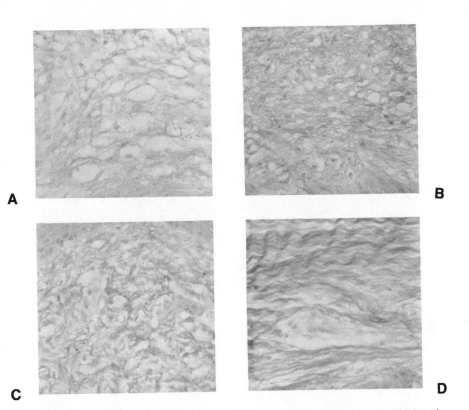

Figure 5.8 Histologic appearances of experimental skin incisions, anterior thighs of healthy men; van Gieson's stain. Postoperative days: **A.** 14; **B.** 21; **C.** 42; **D.** 88. Note the substantially slower healing in the human subject as compared with the rats in Figure 7. *(Courtesy U.S. Army Medical Service, Walter Reed Army Institute of Research.)*

improvement in the quality and compactness of the collagen fibers after the sixth postoperative week, along with a rearrangement and reorientation of those fibers, as a result of the collagen lysis and synthesis that proceed throughout healing.

In man, the rate of collagen accumulation in a simple skin incision is much slower, so that after 88 days there is less collagen than in a comparable rat wound at 42 days (Fig. 5.8). Even after 240 days there is significantly less collagen in the wound than in undamaged skin, and its arrangement has not yet reached its final form. There are few data on the breaking strength or collagen cross-linking of wounds in humans.

301

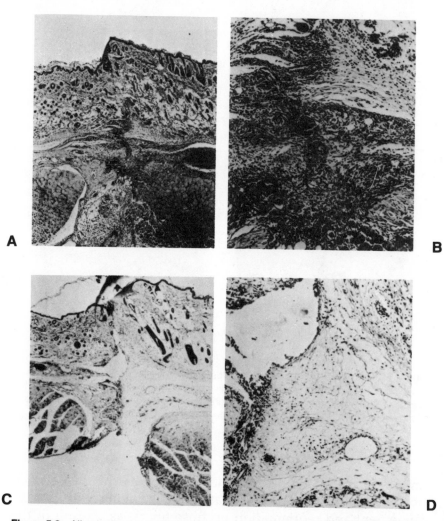

Figure 5.9 Histologic appearances of laparotomy incisions five days postoperatively in control (unburned rats **(A + B)** and burned rats **(C + D). A.** Control rat. Fifth postoperative day. Wound edges are well apposed. Fairly abundant reparative tissue is present in the wound. Hematoxylin and eosin, + 14. **B.** Detail of A, demonstrating numerous fibroblasts and capillaries in the reparative tissue. Hematoxylin and eosin, + 53. **C.** Burned rat. There is a wide gap in the central portion of the reparative tissue. Hematoxylin and eosin, + 14. **D.** Detail of C. Serofibrinous edema at the wound's edges with minimal fibroblastic proliferation and neovascularization. Hematoxylin and eosin, + 53. *(From Levenson SM, Crowley LV, Seifter E, et al.: Effect of environmental temperature and femoral fracture on wound healing in rats. Surg Gynecol Obstet 99:74, 1954 by permission of Surgery, Gynecology, & Obstetrics.)*

Returning to experimental work, a striking impairment has been observed in the repair of primarily closed laparotomy wounds in rats receiving third-degree burns of 35 percent of their body surface (back and flanks). Shock was not a factor here. During the first postoperative week, the incisions of the burned animals were broader and weaker than those of controls (rats subjected to laparotomy but not burned) and were covered by a dry, sanguineous exudate. There was a delay in the appearance and maturation of connective tissue in the laparotomy wounds of the burned rats (Fig. 5.9). A retardation was still evident, though less marked, at the end of the second postoperative week.

Other experiments have shown that the processes of healing dorsal skin incisions and forming reparative granulation tissue in subcutaneously implanted polyvinyl alcohol sponges are slowed in rats who have been subjected to unilateral comminuted, femoral fracture (Fig. 5.10). This effect was even more pronounced in rats with bilateral femoral fractures.

Figure 5.10 Effects of unilateral femoral fracture on healing skin incisions and sponge reparative tissue in s.c. implanted polyvinyl alcohol sponges of pair-fed rats seven days after injury. *(Adapted from Crowley LV, et al.: J Trauma 17:436, 1977, The Williams & Wilkins Co. Baltimore)*

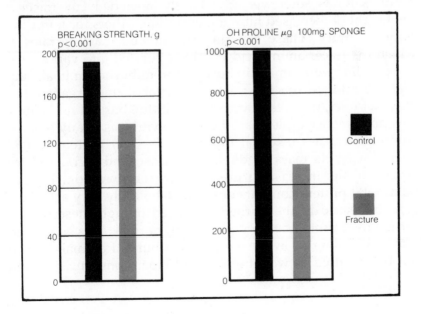

Underlying Mechanisms

Although peripheral circulatory failure was not a factor in the delayed repair observed in the burn and fracture experiments just described, severe, prolonged shock may interfere with wound healing, a result of decreased tissue perfusion and metabolic and immunologic changes. Especially important are the many metabolic and nutritional changes that characteristically follow injury, even in the absence of shock.

Although we will discuss the various metabolites and nutrients separately, it should be emphasized that changes in any one metabolite may affect functional or quantitative changes in other metabolites and influence the responses of certain target organs and tissues. In the final analysis, all must be considered together. A multitude of reactions involving various metabolites proceeds simultaneously in wound repair and although one would like to describe these simultaneously, this is not possible (Fig. 5.11).

Oxygen   The critical role oxygen plays in wound repair and infection is covered in detail in the first two chapters.

Protein Metabolism   A clue to why laparotomy repair is slowed in burned animals was afforded by studies of various tissue proteins in rats; some were given a ^{15}N-labeled glycine tracer at the height of increased nitrogen excretion, others for four days prior to injury. These experiments showed that the rates at which the tracer amino acid was incorporated into various tissue proteins were similar in burned and unburned animals, but that the rates in the most actively metabolizing organs (e.g., liver, GI tract, pancreas) were higher in the burned rats. There was no evidence of decreased protein synthesis in any organs. Although carcass (skeletal muscle and bone) protein turned over slowly, its mass gradually decreased and accounted for almost all the increase in urinary nitrogen excretion. In contrast, total protein contents of the metabolically very active organs increased in the burned rats even though these organs turned over protein more rapidly than normal. This suggested that the healing of liver "wounds" in burned animals would not be impaired as was the repair of laparotomy incisions. In

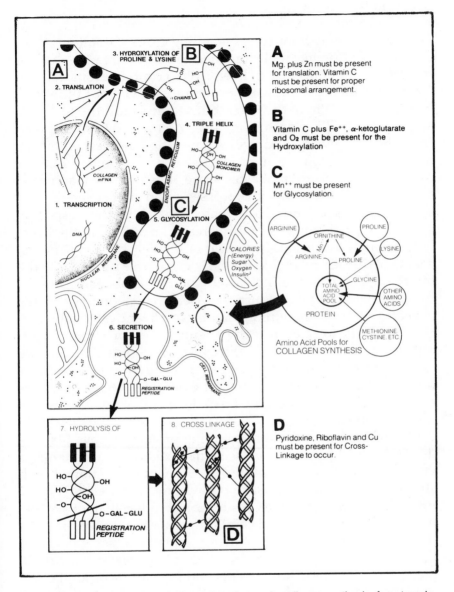

A

Mg. plus Zn must be present for translation. Vitamin C must be present for proper ribosomal arrangement.

B

Vitamin C plus Fe^{++}, α-ketoglutarate and O$_2$ must be present for the Hydroxylation

C

Mn^{++} must be present for Glycosylation.

D

Pyridoxine, Riboflavin and Cu must be present for Cross-Linkage to occur.

Figure 5.11 Diagrammatic representation of steps in collagen synthesis, from translation to secretion, with their nutritional requirements. A proper mix of all nutrients is necessary for each step.

fact, liver regeneration, following partial hepatectomy, is accelerated in burned rats.

The metabolic and functional changes associated with injury are different from those resulting from starvation alone. For example, the metabolic rate decreases in starvation while it increases after injury. Also, liver protein content drops at a rate far greater than does carcass protein in starved but otherwise healthy rats. When they are burned in addition to being starved, loss of liver protein is slowed, as would be anticipated from the ^{15}N glycine and liver regeneration studies. Although the period of negative nitrogen balance after injury is commonly called the catabolic response, the term is inaccurate. Both anabolic and catabolic processes go on after severe injury, but all tissues do not participate equally in the response; catabolism predominates in the carcass, anabolism in the liver.

Albumin catabolism is increased in severely burned patients, a fact not directly related to the early loss of this protein into the injured area, since the increased albumin catabolism goes on for many weeks after the burn. It is clear that albumin synthesis is decreased in ill or injured patients with liver dysfunction and protein synthesis rates in such patients can often be raised with nutritional therapy. There is still controversy regarding the rate of albumin synthesis in injured patients with normal liver function. We have limited information regarding the relative rates of turnover, synthesis, and breakdown of other proteins in injured humans.

The available information regarding protein turnover, breakdown (proteolysis), and catabolism (oxilation) in patients is very limited due to the complexity of the interpretation of such studies where reliance must be placed almost entirely on blood, urine, and fecal data, since tissue biopsy (other than of skeletal muscle, bone marrow, and skin) for research purposes is interdicted in most instances in patients. In studies using constant infusions of ^{15}N glycine or ^{14}C leucine and measurements of plasma flux of these amino acids and rates of incorporation of the labels into urea and CO_2 and their rates of excretion (i.e., urine, respiration), O'Keefe and colleagues and Waterlow and his associates studying patients undergoing elective surgery have concluded that there is a decrease in protein synthesis after injury, with little change in protein breakdown and catabolism. These studies were carried out in the first several days after operation, a time before maximal increases in urinary nitrogen generally occur. Also, patients undergoing elective surgery show considerably less metabolic derangements than patients with accidental trauma. In O'Keefe's study there was an abrupt decline in nutrient intake in the immediate post-operative period when the isotope study was carried out; in studies of Waterlow and associates attempts were made to have the postoperative nutrient intake match the preoperative levels.

Kien et al. studying children with severe burns, some of whom were septic, maintained on high nutrient intakes found that overall protein synthesis and breakdown were increased, the former predominating, as assessed by ^{15}N glycine constant infusion technique studies. Children and adolescents undergoing elective surgery showed decreased protein synthesis, as had adults in the studies of O'Keefe et al. and Waterlow and colleagues. Long et al. studying surgical patients with serious infections found both protein anabolism and catabolism increased, the latter predominating. These findings, then, differed from those of Kien et al., but there were two important variables between the two studies, the ages of the patients and the fact that the children were on relatively high nutrient intakes while the adults were not.

Currently, some investigators are examining how injury affects the urinary excretion of 3-methyl-histidine as an index of muscle protein breakdown. This amino acid is present in muscle protein. Upon breakdown of muscle protein, 3-methyl-histidine is not recycled or oxidized, but is quantitatively excreted in the urine. Thus, measurements of the urinary excretion of 3-methyl-histidine provide an index of the rate of protein breakdown in a muscle, a tissue that has such major role in body protein and amino acid metabolism. The data regarding the effect of serious injury on 3-methyl-histidine is still too fragmentary to come to firm conclusions.

There are a number of studies which suggest an increased breakdown of serum albumin after severe injury. Thermal injury creates severe hypoalbuminemia, especially in the early days after injury. Brown et al. studied thermally injured rats, using the incorporation of 2-^{14}C glycine into albumin injected on the fifth or sixth postburn day as a determinant of protein synthesis. Male rats, 180 to 200 g, fed a laboratory chow, were subjected to 20 percent body surface area scald burns and some were infected immediately thereafter with 10^8 *Pseudomonas aeruginosa* organisms which leads to an expected mortality of 85 to 95 percent. Albumin concentration in the serum decreased significantly after burning, and was lowest in the infected-burned group. The relative specific activity of serum albumin was greatly increased in all burned animals. However, the albumin content of the viscera was also lower in burned animals. In all burned rats, burned skin contained 3.5 times more albumin than unburned skin. The authors concluded that the hypoalbuminemia that follows thermal injury is a consequence primarily of the change in the compartmentalization of body albumin.

More data regarding the turnover of albumin are needed. When liver function is impaired albumin synthesis is decreased, but we do not yet know how albumin synthesis is modified in patients after injury when liver function is not altered. Albumin synthetic rates may at times decrease following injury. This may be related in part to decreased availability of substrate. Skillman and his associates reported that daily postoperative infusion of a 3.5 percent solution of essential and nonessential amino acids led to a greater rate of albumin synthesis than the infusion of 5 percent glucose daily as tested on the fourth postoperative day in patients undergoing elective gastrointestinal surgery (colon resections and gastric surgery).

Data regarding the metabolism of individual amino acids after injury is limited, and the available information deals largely with plasma concentrations. The pattern of change seems different in patients with an uninfected injury from those whose injury is complicated by sepsis. For example, there is a greater increase in plasma alanine in the latter. This has been interpreted as a reflection of impaired gluconeogenesis in septic patients.

It has long been recognized that protein deficiency—including deficits and/or imbalances in such dietary essential amino acids as methionine, cyst(e)ine (essential for newborns, especially prematures) and lysine—interferes with wound repair. Such deficiencies delay almost all aspects of healing, including neovascularization, fibroblast proliferation, collagen synthesis, and wound remodeling.

Proteins and amino acids must be available for cell multiplication and protein synthesis, including the normal synthesis of the enzymes critically involved in the healing processes. The term *essential* as commonly used refers to a *dietary requirement* for the specific amino acid, but *all amino acids are essential in terms of body metabolism.*

The requirement for certain amino acids, such as arginine, is increased following injury to rodents as assessed by wound healing and thymus weight and numbers of thymus lymphocytes. In this circumstance, a previously nonessential (dietary) amino acid may become essential. The same situation may hold for seriously injured humans, but this has not been studied yet.

If protein deficiency is prolonged and/or liver function is severely impaired, serum albumin falls; edema may follow, and the edema itself further interferes with healing. This is of special importance in the healing of anastomoses of the gastrointestinal tract. When edema is present, it should be corrected.

Resistance to infection is seriously lowered in protein-deficient patients, and this can compound wound healing failure (see Chapters 2 and 4).

Carbohydrates and Fats   Dietary carbohydrates and fats are the major energy sources, and adequate amounts of these "nonprotein" calories are required to prevent excessive oxidation of amino acids for caloric needs. If dietary deficits of protein and calories continue, there is a gradual depletion of body protein and development of protein-calorie malnutrition (PCM or marasmus). Isolated protein malnutrition (PM or kwashiorkor) arises when dietary nonprotein calories are adequate but dietary protein is not. The terms "marasmus" and "kwashiorkor" were originated to describe malnutrition syndromes occurring in severely underfed African children. Very recently, the terms have been introduced to describe similar syndromes that may develop in patients with severe injury, infection, prolonged gastrointestinal disorders, or inadequate diet over a prolonged period.

Glucose is a major metabolic fuel, but it is of little value if an insulin deficit prevents its utilization. Popular opinion holds that most of the "poor" wound repair encountered in diabetics is due to microvascular problems associated with the disease; and such vascular impairment certainly interferes with healing. However, recent investigation has shown that rats made diabetic by streptozotocin administration have poor wound-healing capacity despite the fact that they have not developed microvascular complications. The effect is "metabolic." For example, lack of insulin diminishes the ability of fibroblasts and leukocytes to metabolize glucose. When animals with streptozotocin-induced diabetes are given insulin, their wound healing capacity returns to normal. In this experimental situation, the insulin seems especially necessary in the first few days after injury. A secondary effect of an insulin lack is the hyperosmolarity associated with hyperglycemia, and this too interferes with wound repair.

Certain unsaturated fatty acids (arachidonic, linoleic, and linolenic) are essential and must be supplied exogenously. Although linolenic and arachidonic acids can be synthesized by mammals from linoleic, the rates of synthesis are too low to meet metabolic needs. These fatty acids are constituents of triglycerides and phospholipids that are part of cellular and subcellular membranes. The unsaturated fatty acids are also of great importance as essential building blocks for the prostaglandins, which regulate many aspects of cellular metabolism, inflammation, and circulation. Deficiencies in essential unsaturated fatty acids were rarely detected until seriously ill or injured patients were maintained on prolonged parenteral feedings not containing fat. Infants, especially newborns and prematures, are particularly vulnerable, since they have not built up a body store of these essential fatty acids. There is evidence suggesting that requirements for essential fatty acids are increased after severe burns. Experimentally such deficiencies have an adverse effect on wound healing. Unsaturated fatty acids must be given to injured patients if the period of metabolic and physiologic derangements is prolonged, providing them in a proportion of 4 percent to 8 percent of total daily caloric intake (double the minimum recommended intake for healthy individuals). The diets or formulas now given patients via the GI tract almost always contain more unsaturated fatty acids than these suggested amounts. Medium chain triglycerides (MCT) do not supply adequate unsaturated fatty acids. For patients on prolonged parenteral feeding, we recommend infusion of modest amounts of fat emulsion, 500 ml of the currently available 10 percent preparation twice a week.

Hormonal Influences   The nutritional demands caused by injury reflect metabolic responses that are mediated in part by hormones. The roles of increased secretion of catecholamines and adrenal cortical hormones have been studied extensively beginning with the classic studies of Cannon and the later investigations of Selye. Administration of glucocorticoids or ACTH modifies inflammatory reactions and inhibits wound healing. (It has long been known that patients with Cushing's syndrome heal wounds poorly.) Glucocorticoids depress inflammation, decrease fibroblastic proliferation and collagen synthesis, and hinder epithelial migration and contraction. They stabilize cell membranes, prevent release of lysosomal contents and inhibit mitochondrial membrane transport.

Although it is well established that secretion of glucocorticoids is increased early after injury, it is not known whether this is a major factor underlying the impaired wound healing seen in injured animals. In this regard, Ingle and Selye, working independently in experiments with rats kept on maintenance doses of adrenal extracts, found that such rats showed the same metabolic changes after injury as did rats with intact adrenals. They interpreted this as indicating that the adrenal steroids play a permissive role and that an increase in their secretion is not essential to the occurrence of these metabolic reactions to injury. This view was supported by the findings of other investigators with adrenalectomized rats kept on a low maintenance dose of cortisone. However, others have presented evidence indicating that the adrenal glucocorticoids play more than a permissive role, and that the documented increase in their secretion after injury plays a significant role in the metabolic, physiologic, and immunologic changes after injury.

Adrenal medullary hormones—epinephrine and norepinephrine—as well as the norepinephrine secreted by sympathetic ganglia, appear to play a key part in prompting the increased caloric expenditure and altered carbohydrate metabolism that follow a serious injury. The author knows of no studies, however, of the direct effects of postinjury increases in secretion of adrenal medullary hormones on wound repair.

When injury produces hypovolemia, it is at first partly compensated for by catecholamine-induced vasoconstriction which, in turn, diminishes the blood flow and oxygen supply to injured tissue. This O_2 decrement has been demonstrated clinically, although it has not yet been proven to hinder wound repair.

Recent experiments have shown that giving testosterone has no effect on soft-tissue wound repair in rats. Studies were conducted because earlier investigations had shown that the increase in urinary nitrogen excretion that follows injury can be lessened by administration of this androgenic steroid to animals and patients. The question was whether this effect was of any physiologic or clinical benefit, and recent data indicate a negative answer, at least with regard to wound healing. We see no reason to employ testosterone in the period soon after injury, except perhaps to offset excessive glucocorticoid administration (thus using it in the antagonist role it shares with vitamin A).

Pituitary growth hormone has direct stimulatory influences in vitro on DNA synthesis and multiplication of cultured rat fibroblasts, and on DNA synthesis by rat cartilage. The effect of pituitary growth hormone on collagen synthesis may be mediated by insulin. Growth hormone given to normal rats with skin incisions does not affect wound healing; growth hormone given to hypophysectomized rats accelerates healing. Lysyl oxidase activity of the skin is low in unwounded rats hypophysectomized for several months.

Growth hormone did not stimulate skin-wound closure in human volunteers. In this clinical study, though, the hormone may not have been started at the optimal time since it was first administered on the sixth day following wounding, after the early phase of vigorous cell proliferation had passed. In another clinical trial, Wilmore, Pruitt, Mason et al. (1976) recently found that growth hormone administration reduces urinary nitrogen excretion following burns. But whether supplemental growth hormone improves healing in injured animals and patients has not been studied.

ROLE OF NUTRIENTS IN WOUND REPAIR
Water-Soluble Vitamins

Nicholas Lunin (1881), Gowland Hopkins (1912) and Casimir Funk (1912) are generally credited with demonstrating, in experiments with animals receiving purified diets, that in addition to protein, fats, carbohydrates, minerals, and water, certain accessory dietary factors are required to insure growth and health. These factors—vitamins—are needed by the body in "astonishingly small amounts," as Hopkins put it. We do not understand all their functions, but we do know that vitamins influence a wide variety of metabolic and physiologic reactions in health, disease, and injury, and that they affect wound healing in important ways.

Ascorbic Acid   Many centuries before the world knew of ascorbic acid, mariners and explorers were experiencing and describing the ravages of scurvy. Then, in one of the first controlled clinical studies in history, the Scottish physician Lind, in 1753, demonstrated that citrus fruit juices offered a cure—a finding that persuaded the Admiralty to include limes in shipboard rations and thus pinned a nickname on British seamen. This landmark study was conducted with just six pairs of subjects, each receiving a different supplement to the same basal diet. Large numbers are not always needed to establish fundamental principles! But 175 years were to pass before Szent-Györgyi, in the course of studies dealing with biologic oxidation (with no thought at the time of looking for the antiscorbutic substance), isolated and identified hexuronic acid from the adrenal cortex and then from oranges and cabbages. Later, he and Svirbely showed that this carbohydrate derivative had antiscorbutic activity; Waugh and King found identical properties in the vitamin C they had identified in lemon juice; and Haworth and Hurst finally elucidated the compound's chemical structure and accomplished its synthesis.

Unlike other animal species, guinea pigs and primates—including humans—cannot synthesize ascorbic acid because they lack the enzyme needed for the conversion of L-gulonic acid to ascorbic acid. Healthy young men have a total body pool of about 2.3 g of ascorbate—a level they can maintain by ingesting 20 to 30 mg of ascorbic acid per day. In a classic study, Crandon and associates found that although healing of a skin incision in a healthy male surgical resident was not significantly retarded after three months of dietary ascorbic-acid deficiency, it was seriously impaired after six months of the same dietary restriction. Injury, however, increases the requirement for vitamin C dramatically, as will be demonstrated later.

Ascorbic acid—which has a half-life of about 16 days in a healthy man—is an active reducing agent, but there is no unequivocal evidence that it plays a unique role in any specific oxidation-reduction system. It is involved in the reduction of oxygen to superoxide, which is an important intermediate in respiration. In white blood cells, superoxide acts as an antibacterial substance and helps generate other bactericidal agents.

The relationship between vitamin C and the metabolism of the adrenal steroids is unclear, but it has been suggested that ascorbate is involved in the conversion of cholesterol to pregnenolone.

Vitamin C and Healing   The fact that scurvy causes new wounds to heal poorly was recognized in the 16th century or earlier. In the mid-1700s it was noted that scurvy causes old wounds to reopen. The pioneering work of Wolbach and Howe 50 years ago (Fig. 5.12) provided the basis for studies that have now largely defined the clinical and biochemical roles of ascorbic acid in wound repair. The inability of scorbutic animals and humans to heal wounds normally (Fig. 5.13) has been correlated with the almost complete incapacity of animals deficient

Figure 5.12.   Effect of ascorbic acid on collagen synthesis. Mallory's connective tissue stain, × 1000. **Left.** Fibroblast in center of hemorrhagic area (blood clot in extensor thigh muscle) in scorbutic guinea pig. Note minimal extracellular material (collagen) at periphery of fibroblast. **Center and Right.** After ascorbic acid (48 and 72 hours, respectively) administration. Note resorption of hemorrhage and progressive collagen formation. "Collagen is the product of secretory activity of fibroblasts . . ." *(From Wolbach SB: Am J Path, Controlled formation of collagen and reticulum. A study of the source of intercellular substance in recovery from experimental scorbutus 9:689−699, 1933)*

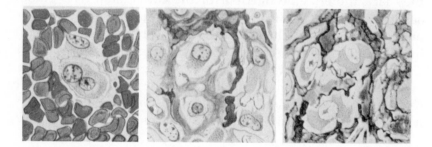

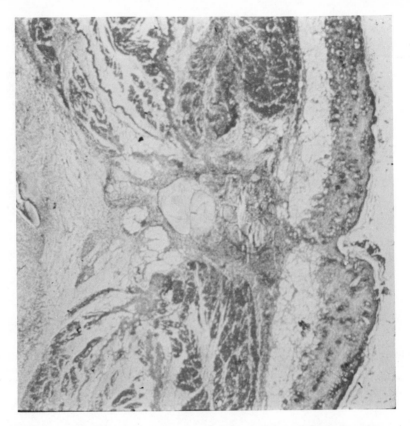

Figure 5.13. Histologic appearance of laparotomy incision of scorbutic guinea pig, seven days postoperatively. Note the considerable hemorrhage in the incision, the separation of the wound edges, and the minimal collagen fibers in the wound.

in ascorbic acid to hydroxylate proline and lysine (see chapters on normal repair and disorders of repair). A vitamin C deficit does not hamper the proliferation of fibroblasts, but it does interfere remarkably with their function.

Electron microscopy reveals a morphologic defect in fibroblasts of scorbutic wounds (Fig. 5.14). In untreated scurvy, there is a general disorganization of ribosomal aggregates on the rough endoplasmic reticulum, but when ascorbic acid is given, ribosome and polysome arrangement becomes orderly. The hydroxylation of lysine and proline in the newly synthesized procollagen proceeds normally, with a consequent in-

315

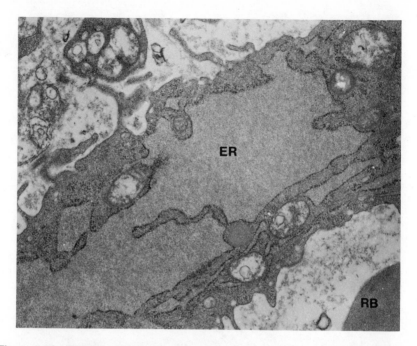

Figure 5.14 Fibrocyte with massively dilated rough endoplasmic reticulum (ER) distended with finely granular material. No mature collagen is seen. RB indicates extravasated red blood cell (× 28,000). *(From Bevelaqua et al.: JAMA 235(17):1876, 1976, copyright © 1976, American Medical Association.)*

crease in the synthesis and secretion of collagen. Fig. 5.14 also illustrates abnormal storage of a substance thought to be unhydroxylated procollagen within the fibroblast of a scorbutic animal.

Because scars are metabolically more active than normal connective tissues for long periods, much more vitamin C is required to sustain them than to maintain developmental collagen. The balance between collagen synthesis and lysis is a delicate one, and any disruption in this equilibrium can cause dissolution of the scar. Certain naturally occurring pteridines can substitute for vitamin C in certain circumstances where rapid collagen synthesis is not needed, but an adequate supply of this vitamin is crucial during the repair process or other situations, such as pregnancy, where collagen synthesis must occur rapidly.

A lack of ascorbic acid leads to increased capillary permeability; to fragility, rupture, and hemorrhage of these vessels; and to a failure to form new capillaries in the healing wound. All this may reflect an inability to synthesize enough basement membrane collagen.

Besides ascorbate, the hydroxylation of proline and lysine requires iron (Fe^{++}), oxygen (O_2) and α-ketoglutarate. It was thought that ascorbic acid acted only as an electron transport substance between ferrous iron and oxygen in the hydroxylation reaction, but more recent evidence shows it to be involved in the activation of prolyl and lysyl hydroxylases as well. These

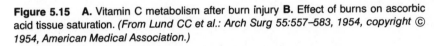

Figure 5.15 **A.** Vitamin C metabolism after burn injury **B.** Effect of burns on ascorbic acid tissue saturation. *(From Lund CC et al.: Arch Surg 55:557–583, 1954, copyright © 1954, American Medical Association.)*

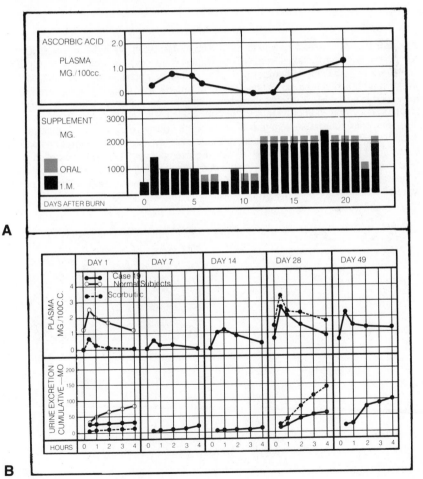

enzymes appear to exist in an inactive subunit form until, in the presence of vitamin C, they polymerize and assume a configuration that permits them to act.

Trauma causes an abrupt drop in plasma ascorbic acid concentrations and in urinary excretion of ascorbate, followed by a decline in ascorbic acid levels in red and white blood cells. The more severe the injury, the greater these reductions. Decreased "tissue saturation" has been indicated by intravenous load tests with ascorbic acid soon after trauma (Fig. 5.15) and has continued for many weeks.

Laparotomy wounds have been found to heal more slowly in burned guinea pigs than the otherwise normal ones, even when the burned animals receive vitamin C in amounts suffi-

Figure 5.16 **A.** Laparotomy wound, seven days postoperatively in an unburned guinea pig receiving 2 mg ascorbic acid daily. Van Gieson's stain, × 460. Note numerous collagen fibers and absence of hemorrhage. **B.** Laparotomy wound, seven days postoperatively, in a burned guinea pig (30 percent body surface, third-degree burns), receiving 2 mg ascorbic acid daily. The laparotomy was made 24 hours after the burn. Van Gieson's stain, × 460. Note hemorrhage and minimal collagen fibers. Note that the histologic picture is indistinguishable from that of the unburned guinea pig that did not receive any ascorbic acid in the postoperative period. **C.** Laparotomy wound, seven days postoperatively, in a burned guinea pig receiving 100 mg ascorbic acid daily after operation. Van Gieson's stain, × 460. Note that giving the burned guinea pig 100 mg ascorbic acid daily in postoperative period results in normal healing of the laparotomy wound. *(From Levenson SM, Upjohn HL, Preston JA, Steer A: Ann Surg 146:357, 1957)*

A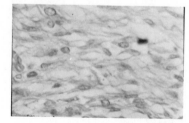

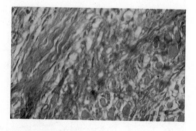 B

C

cient to support normal growth and healing in unburned animals. The poorly healing wounds were histologically indistinguishable from those seen in unburned guinea pigs made scorbutic by a lack of dietary ascorbic acid; there was ample fibroblastic proliferation, but ground substance production was excessive, hemorrhage was persistent, and collagen accumulation was drastically diminished (Fig. 5.16). Large doses of vitamin C (100 mg daily) in the postoperative period prevented such wound changes in burned guinea pigs, however.

No comparable studies of wound repair have been conducted in humans, but a similarly increased need for ascorbic acid—especially in trauma victims—is indicated by the biochemical studies already described. Whether this expanded requirement reflects an accumulation of ascorbic acid at the wound site or a faster rate of vitamin C metabolism after injury, or both, has not been established. Since this vitamin is not stored in great amounts, seriously ill or injured patients may develop a deficiency quickly unless they receive supplementary doses. All the ascorbic acid derangements associated with severe injury can be prevented or reversed with large amounts of vitamin C, and it is now common practice to give extensively burned patients 1 to 2 g per day until their convalescence is well advanced and skin coverage is almost complete. Such daily maintenance doses recommended for severely burned patients are equivalent to 50 to 100 percent of the total amount of ascorbic acid present in the healthy adult. Patients with lesser injuries require 100 to 250 mg daily. There is no evidence whatsoever that doses greater than those required to maintain normal levels of vitamin C in tissues and blood can induce accelerated wound healing.

Vitamin B Complex We have few data on how the B vitamins affect wound repair but, because they serve as cofactors in a variety of enzyme systems, one can surmise that serious deficits in some of them would hamper healing (Table 5.1).

Compared to the many studies on the relationship between ascorbic acid and wound repair, there have been few such investigations of the B complex vitamins. One of that scant number is the experimental work of Bosse and Axelrod, who examined rats placed on diets deficient in riboflavin, pyridoxine or biotin five weeks before they were subjected to

Table 5.1 Vitamins and Their Role in Enzyme Function

Water-soluble	Active Form	Type of Reaction Promoted
Thiamine	Thiamine pyrophosphate	Decarboxylation of α-keto acids
Riboflavin	Flavin mononucleotide Flavin adenine dinucleotide	Oxidation-reduction
Niacin	Nicotinamide adenine dinucleotide Nicotinamide adenine dinucleotide phosphate	Oxidation-reduction
Pantothenic acid	Coenzyme A	Acyl group transfer
Pyridoxol	Pyridoxal phosphate	Amino group transfer
Biotin	Biocytin	CO_2 transfer
Folic acid	Tetrahydrofolic acid	One-carbon transfer
Vitamin B_{12}	Deoxyadenosyl cobalamin	Alkyl group transfer
Lipoic acid	Lipoamide	Hydrogen and acyl group transfer
Ascorbic acid		Cofactor in hydroxylation reactions
Fat-soluble		
Vitamin A		*Visual cycle*
Vitamin D		*Calcium transport*
Vitamin E		*Lipid antioxidant*
Vitamin K		*Prothrombin synthesis*

(From Lehninger AL: Biochemistry. The Molecular Basis of Cell Structure and Function, 2nd ed. Worth, 1975)

open skin wounds. They reported markedly delayed healing in the pyridoxine- and riboflavin-deficient rats and observed that the reparative tissue in those animals, especially in the ones with a pyridoxine deficit, was less dense and more vascular and cellular than that in similarly wounded controls that had been fed a normal diet. No impairment of the closure process was seen on gross examination of the biotin-deficient rats, but histologic studies revealed some retardation of collagen production and less density in the granulation tissue. Also, there was a greater degree of vascularity in the reparative tissues of these animals than in those of the controls.

Overt deficiencies of B vitamins are uncommon in surgical

patients but may arise in those who were seriously mal-nourished before their operation. Megaloblastic anemias sec-ondary to folic-acid or B_{12} deficits are not rare, and Wernicke's syndrome secondary to a thiamine deficiency is occasionally encountered, especially in alcoholics. It should be noted, too, that certain drugs, such as isonicotinic acid hydrazine and es-trogens, increase the body's pyridoxine requirement and that estrogen also increases its need for folic acid.

We know of no *clinical* studies of the effect of the vitamin B complex on wound repair, but the fact that healing problems clearly associated with a B-vitamin deficiency have not been reported suggests either that such deficits would have to be severe before they interfered with the repair process or that their influence is not being recognized.

Severe injury or acute infectious illness causes a decreased urinary excretion of thiamine, riboflavin, and nicotinamide; and tissue saturation tests suggest that the body pools of these vitamins are reduced. Administration of B complex vitamins in amounts five to ten times normal are recommended for seri-ously ill or injured patients. Also, animal experiments indicate that administration of extra nicotinic acid may lessen the early plasma loss caused by burns.

ROLE OF NUTRIENTS IN WOUND REPAIR

Fat-Soluble Vitamins

Deficiencies in fat-soluble vitamins may arise in surgical pa-tients who have experienced prolonged interference with their food intake or with its digestion, absorption, or metabolism. Then, too, there may be instances in which a deficit or excess of some other nutrient—certain trace metals or other vitamins, for example—will interfere with the metabolism of one or more of the fat-soluble vitamins and thereby increase their dietary re-quirement.

Once again, there is very little information on the metabolism of these substances after injury. Interest in vitamin A is mount-ing, not only because of its role in wound healing but because of its influence on a variety of immunologic responses, includ-ing resistance to infection, homograft rejection, tumor growth, and the development of stress ulcers.

Vitamin A   Vitamin A was discovered by McCollum and Davis in 1913 when they found that young rats failed to grow when denied butter fat or egg-yolk fat. That same year, Osborne and Mendel described the experimental eye lesions characteristic of vitamin A deficiency. Steenbock and von Euler then demonstrated that carotene is provitamin A, and Holmes and Corbet in 1937 reported the isolation and crystallization of the vitamin. About that same time, Wald found that vitamin A is the prosthetic group for the conjugated protein called "visual purple," a discovery that explained the connection between diet and night blindness.

One of the first consequences of vitamin A deficiency in animals is a depletion of *vitamin C* reserves; moreover, it seems that *vitamin E* enhances the absorption, storage, and possibly the utilization of vitamin A. (Vitamin E protects vitamin A from oxidation.)

We know that vitamin A is important to vision, reproduction, epithelium maintenance and multiplication, synthesis of glycoproteins and proteoglycans, labilization of lysosomal membranes, and certain immune responses, especially cellular ones. Recent studies have expanded our knowledge of its absorption, transport, and biosynthesis, but our understanding of its mode of action—excepting its special role in vision—is limited.

Some experiments indicate that vitamin A has an accelerating effect on the healing of skin incisions and the formation of reparative granulation tissue in polyvinyl alcohol sponges implanted subcutaneously in normal rats eating a nutritionally complete diet. Supplemental vitamin A obviates to a large extent the impaired healing of incisions and formation of reparative collagen in subcutaneous implanted polyvinyl alcohol sponges in rats with femoral fractures. Also, supplemental amounts have been found to increase the number and size of intraabdominal adhesions in normal mice, while citral, a vitamin A antagonist, reduces such adhesions. Experimentally induced deficiencies of the vitamin retard epithelialization, wound closure, collagen synthesis rates, the prolyl hydroxylase activity of healing tissue, and possibly the cross-linking of new collagen.

The mechanisms underlying these effects are still uncertain. It is believed that a lack of the vitamin depresses the synthesis of sulfated proteoglycans, which are involved in the early phases of wound repair—possibly in the formation of collagen fibrils and fibers. Probably important, too, are the effects of vitamin A on cell membranes. Its ability to labilize lysosomal membranes was demonstrated dramatically by Thomas and Fell. They found that feeding rabbits excessive amounts of the vitamin led to the "floppy ear" syndrome, reflecting the lysis of ear cartilage by lysosomal enzymes released in response to the high vitamin A intake.

Entry of vitamin A into cell membranes is attributed to its lipid solubility, while the presence of alternating double bonds in its molecular structure is thought to facilitate electron transport across the membrane. Glucocorticoids, on the other hand, stabilize cell membranes, as noted earlier. And because vitamin A offsets many of the inhibitory influences of these adrenal steroids on wound repair, it has been suggested that this antagonistic relationship between the two in the healing process is based on their opposite effects on membrane stability. Recent experiments suggest that vitamin A effects the early inflammatory stage of healing and increases the numbers of monocytes/macrophages at the injured site.

Frank vitamin A deficiency is rare in this country (although subclinical deficits are widespread), but not in the "underdeveloped" world, where it is associated with night blindness, xerophthalmia, epithelial metaplasia, increased susceptibility to infection, reduced tolerance to injury or stress, and retarded wound healing. The vitamin A status of humans in generally assessed biochemically in terms of its serum levels and carotene measurements. (Concentrations of the latter precursor nutrient—carotene—may not correlate with an individual's overall state of vitamin A nutrition, however.) Little is known about how vitamin A is metabolized by ill or injured persons or what those patients' specific requirements for the vitamin are, except that they are increased (Fig. 5.17). In the few instances that liver specimens have been analyzed for the vitamin at autopsy, a vitamin A depletion was noted in fatally ill or injured subjects—especially those who had suffered major burns. There are experimental animal studies demonstrating that injury increases vitamin A requirement.

Rats kept on a vitamin A intake barely sufficient to maintain near-normal growth lost considerable weight after relatively

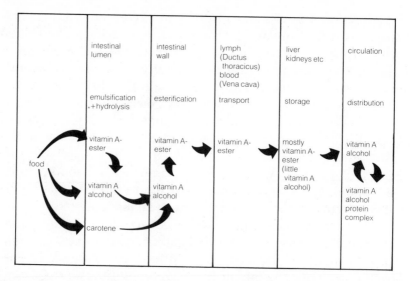

intestinal lumen	intestinal wall	lymph (Ductus thoracicus) blood (Vena cava)	liver kidneys etc	circulation
emulsification +hydrolysis	esterification	transport	storage	distribution
vitamin A-ester	vitamin A-ester	vitamin A-ester	mostly vitamin A-ester (little vitamin A alcohol)	vitamin A alcohol
vitamin A alcohol	vitamin A alcohol			vitamin A alcohol protein complex
carotene				

Figure 5.17 Schematic representation of absorption, storage, and transport of vitamin A. *(From Marks J: A Guide to the Vitamins: Their Role in Health and Disease. Lancaster, England, Technical Publishing Co., 1975.)*

minor wounds (dorsal skin incisions and sponge implants). Their postoperative blood sugar levels were low, they produced less collagen than control animals at comparable postoperative times, and many died. The reduced ability of these mildly A-deficient rats to survive the minor surgical stress may reflect impaired glucose mobilization, perhaps involving interference with corticoid or growth hormone responsiveness.

Rats with subcutaneous abscesses induced by injections of a chemical irritant showed sustained declines in vitamin A concentrations both in the serum and liver. Levels of the vitamin within the abscesses and at their periphery did not differ from those measured in uninjured subcutaneous tissue. Gastrointestinal absorption of vitamin A was not altered in these animals, but its urinary excretion was increased, and its level in the kidney was higher than normal. Supplemental vitamin A prevents the adrenal hypertrophy and thymic atrophy that characteristically follow injury. It also reduces the incidence and severity of stress ulcer.

Large doses of cortisone lead to a rapid depletion of the vitamin in the serum and liver of rats and retard the increase of wound tensile strength. Administration of vitamin A to these animals restores these levels, increases the breaking strength of skin incisions, and improves the rate of epithelialization of open skin wounds. Applications of retinoic acid to open wounds can reverse the retardation in closure induced by salicylates, hydrocortisone, and prednisone.

However, vitamin A administration does not improve the rate of closure in *open* wounds in rats with fractures. The influence of exogenous cortisone on the closure of open skin wounds, therefore, is different from that of fractures—whether this is qualitative or quantitative is unknown. Supplemental vitamin A does improve the impaired healing of skin incisions and the formation of reparative collagen in implanted polyvinyl alcohol sponges in rats with femoral fractures.

Because a large amount of vitamin A is stored in the liver, a deficiency is unlikely to develop after an uncomplicated elective surgical procedure, but undernourished patients should receive supplements before undergoing operation. Prompt supplementation is also advisable in patients with serious injury and those who have undergone operative procedures or developed complications apt to interfere with alimentation for a long period.

As for recommended dosages, we think that a daily supplementation of 25,000 international units—five times the daily intake considered appropriate for healthy adults—is adequate to sustain wound repair even in patients with severe burns. To provide this amount, using the commercially available parenteral vitamin mix would entail administering needless amounts of some of the B vitamins and possibly toxic amounts of vitamin D. Therefore, part of the vitamin A supplementation should be provided through the gastrointestinal tract, since there is no commercially available parenteral preparation of vitamin A alone. But the amounts administered by both routes must be held within the recommended range. Massive daily doses (over 50,000 units), when given for many weeks, have produced instances of acute vitamin A toxicity (visual disturbances, coma, pseudotumor cerebri).

Vitamin D   Since vitamin D deficiency is usually associated with such bone disorders as rickets, the vitamin itself is thought of primarily in connection with fracture repair. However, its role in calcium homeostasis gives it a more general importance, since the calcium ion is required by many enzyme systems, including collagenases.

Dietary vitamin D is hydroxylated, first in the liver, and then in the kidneys (under the influence of parathormone). The hydroxylated vitamin D is essential for synthesis of the transfer protein that binds calcium ion in the intestine and later liberates it in the portal circulation. Part of the absorbed calcium is bound to plasma protein while the rest remains ionized in the blood. Vitamin D also assists renal excretion of the ion and thus helps maintain calcium homeostasis.

For vitamin D to act, adequate dietary protein must be supplied and gut function must permit synthesis of the transport protein and absorption of nutrients. Vitamin D in its active form functions as a hormone.

Because of the great calcium reserves in the bone, neither calcium nor vitamin D deficits are commonly encountered in surgical patients. However, calcium deficits may occur in patients with malabsorption syndromes. In addition, inactive patients tend to lose calcium and phosphorus from their bones. This may have little significance over the short term, but the osteoporotic changes can be quite severe in elderly patients immobilized for protracted periods. Administration of calcium, phosphorus, and vitamin D does not completely reverse the process. Mechanical stress and weight bearing seem to be necessary to maintain bony metabolism and architecture.

Calcium and phosphorus demands are high in patients who have fractures to heal. And because of the efficient homeostatic mechanisms for maintaining blood calcium and phosphorus concentrations within relatively narrow ranges, measurements of those levels may not reflect, for some time, the body's need for calcium and phosphorus supplementation. If calcium and phosphorus are given in the diet,vitamin D must be administered also to assure calcium absorption. The relationship of calcium and magnesium is discussed later.

Stores of vitamin D in the liver are sufficient, as far as we know, to carry the ordinary surgical patient through the immediate postoperative period. But patients with fractures or other severe injuries should receive about 400 to 800 international units of vitamin D per day, one to two times the recommended intake for healthy adults. Evidence of an increased need for the vitamin after injury or during illness is lacking, but there are few objective data in this area.

Vitamin D toxicity has been reported in patients receiving the only commercial parenteral preparation containing both fat- and water-soluble vitamins; patients were given several 10-ml ampules of this formula each day for several weeks, with each ampule supplying 400 international units of vitamin D.

The most important sources of vitamin D are fish liver oils, mammalian liver, and milk because they contain ultraviolet-irradiated steroid precursors of the vitamin. Synthetic vitamins D_2 and D_3 are used in commercial vitamin preparations, while provitamins D (ergosterol) are provided by green vegetables. The provitamins concentrate largely in the skin, where sunlight or some other UV source is required to alter the plant sterol chemically and convert it into vitamin D. Therefore, institutionalized or elderly people who do not get the dietary precursor or sunlight will show a deficiency unless given a vitamin D supplement.

Vitamin K Horvath, McFarlane, and Nein, about 1930 noted that an unidentified fat-soluble food factor was essential to blood clotting. The term "vitamin K" was coined by Dam in 1935 from the initial letter of the German word "koagulation." In that same year, he described the necessity of dietary vitamin K for the synthesis of prothrombin (Factor II). The clinical significance of this finding was revealed by Brinkhaus and his associates three years later in their study of patients with obstructive jaundice or biliary fistulas. Chemical identification of vitamins K, K_1, and K_2 was achieved in 1939.

It has since been established that vitamin K is also involved in regulating the synthesis of clotting factors VII, IX, and X. It had been thought that it played a part in protein synthesis only at the translation stage, but recently it has been shown that the vitamin is essential to post-translation changes of some proteins with calcium-binding properties. The matrix involved in bone calcification contains proteins which require vitamin K for their synthesis, so it is likely that vitamin K is specifically needed for bone repair.

An uncorrected vitamin K deficiency may result in excessive bleeding in the wound, impairing its healing, and predisposing it to infection. In addition to vitamin K_1 ingested in the form of leafy vegetables and liver, the body obtains vitamin K_2 from synthesis by certain gut bacteria. Fat malabsorption prevents the absorption of vitamin K from either source, however, so patients with obstructive jaundice, chronic pancreatitis, or other such disorders may develop a deficiency even if the vitamin is plentiful in their diet and is synthesized by intestinal bacteria. On the other hand, persons taking certain antibiotics and other chemotherapeutic agents for long periods may become K-deficient because of reduced numbers of synthesizing bacteria. Patients with serious liver disease may not be able to synthesize adequate amounts of prothrombin even if sufficient vitamin K is absorbed.

Minimum daily requirements for infants have been estimated at 1 to 5µg/kg body weight (neonates are especially vulnerable to vitamin K deficiency) and at 0.03 µg/kg body weight for adults.

When malabsorption syndromes are present, a daily oral supplement of 50 to 100 µg has been recommended for adults, but for hospitalized patients parenteral administration is preferable; 1 mg per month has been found sufficient when liver function is normal and there are no other significant metabolic disturbances. If vitamin K deficiency (hypoprothrombinemia) is present, 10 to 20 mg IM or IV once or twice daily of menadiol sodium diphosphate, a synthetic water-soluble vitamin K analog, is recommended. For synthesis of prothrombin and the other blood coagulation factors dependent on vitamin K, liver function must be adequate.

Vitamin E Popular claims to the contrary, there are as yet only limited scientific data on vitamin E's role in wound healing. We do know that its action is, in many respects, the reverse of vitamin A's. Where vitamin A labilizes cell membranes, vitamin E stabilizes them. In doing so, particularly in the case of macrophage membranes, vitamin E may possibly inhibit wound repair. It has an antiinflammatory action similar to that of cortisone, an effect that can be ameliorated by vitamin A or anabolic steroids. This is unlikely to be significant clinically, though, unless vitamin E is given in very high doses.

Of the closely related compounds that have vitamin E activity, α-tocopherol is the most active. Discovered by Evans and Bishop in 1923 in rat experiments, the vitamin itself appears to have an antioxidant role, inhibiting the oxidation of unsaturated fatty acids and vitamin A in naturally occurring fats. It has been postulated that vitamin E prevents peroxidation of the unsaturated lipid components of cellular and subcellular membranes, thereby maintaining their integrity.

Evans and Bishop found in their pioneer studies that a deficit of vitamin E leads to a progressive muscular dystrophy and creatinuria, degeneration of germinal epithelium and immobile spermatozoa in male rats, and to abortion of pregnancies in females. A syndrome of edema, skin lesions (papular erythema and seborrhea), and morphologic changes in red cells with increased erythrocytic sensitivity to peroxide and hemolysis has been induced in premature (but not full-term) infants by a diet high in polyunsaturated fatty acids and devoid of vitamin E. These abnormalities quickly responded to vitamin E supplementation. No such clear-cut syndrome stemming from a deficiency in vitamin E has been uncovered in human adults.

The recommended adult daily intake of the vitamin is 10 to 15 mg, depending on the amount of polyunsaturated fats in the diet. It has been advised that tocopherol supplements be given to premature infants and to children suffering from pancreatic cystic fibrosis, biliary atresia, or other conditions characterized by reduced fat absorption. All such conditions, including celiac disease, sprue and excessive mineral oil ingestion, reduce the amount of vitamin E and other fat-soluble vitamins absorbed and call for supplementation of all these.

It is difficult to assign vitamin E a specific role in the wound repair process. There are no studies indicating whether its requirement is altered by serious injury or illness. But since fatty acid deficits have been reported in patients who have been on long-term parenteral nutrition without lipids, it is to be expected that those with serious injuries or disease may develop vitamin E deficiency if supplementary amounts are not given for similarly long periods. Although we recognize the absence of concrete data, we recommend that 20 to 30 mg per day be given to adults in such clinical situations, twice the amount advised for healthy individuals.

ROLE OF NUTRIENTS IN WOUND REPAIR

Minerals

Macrominerals Tissue repair cannot proceed normally when there are excesses or deficiencies of water, sodium, potassium, calcium, chloride, and phosphorus. Calcium is required by many enzyme systems, including tissue collagenases, which are important in soft-tissue wound remodeling. We have so far discussed the effects of calcium and phosphorus only briefly, and then only in relation to vitamin D and the healing of fractures. We will not discuss in any more detail their important metabolic roles or those of sodium, potassium, and chloride since they are described extensively in standard textbooks.

MAGNESIUM This metal, one of the more abundant body minerals, activates a large number of enzymes involved in the energy-producing cycles and protein synthesis, which makes it a factor essential in wound repair. For instance, both cocarboxylase and coenzyme A are active only in the presence of magnesium.

The adult body contains about 25 g of magnesium with most of it stored in the bones combined with phosphate and bicarbonate, and the rest scattered in small amounts throughout all the soft tissues (chiefly intracellularly), where it seems to be enzyme bound chiefly within the mitochondria. The plasma normally contains 0.6 to 1.0 mM/liter (1.4 to 2.4μg/100 ml).

A deficiency in magnesium may stem from chronic diarrhea or from an intestinal fistula, or it may arise in certain renal conditions marked by tubular dysfunction or in postnatal tetany. Patients with short-bowel syndrome, including those with jejunoileal bypasses, are often deficient in magnesium and calcium. The principal clinical features of magnesium deficiency are depression, muscular weakness, vertigo, a proneness to convulsions, and metabolic acidosis.

Clear-cut deficiencies have also been noted in patients on long-term IV hyperalimentation. Often the first sign in such cases is a drop in serum calcium—a secondary effect—since that level is measured much more frequently than serum magnesium. The effect of a magnesium deficit on calcium metabolism has not been fully clarified, although interference with bone calcium mobilization—with or without disruption of parathormone production or function—is clearly a major factor. The influence of a magnesium deficiency on bone repair has not been delineated either, but one would expect significant impairment.

Magnesium concentrations also drop to low levels in chronic alcoholics, probably due to increased excretion and decreased intake. Indeed, it has been alleged that many of the neuromuscular symptoms associated with alcoholism actually reflect a deficit in this element. It is known that wound healing in alcoholics is sometimes retarded, but the nutritional deficiencies in these patients are so numerous and complex that it is impossible to implicate any single factor in the delayed repair.

Trace Minerals   Until recently, little attention was paid to the trace mineral requirements of surgical patients other than for iron and iodine. It was recognized that specific deficiencies could become manifest when a limited intake was combined with such conditions as serious injury or infection, alcoholism, diabetes, or disorders of the digestive system. Recognition of such deficits accelerated with the increasing use of long-term parenteral administration of highly purified nutrients.

Most of the trace metals are involved in enzymatic reactions in one of two ways: as activators or cofactors of specific enzymes, or as integral parts of enzymes, as copper is in lysyl oxidase and manganese in superoxide dismutase. As an activator, the element need not be specific and is replaceable by another. As a cofactor, substitution by another metal usually inactivates the enzyme system.

With one or two exceptions, the symptomatology of trace element deficiencies is ill-defined. The task of connecting a failure in wound healing to a deficit in a specific trace mineral is complicated by many problems, the chief one being the fact that metabolic and nutritional deficiencies are almost never isolated; a patient with one deficiency often has a number of others. Of the many trace metals, iron, zinc, copper, and manganese are perhaps the most important to wound repair.

The body does not store large reserves of most trace metals to draw on in times of need. The elements are generally used and reused, but inevitably some are excreted in urine and feces during normal metabolism, and some are lost from large open wounds, such as extensive deep burns. Urinary excretion of some of the trace minerals increases after injury, and these losses must be promptly rectified from exogenous sources, especially where GI function is impaired or long-term parenteral feeding is required.

ZINC Studies of the effects of supplemental zinc on wound healing have been prompted by observations that urinary levels of the metal increase after a severe injury, while concentrations of it in the blood and hair decrease. The first such investigation, conducted in young men undergoing excision of pilonidal sinuses, was interpreted by some as indicating that zinc administration accelerated wound repair, but the data were not generally accepted as conclusive. Animal experiments since then have shown that where zinc levels are depleted, wound repair is slow, and that when those levels are boosted exogenously, normal healing is restored. A number of other experiments, though, indicate that supplemental zinc has no effect on the repair process when given to animals with normal zinc levels. The same almost certainly holds for humans, but there are conditions, such as serious injury, infection, and digestive-tract disorders, that may give rise to a zinc deficiency, which should be corrected or, better still, prevented.

In wasting diseases that lead to muscle breakdown, zinc is liberated and urinary zinc excretion rises. Plasma concentrations of the metal have been described as low in individuals who have undergone bilateral adrenalectomy despite their corticosteroid therapy—or perhaps because of it—and in these patients extra zinc has been reported to improve the healing of chronic skin ulcers and other wounds.

Zinc is a constituent of several enzymes. Its component status in such enzymes as DNA polymerase means that mitosis is likely to be slow in the presence of zinc deficiency, which thus impedes the cell proliferation required for wound healing.

Aside from its participation in various enzymatic activities, zinc, like the glucocorticoids, stabilizes cellular membranes—probably by inhibiting lipid peroxidases.

Zinc is also believed to play a role in the transport of vitamin A from the liver and the maintenance of normal concentrations of the vitamin in plasma, perhaps by affecting the synthesis of retinol-binding protein.

Following severe injury or administration of glucocorticoids, serum levels of zinc fall and the body's demand for zinc increases. In such situations, a vitamin A deficiency may develop, even though adequate amounts of the vitamin are administered.

Most normal diets provide 10 to 15 mg of the metal per day. It is present in meats, fish, processed cereals and legumes, especially nuts, but not to any great extent in fruits or leafy vegetables. Zinc in plasma is usually bound to albumin and is excreted in feces for the most part; its total body pool in adults is about 2 to 3 g.

For our purposes, though, the important points to remember about zinc are these: When plasma levels fall below $100 \mu g/100$ ml, wound repair problems are likely to arise but can be corrected by administering compounds containing zinc. Giving such supplements to a patient who is not deficient in the metal will not improve healing, however, and could prove detrimental if the amounts administered are excessive. (In animals with plasma zinc levels of around $400 \mu g/100$ ml, in fact, the development of wound strength is impaired.)

IRON Iron (Fe^{++}) is necessary for the hydroxylation of lysine and proline in the formation of collagen, as described in Chapter 1, Normal Repair. Prolonged blood loss, infection, and inadequate intake are the major factors that predispose surgical patients to iron deficiency, which is readily diagnosed by hematologic tests and biochemical measurements of plasma iron constituents. Adequate iron is easily supplied and will prevent or correct a deficit if metabolism of the metal and the production of red cells are not disturbed. But if iron metabolism is deranged, the underlying disorder must be dealt with before the deficiency can be overcome. When a drop in hemoglobin becomes functionally disabling (inadequate oxygen transport and impaired cardiac function), transfusion of erythrocytes is in order.

The amount of iron in a healthy adult is about 4 g: 2.5 in hemoglobin, about 0.3 in tissue (myoglobin, the cytochromes, and ferritin) and 1 in iron stores. Daily losses of the metal in bile, feces, sweat, and urine are small, and iron deficiency is rare among healthy adult men unless they have experienced a serious blood loss.

COPPER   Together with iron, copper is essential to the body's normal output of erythrocytes. It is also a constituent of ceruloplasmin, which catalyzes the oxidation of ferrous ions, ascorbic acid, and aromatic amines by molecular oxygen. It is also a component of many enzyme systems, including lysyl oxidase, the catalyst in the first step toward formation of stable covalent cross-links in collagen. It is this series of cross-linking reactions that gives strength and stability to connective tissue and scars.

Thus, we can deduce that a serious copper deficiency hampers wound repair in at least two critical ways. First, it disrupts the process of erythropoiesis, possibly causing an anemia severe enough to interfere with oxygen transport and therefore with collagen synthesis. Second, it hinders the formation of lysyl oxidase, and this leads to inadequate collagen cross-linking and diminished wound strength.

Penicillamine administration over a long time, such as in the treatment of patients with Wilson's disease, is likely to impair collagen cross-linking, not only by its direct reaction with lysylaldehyde, as described in Chapter 1, but possibly by chelating copper and increasing its excretion, thereby interfering with lysyl oxidase activity by inducing a copper deficit.

Total body copper in a normal adult ranges from 100 to 150 mg, with the liver showing a higher concentration than other tissues. The normal adult diet provides about 2 mg a day, green vegetables, oysters, liver, and many kinds of fish being good sources. Almost all the metal circulating in plasma is bound to ceruloplasmin, which is not excreted via the urinary tract. Most copper is therefore excreted in the feces.

Infants, especially those who are premature or suffer from a severe protein-calorie deficit, may develop a copper deficiency manifested as chronic diarrhea and anemia. Also, Menkes' syndrome, a rare genetic condition that blocks absorption of the metal, leads to mental retardation, hypothermia, skeletal changes, degeneration of the aortic elastica and a failure to keratinize hair, which may become kinky.

Copper deficiency was rarely reported in adults until long-term intravenous alimentation was introduced. Prolonged parenteral nourishment should include supplementary amounts of the metal. As far as we know, no clinical cases of impaired wound healing have been traced directly to a copper deficiency

334

except possibly in patients receiving penicillamine for Wilson's disease. But here again we face the familiar problem of trying to implicate a single nutritional deficit in a wound failure, while recognizing that it is almost always accompanied by many other deficits in seriously ill, injured, or malnourished patients.

MANGANESE Manganese functions as an activator of such enzymes as the phosphatases, kinases, decarboxylases, glycosyltransferases, and arginase. Of importance to the repair process is the role of these manganese-activated enzymes in the synthesis of glycosaminoglycans, and their involvement in the addition of carbohydrate moieties to peptide chains of specific glycoproteins. It is believed that a manganese deficit would affect the formation of connective tissue and thus interfere with wound healing. Evidence for this is the development of "slipped tendons" by chicks fed diets deficient in manganese.

Foods rich in this element include whole cereals, legumes, and leafy vegetables. Tea is an especially good source, containing about 20 μmol per cup, but meat, milk, and refined cereals are not. The average Western diet provides 2 to 9 mg a day. Manganese deficiency, which can be produced experimentally in many laboratory animals, may also occur naturally in cattle grazing in peat pastures poor in the metal. The features of this condition are impaired growth and reproduction, anemia, bone changes, and disturbances of the nervous system. As far as is known, only one clinical case of manganese deficiency has been reported: a patient who exhibited hypocholesterolemia, weight loss, dermatitis, and changes in hair and beard color, along with other nonspecific symptoms.

MOLYBDENUM Molybdenum occurs in association with riboflavin enzymes. The actions of molybdenum, copper, and zinc are closely interrelated in the process of red cell production and other metabolic functions, and these interrelationships seem likely to affect wound repair, although no case of poor healing has yet been traced to a molybdenum deficit so far as we know.

COBALT Cobalt is an essential part of vitamin B_{12}. Cobalt may also serve as a nonspecific divalent cation of some enzyme systems. The administration of vitamin B_{12} appears to supply the necessary amounts of cobalt, and this is the preferred method of cobalt administration. Cobalt toxicity is a known clinical entity. Therefore, cobalt administration, other than vitamin B$_{12}$, is not recommended at this time.

CHROMIUM   Only the trivalent form of chromium is biologically active. A deficiency of chromium interferes with carbohydrate metabolism in man and animals, and so may impede healing as well. Deficits in laboratory animals have retarded the removal of ingested glucose, while in some diabetic patients and others with glucose intolerance, (especially children with protein-calorie malnutrition) chromium supplements have been accompanied by improved glucose tolerance.

SELENIUM   Selenium was first recognized as a possible essential trace element in 1957. Studies have demonstrated that dietary necrotic liver disease is induced in rats only when there are three concurrent deficiencies: vitamin E, sulfur-containing amino acids, and selenium. Clinically, a selenium deficit may be present in severe protein malnutrition in children (kwashiorkor).

This element appears to act in concert with vitamin E to protect cell membranes. It is probable that excessive amounts of selenium impede healing, as do other membrane stabilizers, such as cortisone and vitamin E, in high doses. Although selenium intoxication and deficiency are important matters in animal husbandry in some areas, neither has been described in man and there is no evidence that they affect wound healing in patients.

OTHER TRACE MINERALS   As for the rest, some trace minerals like vanadium and tin are known to be dietary requirements in growing rats, but little is known about their biochemistry and nothing about their possible effects on wound healing. Premature infants fed parenterally for long periods are the patients most at risk of any as yet unidentified deficiencies in these or other trace minerals.

NUTRITION AND WOUND INFECTION

The problems of wound infection are inextricably bound to those of wound healing: When healing is impaired, infection is

336

more common; when infection is present in the wound or even at a distance from the site, healing is often delayed.

An association between infection on the one hand and metabolism and nutrition on the other has been recognized for centuries. There is a synergistic interaction between metabolic and nutritional abnormalities and infection. The synergism works both ways: malnutrition increases one's susceptibility to infection, and infection exacerbates malnutrition.

Whether or not clinical infection develops depends on (1) the nature and number of the contaminating pathogen(s) and (2) the relative resistance of the host. Host defenses encompass inherited and acquired mechanisms that are both immunologic and nonimmunologic and that act locally and systemically (see Chapter 4). Variables that condition this resistance include some that are related to wounds per se: the number and type of contaminating microbes, the presence or absence of foreign bodies and necrotic tissue, the status of the patient's blood supply in general and at the wound site, the adequacy or inadequacy of the medical and surgical care and the severity of the injury or illness that is challenging the patient's resistive mechanisms (see Chaps. 3 and 4).

Undermined Defenses

Extensive injury lowers resistance to infection, especially if it is accompanied by shock. The metabolic abnormalities that follow severe injury or disease further erode host resistance in ways that become quickly apparent. Specifically, posttraumatic dysnutrition alters:

Immunologic functions—humoral and cell-mediated, specific and natural

Inflammatory reactions—the number, types, and functions of the leukocytes, and the character of the vascular and chemical responses

Cellular and tissue integrity, wound repair processes and tissue regeneration

Intestinal microflora

Neuroendocrine and psychologic factors

Responses to a wide variety of drugs

Certain peptides and proteins that appear in the sera of seriously ill and injured patients interfere with polymorphonuclear leukocyte and RES functions, chemotaxis, and the action of certain antibiotics.

There is growing evidence that the levels of some immunologic factors—certain serum immunoglobulins, for example, particularly IgG—drop after a severe injury. This may occur before serious nutrition disorders appear. Methyl prednisone has been shown clinically to increase the catabolism of IgG during drug administration and to decrease its synthesis, then and for some time afterward.

Complement function is disrupted and T lymphocyte function depressed following injury. The first effect may explain the impaired inflammatory reaction after injury, while both may account for the increased susceptibility to infection. The function of the reticuloendothelial system (RES) is depressed ("blocked") after severe injury, especially if shock has been present. Which of these effects is a direct effect of injury and which from dysnutrition is not clear.

The Role of Nutrients

All these changes are intensified if the nutritional needs of the patient are not met and dysnutrition results. That *protein depletion* inhibits certain antibody responses was demonstrated by Cannon and his associates. And protein-calorie undernutrition appears to interfere with some granulocytic activities, including phagocytosis and the intracellular killing of bacteria, and possibly some other functions of wound macrophages (Table 5.2 and Fig. 5.18).

Leukocytes derive energy from sugars and oxygen to ac-

Table 5.2 Transformation under Phytohaemagglutinin Stimulation of Lymphocytes from Children with PCM and Controls

Cells	P.C.M. (Mean %)	Controls (Mean %)	Difference		
			D	t	P
Untransformed	32.47±14.0	4.54±1.36	27.93	5.82	<0.001
Blastoid	66.28±13.48	90.92±1.47	24.64	5.33	<0.001
Mitotic	1.26± 1.01	4.53±0.98	3.27	4.61	<0.001

(From Smythe PM, Brereton-Stiles GG, Grace HJ, et al.: Lancet 7731:939, 1971)

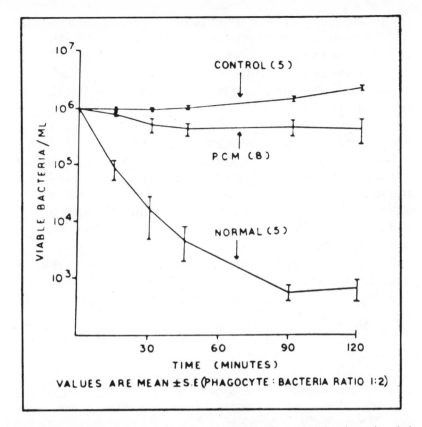

Figure 5.18 Bactericidal activity of leukocytes isolated from normal and protein-calorie deficient PCM children. Controls are tubes containing no leukocytes. *(From Selvaraj RJ, Bhat KS: Am J Clin Nutr 25:166, 1972, copyright © 1972 by the American Society for Clinical Nutrition.)*

complish migration and chemotaxis, phagocytosis, protein synthesis, and the reduction of oxygen to superoxide and other bactericidal compounds. Elevated concentrations of blood and tissue glucose impede chemotaxis, while low levels reduce the availability of energy sources.

Although the pattern we discern here is still incomplete, provision of adequate insulin and maintenance of normal or near-normal blood glucose levels are important to the control of infection. This suggests that in situations where the possibility of a wound infection poses a severe hazard to a diabetic patient, the surgeon ought to control carbohydrate metabolism by constant infusions of both glucose and insulin. He must be alert, though, to the patient's changing insulin requirements as the infection improves or deteriorates. A dosage that might be beneficial one day often proves excessive a few days later if the infection has begun to come under control.

Deficiency of the *essential fatty acids* is accompanied by decreased resistance to infection in experimental animals, and is likely the case in humans.

Vitamin C deficiency modifies the inflammatory reaction to a wounding injury and interferes with the walling off of an infected area by inhibiting collagen formation and impeding neutrophil functions. Additionally, ascorbic acid is used by the granulocytes to produce superoxide, an important link in the chain of oxidative killing of microorganisms. Further, ascorbic acid is required for normal complement metabolism and function (Fig. 5.19).

Deficiencies of the B complex vitamins, notably pyridoxine, pantothenic acid, and folic acid, inhibit antibody formation and also certain white cell activities, including bacterial killing (Fig. 5.20).

Figure 5.19 **A.** Control; normal guinea pig. Lesion 18 days after s.c. inoculation of *S. aureus*. Circumscribed abscess with narrow, orderly zone of normal connective tissue, hematoxylin and eosin, × 36. **B.** Scorbutic guinea pig; scorbutic diet 28 days. Lesion 18 days after *S. aureus* SC inoculation. Large abscess with disorderly connective tissue reaction and destruction of muscle layers. Hematoxylin and eosin, × 36. *(From Meyer E, Meyer MB: Bull Johns Hopkins Hosp 74:98, 1944 copyright 1944 by The Johns Hopkins University Press.)*

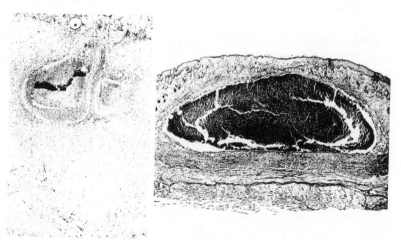

A   B

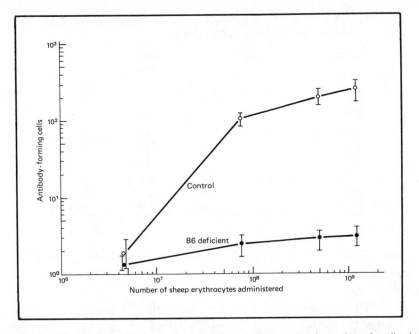

Figure 5.20 Effect of dosage of sheep erythrocytes upon the formation of antibody-forming cells (AFC) determined four days after administration of erythrocytes. AFC are given as average ± SE. Each point represents four to six rats. *(From Kumar M, Axelrod AE: J Nutr 96:53, 1968 © J. Nutr., American Institute of Nutrition.)*

Vitamin A clearly is crucial to host resistance to infection, since it potentiates certain cell-mediated immune responses and perhaps antibody production. Supplemental amounts given to mice on a normal diet increase their resistance to Moloney sarcoma virus, C3H-BA mammary carcinoma and vaccinia—probably reflecting the influence of vitamin A on the thymus and adrenal glands (Table 5.3). When healthy rodents are subjected to a variety of stressors—casting, wounding, or viral challenge, for instance—the consequent decrease in thymus size and increase in adrenal size were lessened when they were given vitamin A supplements.

Vitamin A acts as an immune adjuvant and steroid antagonist in rodents. It seems to increase the available numbers of antibody-forming cells and lymphocytes of thymic origin. It does not antagonize the protective effect of large doses of cor-

Table 5.3   Effect of Supplemental Vitamin A on Tumor Development in Mice Injected with Moloney Sarcoma Virus

Group	Inoculum	Incidence (%)	Latency Period	Regression
Control	10^{-1}	100	6.8	50
Vitamin A		75	9.4	90
P Value		0.01	0.001	0.001
Control	10^{-2}	100	8.5	50
Vitamin A		62	10.1	80
P Value		0.01	0.001	0.001
Control	10^{-3}	40	9.0	70
Vitamin A		35	10.2	100
P Value		0.3	0.01	0.001

ticosteroids on skin allografts, but it may protect against septicemia and death following some bacterial, fungal, and viral challenges.

Iron deficiency may hinder intracellular bacterial killing, perhaps by diminishing the activity of myeloperoxidase, an iron-dependent enzyme. This effect is possibly offset, however, by a retardation in bacterial multiplication due to the deficiency in iron and transferrin. A correlation between serum albumin and serum transferrin levels has been found in surgical patients.

Zincuria and depleted concentrations of tissue zinc may follow injury, and there is evidence indicating that such declines may reduce host resistance to infection. The interrelationship between zinc and vitamin A suggests that deficiencies of both probably have additive effects in decreasing host resistance.

Slowed or otherwise abnormal healing predisposes a wound to infection; and, as emphasized throughout this chapter, healing is impaired in seriously injured animals and patients if the metabolic and nutritional demands imposed by the trauma are not met. When an infection develops, it lowers the metabolic and nutritional status of the patient even further. Appetite and food intake decline; gastrointestinal, hepatic, and other organ functions may become abnormal; and a spectrum of metabolic reactions similar in many respects to those following injury emerges. The result, then, can be a vicious cycle, which, if not interrupted, will lead to a protracted convalescence and possibly death.

Optimal patient care must include measures to prevent or minimize metabolic and nutritional disturbances, and to treat them promptly when they arise. Emphasis should be on prevention whenever possible.

Although the metabolic derangements that follow serious injury and infection are not due primarily to dietary changes, their intensity and duration, including those of negative nitrogen balance and body protein loss, are modulated significantly by food intake. But the simple provision of food, by whatever route, is not, in itself, sufficient. Nutritional care must be integrated into the patient's total care that also includes medical, surgical, chemotherapeutic, immunologic, psychologic, and environmental measures. No attempt is made in this chapter to fully detail the nutritional prophylaxis and treatment of injured, infected, or acutely ill patients. However, some sound guidelines and general principles regarding their nutritional care with particular reference to the repair of wounds are suggested.

Prophylactic measures should be started early, and vigorously pursued, because appropriate dietary intervention can minimize, and often prevent, the rapid and progressive nutritional depletion that still too frequently attends severe injury or acute disease. The physician must also modify the underlying clinical disorder in as favorable a manner as possible. We know that the requirements of seriously injured and ill patients are greater than those of healthy individuals, and that dietary intakes should be started early and increased at a fairly rapid rate. Although we do not yet know the optimal quantitative relationships of the various metabolites, that does not prevent us from providing excellent metabolic and nutritional support.

In the first few days after an operation or severe injury, no strenuous attempt should be made to meet completely the previously healthy patient's caloric and protein needs. The major priorities at this time are the prevention of treatment of shock, and the maintenance of fluid and electrolyte balances and blood volume. Some have recommended infusions of amino acids during these early days. Extra measures of vitamins A, B complex, and C should be given during this period because they do not interfere with other therapies and may forestall early deficiencies. Gastrointestinal function is often impaired at this time, especially if the patient has very extensive injuries, has been in shock, or has had an intraabdominal injury or operation. So overvigorous oral or tube feeding at this time is apt to result in nausea, vomiting, gastric dilation, or ileus.

Within the first week after trauma, though, the surgeon should begin to implement a comprehensive and progressive dietary program. Acutely sick or injured patients usually have a poor appetite and, if left to themselves, will simply not eat enough to satisfy their wounded bodies' demands. Therefore, when the GI tract is functioning properly, they should be encouraged to eat, and here the dietitian has an important role in preparing tasty food attractively served. The use of liquid formulas is often the best way to ensure adequate oral ingestion of the required nutrients. At times, feeding via a small nasogastric tube or by jejunostomy is indicated. The intake must be increased gradually, often over a week or two, to minimize gastrointestinal upsets.

Parenteral supplementation is required not infrequently by severely injured patients, but our experience indicates that prolonged IV feeding is not usually needed by injured patients unless they have suffered damage to the GI tract or have developed severe sepsis or some other complication that interferes with gut function. In such cases, complementary or sole use of the parenteral route is in order. The decision to use parenteral feeding should be made *early*. A good rule of thumb is that if, by the fourth or fifth day after an operation or injury, one cannot confidently expect to begin adequate nourishment by the oral or nasogastric tube routes in the immediate future, one should institute adequate parenteral nutrition.

When uninjured malnourished patients enter the hospital, prompt steps should be taken to improve their nutritional state. Effective treatment depends on recognizing and correcting the underlying cause of the problem and in providing proper nutrition (Fig. 5.21). The methods and timing of nutrient supply in these cases depend on the clinical situation. If an operation is required on an urgent or emergency basis, efforts should be directed primarily to replacing depleted supplies of red blood cells, plasma proteins, water, electrolytes, vitamins, and carbohydrates by parenteral routes, but little can be done at that

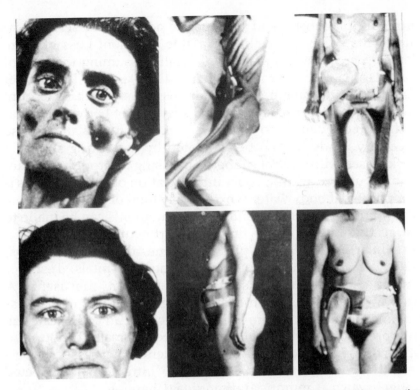

Figure 5.21 Woman with ulcerative colitis just after an ileostomy and colon resection (upper row) and several months later (bottom row). Note the severe malnutrition at the time of operation and the marked improvement in nutritional status postoperatively *(From Brooke, BN. In Turell R (ed): Diseases of the Colon and Anorectum. Philadelphia, Saunders, 1969)*

time to correct generalized tissue protein or essential fatty acid deficiencies. If surgical intervention is not urgent, the patient's nutritional status can be significantly improved by a gradual and progressive dietary program combining oral, tube, and parenteral feedings over a period of weeks. Patients with serious liver or renal disease present special problems, some of which will be mentioned briefly.

Diagnosis of Nutritional Problems

The clinician's awareness of the possibility and extent of nutritional disturbances in injured patients is a prerequisite for appropriate diagnostic and therapeutic actions and serial measurements of body weight are a sine qua non! Loss of more than 10 percent of normal body weight (assuming the patient was reasonably close to his or her "ideal" weight) is a danger signal. The interpretation of weight loss must take into account the possible presence of abnormal amounts of body water (dehydration or edema), so an assessment of water balance is also necessary. Body fat can be estimated by measuring skin-fold thicknesses with special calipers and using appropriate nomograms, but here again, proper interpretation of these findings is complicated if body water is excessively high or low.

A number of different isotope measurements can be made to gauge the various body fluid compartments (intra- and extracellular), red cell mass, plasma volume, and lean body mass, but these are not used routinely in most hospitals. Tests for plasma albumin and transferrin concentrations are useful. A drop in these levels often signals a significant nutritional disturbance, although severe liver dysfunction can complicate the interpretation of these values as indices of malnutrition. Another useful clue to nutritional disorders is depressed hypersensitivity reactions—for example, to intradermally injected antigens such as mumps and candida (Chap. 4).

Assessment of vitamin deficiencies in hospital patients generally depends more on chemical measurements of blood and urinary levels, and tissue saturation than on clinical observations. The same is true for trace mineral abnormalities or unsaturated fatty acid deficits.

An estimate of the caloric expenditure of certain seriously ill or injured persons can be made without expensive and sophisticated equipment. Respiratory minute volume correlates closely with metabolic rate, provided the patient does not have metabolic acidosis or alkalosis, or other disturbances that affect the respiratory center. In those patients with normal breathing function, therefore, serial determinations of respiratory minute volume, combined with careful serial measurements of weight and assessments of water balance, will provide practical information on their metabolic needs, and therefore a rational basis for their nutritional care.

In most instances, the surgeon will base his estimate of a patient's caloric expenditure on past experience—as described, for example, by Kinney (1975): A patient undergoing uncomplicated major elective intraabdominal surgery experiences only a modest (about 10 percent) increase in metabolic rate, while a patient with an uncomplicated injury, such as femoral fracture, has an increase of about 20 percent. In contrast, the metabolic rate of a patient with an infection, such as peritonitis, climbs by 20 to 40 percent; and one with an extensive third-degree burn may have a prolonged increase of 50 to 100 percent. Fever, in and of itself, increases the metabolic rate by about 10 percent for each degree C.

Dietary Needs

The food, provided by whatever route, should constitute a complete metabolic mix, containing high-quality protein (or appropriate proportions of amino acids), carbohydrates, minerals, water, essential fatty acids, and vitamins. The calorie-nitrogen ratio should be about 120 to 150:1 during the early weeks following severe injury and then raised to 200 to 255:1 during convalescence as the patient goes into positive nitrogen balance.

Severely injured children can be kept in excellent nutritional condition by feeding them one to one and a half times their normal caloric and protein intakes. Seriously injured women have been well maintained on diets supplying them with about one and a half to two times their normal total calorie requirements and from two to three times their normal protein requirements. Young men, though, should be provided with three to four times their normal protein intake and about one and a half to two and a half times their normal calorie needs to minimize their body protein and urinary nitrogen losses following severe trauma.

Patients often require extra insulin during the early postinjury period to metabolize the carbohydrates administered in these diets and to prevent hyperglycemia and glycosuria. Their lipid metabolism is usually unimpaired, however, and the author generally supplies 30 to 40 percent of the calories in the form of fat. Long, Wilmore, and their colleagues have reported a marked difference in the protein-sparing effects of carbohydrates and fat. As carbohydrate intake increased, they found a correspondingly greater protein-sparing effect, as gauged by nitrogen balance measurements, and this effect reached its

347

maximum when all nonprotein calories were supplied by carbohydrate. In contrast, increases in the dietary fat content had little effect on the nitrogen balance of patients on isocaloric regimens. These findings suggest a vast difference between the relative protein-sparing effects of carbohydrate in healthy and seriously ill or injured patients, because its effect in healthy persons is only modestly greater than that of fat. Further study of the effect of fats and carbohydrates on protein metabolism is needed, not only because new findings will help us plan optimal oral or parenteral diets, but because they will contribute to our understanding of the metabolic and nutritional problems in the sick and injured.

Whatever answers are forthcoming concerning the optimal carbohydrate-fat ratio, it remains necessary to provide, orally or parenterally, some unsaturated fatty acids in the form of triglycerides. This requirement is especially important in neonates, particularly the premature, but it must be met, too, in older children and adults. The author recommends that at least 4 to 8 percent of the total calories provided be in the form of polyunsaturated fats. Infusion of 500 ml three times a week of the commercially available 10 percent fat emulsion will meet this need for patients nourished parenterally for long periods.

Although the vitamin demands raised by serious injury are not fully understood, the author advises giving 5 to 10 times the normal recommended intake of B vitamins, 20 to 40 times that of vitamin C, and 5 times that of vitamin A. The usual recommended intake of vitamin E should be doubled or tripled, and an increased need for vitamin K can be anticipated in patients with malabsorption. Vitamin D should be given daily in amounts one to two times the normal intake. Adequate macro and trace minerals must be supplied. Supplying the latter by way of the gastrointestinal tract is easy, but supplying trace minerals parenterally is difficult as will be described later.

Hormonal therapy (other than insulin) has no established place in the routine nutritional treatment of previously healthy injured patients.

Special Nutritional Problems

The difficulty of meeting the protein requirements of seriously injured patients is compounded if they have serious liver and/or renal dysfunction. Under such circumstances, the amount of protein given must generally be sharply curtailed and special attention paid to its quality. Intake for a patient with oliguric renal failure, for example, should be limited to about 20 to 25 g of very high-quality protein or a mixture consisting chiefly of the essential amino acids; these include valine, leucine, isoleucine, threonine, phenylalanine, methionine, tryptophan, lysine, and histidine. For premature infants especially, but also for other newborns, cyst(e)ine is also essential. In addition, arginine may be required by injured patients.

Liver dysfunction may necessitate a reduction in protein intake to prevent encephalopathy. Some evidence strongly suggests that administration of branched-chain amino acids and a reduction in the aromatic amino acids supplied are useful in such patients, but this work is still in the investigational stage. Also, as precursors of essential amino acids, α-keto and α-hydroxy acids may be useful to minimize nitrogen intake and lessen the rate of blood urea rises in patients with renal or liver dysfunction.

Special Oral or Tube Diets   Amino acid diets are called for when protein digestion is impaired significantly (by severe pancreatic dysfunction, for example) or when minimal stimulation of the pancreas is desirable (such as during recovery from acute pancreatitis). In the latter case, the formula should be fed through a nasojejunal tube. Patients given these so-called elemental diets also experience an abrupt drop in their fecal bulk and nitrogen excretion. The physician should be aware that the osmolarity of such feeding is high when given in the "final" dilutions required to supply adequate calories and amino acids with acceptable levels of water intake. Therefore it is important to start such feedings in an isotonic dilution and gradually increase their tonicity to avoid GI upsets.

When reducing fecal bulk is a primary aim, and when protein digestion is not impaired, patients should be fed protein of high quality and very low residue, such as egg albumin.

When digestion or absorption of the usual triglycerides is impaired, certain patients can utilize medium-chain triglycerides, which are absorbed largely into the portal blood system rather than the lymph system. As mentioned, these are deficient in unsaturated fatty acids.

Patients who are lactose-intolerant due to an intestinal deficiency in lactase should not be given milk but should be given foods containing carbohydrates other than lactose.

Glucose polymers, sucrose, for instance, which are hydrolyzed and absorbed rapidly, obviate hyperosmolar effects because their osmolarity per calorie delivered is far lower than that of glucose—five times lower in one commercially available preparation. Many patients with nonspecific chronic diarrhea respond well to diets containing these polymers, which are also very useful when total fluid intake must be limited, such as in patients with oliguric renal dysfunction.

Parenteral Feeding   Certain considerations that are fundamental for oral feeding hold as well for parenteral nutrition. Each infusion should be as nutritionally complete as possible, and it should be given at a rate suitable for its best utilization.

The caloric, protein, and amino acid needs of most patients can be fulfilled with the IV preparations now available. However, no special mixture of branched-chain amino acids or α-keto and α-hydroxy analogues are available commercially. There is a preparation of essential amino acids available for patients with renal dysfunction.

The ingredients of current parenteral preparations in the United States are 1) mixtures of free amino acids, 2) mixtures of free amino acids and peptides (the result of acid or enzymatic hydrolysis of proteins), 3) glucose, 4) electrolytes, 5) fat emulsions, 6) human serum albumin and a mixture of albumin and certain globulins (treated to inactivate any contaminating serum hepatitis virus), 7) vitamins, 8) red blood cells and whole blood, and 9) water.

In Europe, xylitol and sorbitol replace some of the glucose generally given in the United States, and fat emulsions are used more often to provide a large share of the calories.

Free amino acids have some advantages over protein hydrolysates; these include: 1) reproducibility of the preparations, 2) all the amino acids are metabolized but some of the peptides may not be, 3) the hydrolysates have more ammonia and are less suitable for use in patients with liver disease, 4) special mixtures of amino acids can be provided to meet special needs of particular types of patients, e.g., those with severe renal or hepatic dysfunction. There may, however, be as yet unidentified roles for certain peptides or it may be easier to supply certain amino acids in metabolizable peptide form than in the free form, e.g., for solubility reasons.

When hypoproteinemia poses a specific indication for inducing a rapid rise in the plasma protein level, for instance, to reduce edema in an anastomosed GI tract or other wound, the problem is best solved by infusing commercially prepared protein fractions. The infused albumin when given in adequate amounts can raise and maintain serum albumin faster than this can be accomplished by depending on hepatic synthesis from infused amino acids.

Significant anemia can be corrected with erythrocyte transfusions, but one *should not overtransfuse* an anemic patient with the expectation of improving his general nutrition. The nitrogen in the infused red cells enters the total nitrogen pool only when those cells are destroyed, and the average survival time for freshly drawn and transfused red cells is about 120 days, even in severely injured patients (excepting those with hemorrhage, burns, or infections). The longer erythrocytes are refrigerated (not frozen) in a blood bank, the shorter their life span after transfusion. But in no case should excessive infusions of red cells be employed for nutritional purposes, because the risks in this maneuver far outweigh any possible benefits.

No commercially available parenteral preparation contains all the trace minerals required by patients being fed parenterally for long periods. Blood and plasma infusions, when given for other reasons, supply some of these needs, but generally in insufficient amounts. At present, therefore, each hospital pharmacy has to make up its own mixture of trace minerals, an unfortunate situation that denies many patients the supplements they require. An added difficulty is that our knowledge is still incomplete regarding the requirements after injury for a number of "essential" trace minerals.

Environmental Factors

Much of the body heat is lost by radiation. There have been a number of studies in which attempts have been made to reduce the metabolic rate and nutritional demands of injured animals and patients by altering the ambient temperature. These have been based on the view that patients lose considerable body heat because hospital room temperatures are often kept at levels below the zone of thermal neutrality (i.e., the ambient temperature at which metabolic rate is at its lowest).

The increase in urinary nitrogen excretion observed in rats with burns (Caldwell) or with femoral fractures (Cuthbertson) is considerably lessened when the animals are adapted to a higher-than-normal ambient temperature (30 C vs. 22 C) prior to injury and maintained at that temperature afterward. Moreover, this same effect has been found in rats maintained at 22 C before injury and then transferred to a 30 C environment immediately after it. A moderate shortening of the time required for the closure of open skin wounds in rats (Cuthbertson), as well as improvements in the healing of skin incisions and the formation of reparative granulation tissue in implanted sponges (Fig. 5.22), has also been noted at the higher room temperature (Crowley).

Clinical data concerning the influence of temperature on the metabolic changes after injury and wound healing are inconclusive. In patients with closed limb fractures, Cuthbertson found that those kept at 30 C excreted less urinary nitrogen than ones kept at 22 C. But Wilmore and his associates believe that the difference observed in metabolic reactions at 30 C and 22 C does not reflect "benefits" conferred by the higher temperature but rather the adverse effects of the lower one, since 22 C is below the zone of thermal neutrality. The latter group found that oxygen consumption was unaffected by ambient temperatures in the range of 25 C to 31 C in controls and patients with burns of less than 40 percent of total body surface, but that it declined modestly in patients with larger burns when they were in the warmer environment.

Earlier, Barr et al. (1968) had reported that burn patients treated in an atmosphere of warm, dry air (32 C, 20 percent relative humidity) showed significantly lower metabolic rates than those treated in a cooler and more humid environment (22 C, 45 percent relative humidity). Their patients were treated by exposure, without ointments or dressings. Similarly treated burn patients showed lesser increases in albumin catabolism and urinary nitrogen excretion when kept in the warmer, drier environment.

Burn patients were permitted by Arturson (1976) to control their environment temperature by regulating infrared heaters. Patients of both sexes, 15 to 61 years of age, with burns involving 23 to 55 percent of body surface were studied; no mention is

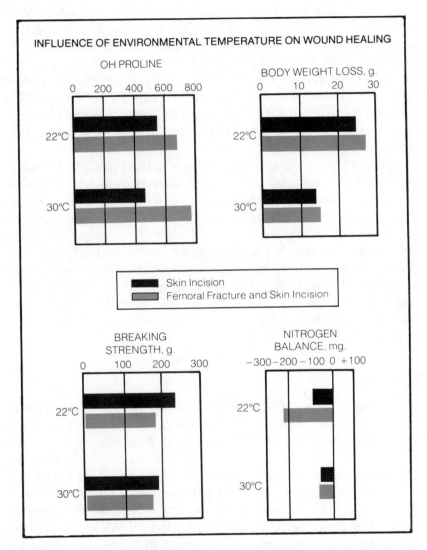

Figure 5.22 Effect of transfer to a warm environment (30 C) immediately after operation on body weight, nitrogen balance and wound healing of rats with and without femoral fracture (seven days postoperatively).

made of depth of burns. The metabolic rate, corrected for rectal temperature, was independent of the size of the burn and the time after injury. No "hypermetabolism" was found, that is, metabolic rate was not increased when the patient was asleep. However, ". . . all kinds of psychic disturbances, as well as pain, shivering, etc., increased the metabolic rate 30 to 40 percent above the value obtained when the patient was asleep." As far as we are aware, Wilmore and his associates studied their patients awake, and thus the results of the two studies may not be so different. Also, Arturson corrected the observed caloric expenditure to a rectal temperature of 37 C while Wilmore et al. did not.

Although these and several other studies have produced no consistent evidence as to the effects of environmental temperatures on metabolic and physiologic responses to injury, it is an area that deserves further investigation. For the present, we concur in the practice of allowing patients to select the room temperature at which they are most comfortable. In general, this means an environment warmer than the nurses and physicians would choose for their own comfort, particularly in the case of burn patients. But it may be that in making their selection, patients choose the ambient temperature at which their metabolic rates are lowest.

Exercise

It is important to encourage early ambulation and exercise as soon as the patient's condition permits, not only to prevent the many complications of inactivity and bed rest, but for the quickest restoration of appetite and strength. From the metabolic and nutritional point of view, it should be noted that when healthy young men in nitrogen equilibrium are immobilized in bed, with plaster casts extending from their toes to axillae and maintained on the same dietary intake as prior to immobilization, their urinary excretion increases by about 1 g each day. When previously well young men with femoral fractures, treated by traction and eating more than their "normal" requirement, do calisthenic exercises (upper extremities and uninjured leg), starting promptly after injury, their urinary nitrogen excretion is reduced and the period of negative nitrogen balance is shortened.

SUMMARY

The metabolic and nutritional derangements of injured and ill patients are complex matters, but the purpose of this chapter has been a simple one: to direct the surgeon's attention to the signals that patients and their wounds are transmitting.

One cannot make hard and fast rules about the quantitative requirements for calories, proteins, or other nutrients for each individual. Patients set their needs in terms of their altered metabolism and the task their injuries have imposed on their reparative mechanisms.

The surgeon then exercises his skill and art in determining which patients will need supplemental nutritional support and when, so that he can provide it before an actual imbalance or deficiency retards healing and predisposes to infection. Also, the surgeon must be quick to recognize when patients and their wounds are showing the effects of "posttrauma dysnutrition," identify the source of the problem, and move to correct it.

To achieve these goals, the surgeon must know how a normal wound heals and how patients respond metabolically to injury, not just in theory, but in practice. He must become a student of each wound, observing it, reviewing its history and reflecting on its progress. The surgeon can respond to the nutritional demands of patients and their wounds only after he has painstakingly instructed himself in the first-hand evaluation of the healing process and the metabolic changes associated with injury and illness. Finally, it should be emphasized that nutritional prophylaxis and therapy must be integrated into the total care program for each patient.

REFERENCES

Arturson G: Hypermetabolism and its treatment in patients with burns. Eighth Annual Meeting, American Burn Association, San Antonio, Tex., Abs. No. 26, April 1–3, 1976

Barr PO, Liljedahl SO, Birke G, et al.: Oxygen consumption and water loss during treatment of burns with warm dry air. Lancet 1:164–168, 1968

Bevelaqua et al.: Scurvy and hemarthrosis. JAMA 235 (17):1876, 1976

Brooke, BN: Surgical aspects of ulcerative colitis. In Turell R (ed): Diseases of the Colon and Anorectum. Philadelphia, Saunders, 1969, Ch. 34

Kinney JM: Energy requirements of the surgical patient. In Ballinger WF, et al. (eds): Manual of Surgical Nutrition, Committee on Pre- and Post-operative Care, American College of Surgeons. Philadelphia, Saunders, 1975

Kumar M, Axelrod AE: Cellular antibody synthesis in vitamin B_6-deficient rats. J Nutr 96:53, 1968

Lehninger AL: Biochemistry. The Molecular Basis of Cell Structure and Function, 2nd ed. New York, Worth, 1975

Levenson SM: Some challenging wound healing problems for clinicians and basic scientists. In Dunphy JE, Van Winkle W Jr (eds): Repair and Regeneration. New York, McGraw-Hill, 1969, Ch. 21

————: Pathophysiology of burns. In Lynch JB, Lewis R (eds): Symposium on Treatment of Burns. St. Louis, Mosby, 1973, Ch. 3

————, Watkin DM: Protein requirements in injury and certain acute and chronic diseases. Fed Proc 18:1155, 1959

————, et al.: The effect of thermal burns on wound healing. Surg Gynecol Obstet 99:74, 1954

————, Geever EF, Crowley LV, et al.: The healing of rat skin wounds. Ann Surg 161:293, 1965

————, Upjohn HL, Preston JA, Steer A: Effect of thermal burns on wound healing. Ann Surg 146:357, 1957

Lund CC, Levenson SM: Burns. In Cole WH: Operative Technique. New York, Appleton, 1949, Ch.3

Lund CC, et al.: Ascorbic acid, thyamine, riboflavin and nicotinic acid in relation to acute burns in man. Arch Surg 55: 557–583, 1947

Marks J: A Guide to Vitamins: Their Role in Health and Disease. Lancaster, Eng., Technical, 1975

Meyer E, Meyer MB: The pathology of staphylococcus abscess in vitamin C deficient guinea pigs. Bull Johns Hopkins Hosp 74:98, 1944

Selvaraj RJ, Bhat KS: Metabolic and bactericidal activities of leukocytes in protein calorie malnutrition. Am J Clin Nutr 25:166, 1972

Smythe PM, Brereton-Stiles GG, Grace HJ, et al.: Thymolymphatic deficiency and depression of cell-mediated immunity in protein-calorie malnutrition. Lancet 20:939, 1971

Wilmore DW, Mason AD Jr, Pruitt BA Jr: Impaired glucose flow in burned patients with gram-negative sepsis. Surg Gynecol Obstet 143:720–724, 1976

Wolback SB: Controlled formation of collagen and reticulum. A study of the

356

source of intercellular substance in recovery from experimental scorbutus. Am J Path 9:689–699, 1933

——, Howe PR: Intercellular substances in experimental scorbutus. AMA Arch Pathol 1:1–24, 1926

BIBLIOGRAPHY

General

Ballinger WF, Collins JA, Drucker WR, Dudrick SJ, Zeppa R (eds.): Manual of Surgical Nutrition, by the Committee on Pre- and Postoperative Care, American College of Surgeons, Philadelphia, W. B. Saunders Company, 1975

Benedict FG: A Study of Prolonged Fasting. Carnegie Institute of Washington Publications, Washington, D.C. p. 203, 1915

Cannon WB: Wisdom of the Body. New York, Norton, 1932

Cuthbertson DP: The Biochemical Response to Injury. In Stoner HB, Threlfall CJ (eds.): The Disturbance of Protein Metabolism following Physical Injury. Springfield, Ill., Thomas, 1960, 193–216

DuBois EF: Metabolism in fever and in certain infections. In Barker LF (ed.): Endocrinology and Metabolism. Vol. IV, D. New York, Appleton, 1922, pp 94–151

Goldbith SA, Joslyn MA (eds.): Milestones in Nutrition. Westport, Conn.: Avi, 1964

Goodhart RS, Shils M: Modern Nutrition in Health and Disease, 5th ed. Philadelphia, Lea & Febiger, 1973, p. 1153

Hippocrates: The Genuine Works of Hippocrates (translated from the Greek by Francis Adams). Baltimore, Williams & Wilkins, 1939

Hunt TK: Fundamentals of Wound Management in Surgery, Wound Healing: Disorders of Repair. South Plainfield, N. J. Chirurgecom, 1976

Hunt TK, Van Winkle W Jr: Fundamentals of Wound Management in Surgery, Wound Healing: Normal Repair. South Plainfield, N. J., Chirurgecom, 1976

Keys A, Brozek J, Henschel A, Michelson O, Taylor HL: The Biology of Human Starvation. Minneapolis, University of Minnesota Press, 1950

Kleiber M: The Fire of Life—An Introduction to Animal Energetics. New York, John Wiley, 1961.

Lehninger AL: Biochemistry. The Molecular Basis of Cell Structures and Function, 2nd ed. New York, Worth, 1975

Levenson AM: Some challenging wound healing problems for clinicians and basic scientists. In Dunphy JE, Van Winkle W (eds.): Repair and Regeneration. New York, McGraw-Hill, 1969

Lusk G: The Elements of the Science of Nutrition. Philadelphia, Saunders, 1906

Moore FD: Metabolic Care of the Surgical Patient. Philadelphia, Saunders, 1959

Olson RE (ed.): Protein-Calorie Malnutrition, a Nutrition Foundation Monograph. New York, Academic Press, 1975, p. 467

Peacock EE, Van Winkle W Jr: Surgery and Biology of Wound Repair, 2nd ed. Philadelphia, Saunders, 1976

Present Knowledge in Nutrition, 4th ed. Washington, D.C., The Nutrition Foundation, 1976, p 624

Seyle H: Stress. London, Butterworth, 1976

Suskind R, Amacher P: Role of Malnutrition in Immune Responses. New York, Raven Press, 1976

Metabolic Reaction to Injury

Albright F: Cushing's syndrome and its connection with the problem of the reaction of the body to injury. Harvey Lectures 38:123–186, 1943

Ballantyne FC, Fleck A: The effect of environmental temperature (20° and 30°) after injury on the catabolism of albumin in man. Clinica Chimica Acta 46:139, 1973

Birke G, Liljedahl SO, Plantin LO, Wetterfors J: Albumin catabolism in burns and following surgical procedures. Acta Chir Scand 118:353–366, 1959–60

Blocker TG Jr, Levin WC, Perry JE, et al.: The influence of the burn state on the turnover of serum proteins in human subjects. Arch Surg 74:792, 1957

Brown WL, Bowler EG, Mason AD Jr, Pruitt BA Jr: Metabolism in burned rats. Am J Physiol 231:476–82, 1976

Burke J: Personal Communication

Caldwell FT Jr: Clinical aspects of the temperature regulation. In Ballinger WF, et al. (eds): Manual of Surgical Nutrition, Committee on Pre- and Postoperative Care, American College of Surgeons, Philadelphia, Saunders, 1975

Clowes GHA, Jr (ed): Symposium on response to infection and injury, I and II. Surg Clin North Am, 56(4):801 and 56(5):997, 1976

Crane CW, Picou D, Smith R, et al.: Protein turnover in patients before and after elective orthopedic operations. Brit J Surg 64:129, 1977

Cuthbertson DP: The disturbance of metabolism produced by bony and non-bony injury, with notes on certain abnormal conditions of the bone. Biochem J 24:1244–1263, 1930

Davies JWL, Ricketts CR, Bull JP: Studies of plasma protein metabolism. Part I. Albumin in burned and injured patients. Clin Sci 23:411–423,1962

Egdahl RH: Pituitary-adrenal response following trauma to the isolated leg. Surgery 46:21, 1959

Gamble JL: Physiological information gained from studies on life-raft rations. Harvey Lectures 42:247, 1947

Hume DM: Endocrine and metabolic response to surgery In Schwartz, S (ed): Principles of Surgery. 2nd ed. New York, McGraw-Hill, 1974

Ingle D: The role of the adrenal cortex in the etiology of disease. J Clin Endocrinol 14:1272–1274, 1954. Also Seyle H, Heuser G (eds): Stress, New York, MD Publications, 1955/56

Kien CL, Young VR, Rohrbaugh DK et al.: Increased rates of whole body protein synthesis and breakdown in children recovering from burns. Ann Surg 187:383–391, 1978

358

Kinney JM: Energy requirements of the surgical patient. In Ballinger WF, et al. (eds): Manual of Surgical Nutrition, Committee on Pre- and Postoperative Care, American College of Surgeons. Philadelphia, Saunders 1975

Levenson SM, Crowley LV, Oates JF, Glinos AD: Injury, wound healing and liver regeneration. Proc. Sec. Army Sc Conf. 2:109–122, 1959

Levenson SM, Einheber A, Malm, OJ: Nutritional and metabolic aspects of shock. Fed Proc 20:99–140, 1961

Levenson SM, Pirani CL, Braasch JW, et al.: The effect of thermal burns on wound healing. Surg Gynecol Obstet 99:74–82,1954

Levenson SM, Upjohn HL, Preston JA, Steer, A: Effect of thermal burns on wound healing. Ann Surg 146:357–368, 1957

Long CL, Spencer JL, Kinney JM, Geiger, JW: Carbohydrate metabolism in man. J Appl Physiol 31:110–116, 1971

Long CL, Jeevarandam M, Kim BM, et al.: Whole body protein synthesis and catabolism in septic man. Am J Clin Nutr 30:1340, 1977

Long CL, Young VR, Kinney JM, et al.: Metabolism of 3-methylhistidine in man. Fed Proc 33:691a, 1974

Long CL, Schiller WR, Blakemore WS, et al.: Muscle protein catabolism in the septic patient as measured by 3-methylhistidine excretion. Am J Clin Nutr 30:1349, 1977

Moore FD, Brennan MF: Surgical injury: body composition, protein metabolism, and neuroendocrinology. In Ballinger, WF, et al. (eds): Manual of Surgical Nutrition, Committee on Pre-and Postoperative Care, American College of Surgeons. Philadelphia, Saunders, 1975, chap. 9

Mouridsen HT: Turnover of human serum albumin before and after operations. Clin Sci. 33:345–354, 1967

O'Keefe SJD, Sender PM, James WPT: "Catabolic" loss of body nitrogen in response to surgery. Lancet 2:1035–1038, 1974

Sender PM, Waterlow JC: Protein turnover in injury. In: Richards JR, Kinney JM, (eds): Nutritional Aspects of the Critically Ill, Churchill Livingstone, London, 1977 p. 177

Seyle H: "Conditioning" versus "Permissive" actions of hormones. J Clin Endocrinol. 14:122–127, 1954. Also in Seyle H, Heuser G (eds.): Stress, New York, MD Publications, 1955/56

Ascorbic Acid

Crandon JH, Lund CC, Dill DB: Experimental human scurvy. New Engl J Med 223:353–369, 1940

Hodges RE, Baker EM, Hood J, Sauberlich HE, March SC: Experimental scurvy in man. Am J Clin Nutrition 22:535–548, 1969

King CG, Burns JJ (eds): Second conference on vitamin C. Ann N Y Acad Sci, 258: 1975

Levenson SM, Green RW, Taylor FHL, et al.: Ascorbic acid, riboflavin, thiamine and nicotinic acid in relation to severe injury, hemorrhage and infection in the human. Ann Surg 124:840–856, 1946

Lind J: In Stewart CP, Guthrie D (eds): Treatise on Scurvy. Containing a Reprint of the First Edition of A Treatise of the Scurvy with Additional Notes. A Bicentenary Volume. Edinburgh, The University Press, 1953

Lund CC, Levenson SM, Green RW, et al.: Ascorbic acid, thiamine, riboflavin and nicotinic acid in relation to acute burns in man. Arch Surg 55:557–583, 1947

Pirani CL, Levenson SM: Effect of vitamin C deficiency on healed wounds. Proc Soc Exper Biol Med 82:95–99, 1953

Ross R, Benditt EP: Wound healing and collagen formation. II. Fine structure in experimental scurvy. J Cell Biol 12:533–51, 1962

Wolback SB, Howe PR: Intercellular substances in experimental scorbutus. Arch Pathol 1:1–24, 1926

Vitamin A

Chernov MS, Hale HW, Wood H: Prevention of stress ulcers. Am J Surg 122:674–677, 1971

Shaffer PA, Coleman W: Protein metabolism in typhoid fever. Arch Intern Med 4:538–600, 1909

Skillman JJ, Rosenoer VM, Smith PC, Fang MS: Albumin synthesis in post-operative patients, New Engl J Med 295:1037–1042, 1976

Sterling K, Lipsky SR, Freedman LJ: Disappearance curves of intravenously administered I[131] tagged albumin in the post-operative injury reaction. Metabolism 4:343–349, 1955

Waterlow JC, Golden M, Picou D: The measurement of rates of protein turn-over, synthesis and breakdown in man and the effects of nutritional status and surgical injury. Am J. Clin Nutr. 30:1333–1339, 1977.

Williamson DH, Farrell R, Kerr A, et al.: Muscle protein catabolism after injury in man, as measured by urinary excretion of 3-methylhistidine. Clin Sci Mol Med 52:527–534, 1977

Wilmore DW, Mason AD, Jr, Pruitt BA, Jr: Impaired glucose flow in burned patients with gram-negative sepsis. Surg Gynecol Obstet 143:720–724, 1976

Vitamins, General

Follis RH, Jr: In Deficiency Disease. Springfield, Ill, Thomas, 1958, p 125

Hopkins FG: Feeding experiments illustrating the importance of accessory food factors in normal dietaries. J Physiol 44:425–460, 1912

Marks J: A Guide to the Vitamins: Their Role in Health and Disease. Lancaster, England, Technical Publishing Co, 1975

Hunt TK, Ehrlich HP, Garcia JA, Dunphy JE: Effect of vitamin A on reversing the inhibitory effect of cortisone on healing of open wounds in animals and man. Ann Surg 170:633–641, 1969

McCollum EV: A History of Nutrition. Boston, Houghton Mifflin, 1957

Moore T: Vitamin A. Amsterdam, Elsevier, 1957

Rai K, Courtemanche AD: Vitamin A assay in burned patients. J Trauma 15:419–424, 1975

Seifter E, Crowley LV, Rettura G, et al.: Influence of vitamin A on wound healing in rats with femoral fracture. Ann Surg 181:836–841, 1975

Smith JC Jr, McDaniel EG, Fan FF, Halsted JA: Zinc: A trace element essential in vitamin A metabolism. Science 181:954–955, 1973

Fell HB, Thomas L: Comparison of the effects of papain and vitamin A on cartilage. J Exper Med 111:719–744, 1960

Trace Minerals

Burch RE, Sullivan JF (eds.): Symposium on trace elements. Med Clin North Am 60(4): 655, 1976

Chvapil M: Zinc and wound healing. In Zederfeldt B (ed): Symposium on Zinc. Lund, Sweden, A. B. Tika, 1974

Prasad A (ed): Trace Elements in Human Health and Disease, Vol. I. Nutrition Foundation Monograph Series. New York, Academic Press, 1976, p 470

Underwood EJ: Trace Elements in Human and Animal Nutrition, 3rd ed. New York, Academic Press, 1971

Wound Healing and Wound Infection

Alexander JW: Emerging concepts in the control of surgical infections. Surgery 75:934–946, 1974

Axelrod AE: Modern nutrition in health and disease. In Goodhart RS, Shils ME (eds): Nutrition in Relation to Acquired Immunity. Philadelphia, Lea & Febiger, 1973; pp 493–505

Beisel WR: Metabolic response to infection. Ann Rev Med 26:9–20, 1975

Cannon PR: Recent Advances in Nutrition with Particular Reference to Protein Metabolism. Kansas University Press (No. 14 of the Porter Lecture Series), Laurence, Kansas, 1950

Cohen BE, Cohen IK: Vitamin A: adjuvant and steroid antagonist in the immune response. J Immunol 3(5):1376–1380, 1973

Dubos RJL: The micro-environment of inflammation or Metchnikoff revisited. Lancet 2:1–5, 1955

Howard RJ, Simmons RL: Acquired immunologic deficiencies after trauma and surgical procedures. Surg Gynecol Obstet 139:771–782, 1974

Koros AMC, Axelrod AE, Hamill EC, South DJ: Immunoregulatory consequences of vitamin deficiencies on background plaque-forming cells in rats (39388). Proc Soc Exper Biol Med 143:322–326, 1976

Kulapongs P, Suskind R, Vithayasia V, Olson RE: Cell-mediated immunity and phagocytosis and killing function in children with severe iron deficiency anemia. Lancet 2:689–691, 1974

Law DK, Dudrick SJ, Abdou NI: The effects of protein calorie malnutrition on immune competence of the surgical patient. Surg Gynecol Obstet 129:257–266, 1974

Lederer WH, Kumar M, Axelrod AE: Effects of pantothenic acid deficiency on cellular antibody synthesis in rats. J Nutrition 105:17–25, 1975

361

Lennard ES, Alexander JW, Craycraft TK, MacMillan BG: Association in burn patients of improved antibacterial defense with nutritional support by the oral route. burns, including thermal injury. Burns 1:98, 1975

MacLean LD, Meakins JL, Taguchi K, et al.: Host resistance in sepsis and trauma. Ann Surg 182:207–217, 1975

Meyer E, Meyer MB: The pathology of staphylococcus abscess in vitamin C-deficient guinea pigs. Bull Johns Hopkins Hosp 74:98–118, 1944

Morris JJ, et al.: Effect of Antimicrobial Agents upon Wound Healing. Antimicrobial Agents and Chemotherapy, 7th Interscience Conference on Antimicrobial Agents and Chemotherapy. Chicago, American Society for Microbiology, 1968

Munster AM, Eurenius K, Katz RM, et al.: Cell-mediated immunity after thermal injury. Ann Surg 177:139–143, 1973

Pruitt BA, Jr: Infections caused by pseudomonas species in patients with burns and in other surgical patients. Am J Clin Nutrition 29:758–761, 1976

Schlesinger L, Ohlbaum A, Gre L, Stekel A: Decreased interferon production by leukocytes in marasmus. Am J Clin Nutr 29:758–761, 1976

Scrimshaw NS, Taylor CE, Gordon JE: Interactions of Nutrition and Infection. Monograph Series No. 57, Geneva, World Health Organization, 1968

Seifter E, Zisblatt M, Levine N, Rettura G: Inhibitory action of vitamin A on a murine sarcoma. Life Sciences 13:945–951, 1973

Sirisinha S, Edelman R, Suskind R, Charupatana C, Olson RE: Complement and C3-proactivator levels in children with protein-calorie malnutrition and effect of dietary treatment. Lancet 1:1016–1020, 1973

Smythe PM, Brereton-Stiles GG, Grace, HJ, et al.: Thymolymphatic deficiency and depression of cell-mediated immunity in protein-calorie malnutrition. Lancet 2:939–943, 1971

Vitale JJ, Good RA (eds): Nutrition and Immunology, Vol. 28, Special Publications Department, Am J Clin Nutrition, June, 1974, p 47

Warden GD, Mason A, Jr, Pruitt BA, Jr: Suppression of leukocyte chemotaxis in vitro by chemotherapeutic agents used in the management of thermal injuries. Ann Surg 181 (3):363–369, 1975

Weinberg ED: Iron and susceptibility to infectious disease. In the resolution of the contest between invader and host, iron may be the critical determinant. Science 184:952–956, 1974

Environment

Arturson G: Hypermetabolism and its Treatment in Patients with Burns. Eighth Annual Meeting, American Burn Association, San Antonio, Texas, Abs. No. 26, April 1–3, 1976

Barr PO, Liljedahl SO, Birke G, et al.: Oxygen consumption and water loss during treatment of burns with warm dry air. Lancet 1:164–168, 1968

Caldwell FT, Jr: Changes in energy metabolism during recovery from injury. In Porter R, Knight J (eds): Energy Metabolism in Trauma, Ciba Symposium, London, J. and A. Churchill, 1975, pp 23–38

Campbell RM, Cuthbertson DP: Effect of environmental temperature on the metabolic response to injury. Quart J Exper Physiol 42:114–129, 1967

362

Crowley LV, Kriss P, Seifter E, et al.: Nitrogen metabolism and wound healing in rats: Effects of femoral fracture, testosterone and environmental
temperature. Fed Proc 31, Abs. No. 2897, 1972, and J Trauma (in press).
Wilmore DW, Long JM, Mason AD, Jr et al.: Catecholamines: mediator of the
hypermetabolic response to thermal injury. Ann Surg 180:653–669, 1974

Exercise

Cuthbertson DP: The influence of prolonged muscular rest on metabolism.
Biochem J 23:1329–1345, 1929
Whedon GD, Deitrick JE, Shorr E: Modification of the effects of immobiliza-
tion upon metabolic and physiologic functions of normal men by the use
of an oscillating bed. Am J Med 6:684–711, 1949
Vail E: The Influence of Exercise on Nitrogen Metabolism Following Severe
Trauma in Adult Male Patients. M.S. Thesis at Medical College of Vir-
ginia, Richmond, 1952.

6

TECHNICAL FACTORS IN WOUND MANAGEMENT

Richard F. Edlich

George Rodeheaver

John G. Thacker

Milton T. Edgerton

Every surgical wound is the result of a finite energy exchange that causes tissue disruption. The dynamics of this exchange of energy will determine the magnitude of injury. Disruption of the body covering leaves the once-sterile underlying integument exposed to contamination. The contaminants are derived either from the victim (endogenous) or the energy source (exogenous). Bacteria are one of the contaminants, making the care of the wound an exercise in microbiology. Other contaminants, such as dirt, may also reside in the recesses of the wound, especially in accidental injuries.

In his quest to reconstitute the embattled tissue, the surgeon must appreciate the consequences of its devastation. The mechanism of injury provides reliable indications of its ravages. Whether the tissue injury will be limited to the initial wounding depends upon the outcome of the interaction between the contaminants and the injured tissue. In the event that contaminants are reactive, a relatively insignificant wound may become a catastrophe. This circumstance can be averted by the implementation of a well-devised and executed surgical plan. Some fundamental technical skills needed to achieve this goal are described in this chapter.

DETERMINANTS OF INFECTION

Mechanisms of Injury

I believe that the tendency will always be in the direction of exercising greater care and refinement in operating, and that the surgeon will develop increasingly a respect for tissues, a sense which recoils from inflicting, unnecessarily, insult to structures concerned in the process of repair.

William S. Halsted, 1913

In the language with which a surgeon labels the world around him, he often unconsciously separates the concept of accidental traumatic tissue injury from that which is a result of surgical operation. This division of thought may provide the surgeon with a false sense of confidence that the consequences of traumatic injury are indeed distinct from those of operation. However, the consequences of traumatic injury and operation are identical in most respects.

The outcome of both injury and surgery can be predicted by applying concepts of energy, force, and work that were first appreciated in the 16th century. Surgical division of tissue simply employs various forms of energy transfer, mechanics, and electrical radiance in a planned procedure to elicit an anticipated result. Although accidental traumatic injury is caused by the same energy sources, the incident is unexpected, unplanned, and uncontrolled. *If the surgeon does not appreciate and control the sources of energy he employs, an operation becomes a form of assault similar in nature to a traumatic injury.* The "complete" surgeon must harness and control the sources of energy and appreciate their potentially destructive effects. He must also be aware of the consequences of applying uncontrolled amounts of energy to tissues, as occurs in accidental injury, and treat the resultant wounds appropriately. Clinically, one of the most important consequences of any wounding process is that the divided edges of the wound are vastly more susceptible to infection than unwounded tissue. The magnitude of this enfeebled resistance to infection will vary with the mechanism of wounding.

Mechanical Energy   There are three mechanical forces that can lead to soft-tissue injury: shear, tension, and compression.

When performing surgery, the surgeon applies a carefully controlled force of planned magnitude to divide tissue. The force, which is shearing in nature, is delivered to the tissues by a scissors or scalpel.

In most traumatic soft-tissue injuries, this same type of force of an uncontrolled magnitude is applied to tissue by a piece of glass, a metal edge, or knife. In such a case, shear forces of equal magnitude are applied to this tissue in opposite directions in two adjacent parallel planes separated by a small distance. The amount of tissue volume contacted by sharp devices such as a scalpel or piece of glass is extremely small and consequently very little total energy (< 100 joules) is required to produce tissue failure.

THE SCALPEL   When cutting tissues, the surgeon must employ a scalpel that divides tissue with the least trauma. The performance of a scalpel blade is best judged by its sharpness, durability and resistance to breakage.

The sharpness of the blade is dependent on the radius of curvature of its ultimate edge (Fig. 6.1). The ultimate edge of the scalpel is generated by a series of grinding processes which

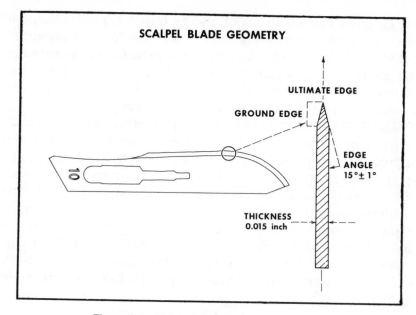

Figure 6.1 Physical design of the scalpel blade.

expose the blade to wheels of different coarseness (grit). The mechanics of the grinding process influence the configuration of the ultimate edge and the performance of the blade.

In combination grinding, each side of the blade is ground separately. Each grinding step generates a curl of wire that is removed by buffing. A side effect of the buffing process is the rounding of the ultimate edge, diminishing blade sharpness (Fig. 6.2A).

In rotary grinding, both sides of the blade are ground simultaneously, after which they are polished. The ultimate edge of a blade made by this process is a symmetrical and triangular edge coming to a point (Fig. 6.2B). When equal force is applied, blades ground by the rotary process can cut to a greater depth than blades ground by the combination process.

The scalpel's susceptibility to breakage is particularly important to the surgeon operating near bone. If the surgeon inadvertently presses the tip of the blade against a bony surface, the blade may fracture. The detached segment behaves as a missile becoming lodged in the tissues. The search for this embedded foreign body is usually fruitless, and it becomes a constant reminder to the surgeon, and occasionally to the patient, of the operative procedure. The durability of the scalpel can be en-

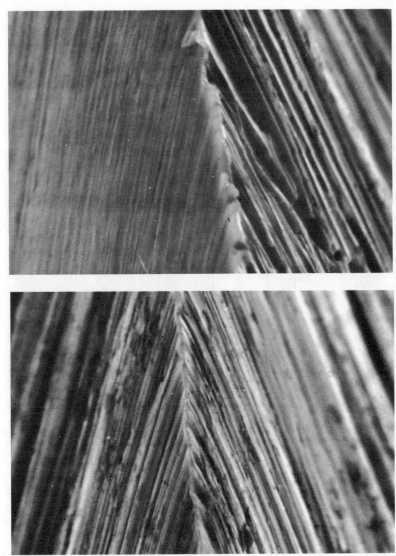

Figure 6.2 Electron photomicrograph (5000×) of the ultimate edge of a scalpel blade. **A.** In combination grinding, the ultimate edge of the blade is rounded and uneven. **B.** The ultimate edge of the blade generated by rotary grinding is a symmetrical, triangular edge coming to a point.

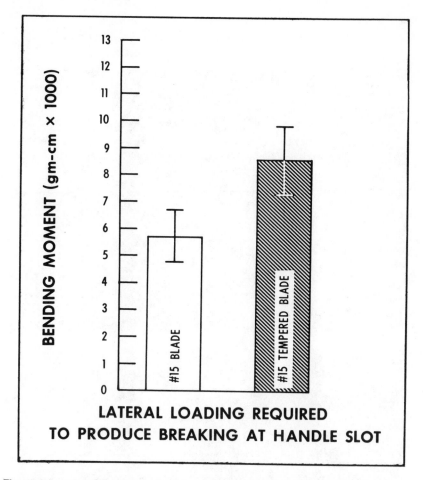

Figure 6.3 Lateral loading required to produce breaking at handle slot. By tempering the blade, its resistance to breakage is increased by nearly 50 percent.

hanced about 50 percent by tempering the blade after the edge has been created. (Fig. 6.3).

The configuration of the cutting edge of a scalpel blade is designed to accomplish a specified surgical task using a pre-scribed technique. The cutting edge of the No. 10 blade is pre-dominantly straight except for its curved distal end. When the surgeon cuts the skin with the No. 10 blade, the knife is held like a violin bow so that the long, straight cutting edge of the blade contacts the skin. One sweep of the blade results in a deep straight incision (Fig. 6.4A). When a No. 15 blade is held in this manner the design of the blade prevents the cutting edge from making contact with the skin (Fig. 6.4C). The design of a No. 15 blade permits the surgeon to cut short incisions that often must follow irregular anatomic landmarks with precision. With No. 15 blades, the curved portion of the blade accounts for the major portion of the cutting edge. The surgeon can gain optimal control of this blade by holding its knife handle as a pencil (Fig. 6.4B). In so doing, the curved portion of the blade cuts the skin. When the surgeon uses a No. 10 blade in this manner, proper control is lacking and usually a jagged incision is cut (Fig. 6.4D).

While the decision to discontinue the use of a scalpel blade during an operation is usually related to blade dulling, some surgeons discard a blade after it contacts what they believe to be a source of contamination. A ritual practice in surgery has been to discard the sharp scalpel blade following its use on skin fearing that its surface may possibly be contaminated and will carry organisms into the depths of the wound. This fear is unfounded. Jacobs (1974) found that scalpels cultured subsequent to cutting skin are almost always sterile. *Therefore, the custom of discarding a sharp scalpel blade following its use on skin should no longer be mandatory.*

Despite all the technical advances in scalpel design, the ultimate performance of the scalpel rests with the surgeon's technical skill. The experienced surgeon who is cognizant of scalpel performance and the anatomy of tissue can cut to the desired depth with one sweep of the blade. The resultant wound is resistant to the development of infection (Fig. 6.5). The surgeon who does not appreciate the potential of his instrument and is unfamiliar with the structural configuration of the tissue will generally cut with multiple strokes of the knife. Such repeated passages of the scalpel through tissue damage local vasculature, weaken host defenses, and invite infection.

TRAUMATIC COMPRESSION When a soft-tissue wound is caused by a collision of two bodies, the mechanisms of injury are predominantly compression and/or tension rather than shear. In impact injuries resulting from the collision of a flat body against soft tissue without underlying bone, the mechanism of injury is mainly tension. Tensile stresses in soft tissue are caused by two forces of equal magnitude applied in opposite directions to the tissue. In impact injuries due to a collision of a flat body against

371

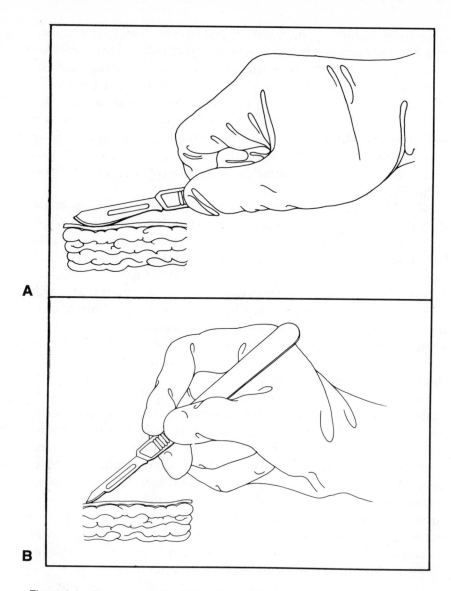

Figure 6.4 Recommended techniques for cutting skin with a No. 10 blade **(A)** and No. 15 blade **(B)**.

soft tissue overlying bone, tissue failure is secondary to compressive forces consisting of two equal forces oriented towards each other. In either case, injury occurs when tensile or compressive forces exceed the yield stress of tissue.

372

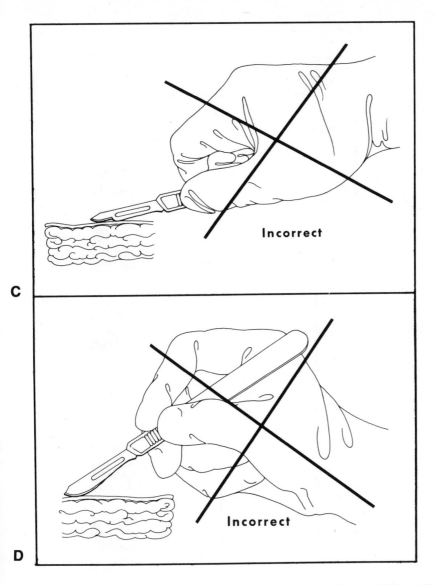

Figure 6.4. (cont.) Incorrect surgical techniques for cutting skin with a No. 15 blade **(C)** and a No. 10 blade **(D)**.

When the forces creating the wound are primarily compressive or tensile in nature rather than shear, the host defenses are even more weakened and susceptible to infection. The energy required to injure tissue by these forces is considerably greater

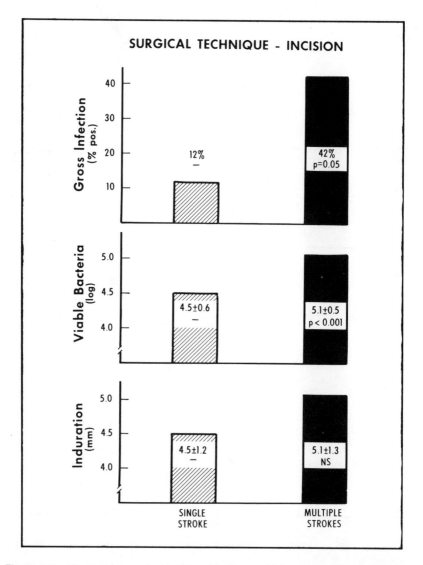

Figure 6.5 After making surgical incisions by either a single sweep of the scalpel blade, or multiple strokes of the blade, the experimental guinea pig wounds were subjected to a comparable level of *S. aureus*. The inflammatory response (gross infection, induration) of the contaminated wounds made by a single sweep of the knife were significantly less than that in wounds made by multiple strokes. The viable bacterial counts of the wounds were proportional to their inflammatory responses.

374

than for shear forces since the energy is distributed over a larger volume.

The amount of energy absorbed by tissue during an impact can be calculated by the following equation:

$$T = \frac{MV^2}{2}$$

where   T = kinetic energy (joules)
        M = Mass (kg)
        V = relative velocity between the objects that impact (m/sec).

The extent of compressive or tensile injuries will vary with the size (mass) of the object impacting the body surface and its velocity when it makes contact. Changes in the relative velocity (V) of the object that impacts has a greater influence on the level of kinetic energy (T) than do variations in the mass (M) of the object.

Even when the impact injury results from the collision between two relatively slow moving objects (<5 meters/sec), the damage to the host's defenses are substantial. The striking of the victim's head against the dashboard in an automobile collision is a case in point. If the energy level absorbed is sufficient to lacerate the skin, the wound's defenses are markedly impaired. The wound then becomes susceptible to infection by bacteria from either endogenous or exogenous sources. In such wounds, antibiotics can suppress the growth of bacteria, but not to the same degree as in tissue not subjected to impact.

A collision between a missile and the human body represents a considerably higher level of energy absorption per unit volume of tissue. The rapid speed with which the energy is transferred also contributes to the magnitude of injury. One of the main themes of military surgical history is this collision between man and metal. As tissues are struck by a missile, a combination of shear, tensile, and compressive forces interact to produce a relatively predictable amount of destruction. At speeds up to 300 meters/sec, the "low-velocity" projectile penetrates the target making a deep narrow tract (Table 6. 1). In such injuries, the tissue damage is confined to the immediate pathway of the bullet.

Table 6.1 Differences in Impact According to Bullet Caliber

Type	Weight (grains)	Muzzle Velocity (m/sec)	Energy at Muzzle (joules)	Energy at 100M (joules)
Rifle Cartridges				
22-250 Remington	55	1143	2303	1675
270 Winchester	100	1060	3646	2831
6MM Remington	80	1058	2900	2260
243 Winchester	80	1042	2816	2195
300 Winchester	150	1002	4888	3932
25-06 Remington	120	950	3360	2804
30-06 Springfield	150	905	3850	3006
22 Hornet	45	819	980	565
458 Winchester Magnum	500	649	6765	5423
32 Remington	170	646	2343	1631
30 Carbine	110	603	1311	843
Pistol and Revolver Cartridges				
22 Long	29	378	134	81
357 Magnum	158	376	725	489
22 Short	27	352	108	69
45 Colt	255	262	556	461
44 S&W Special	246	230	420	359
32 Short Colt	80	227	136	84
38 Special	200	194	243	213

When a high-velocity projectile (>1000 meters/sec) strikes, considerably more energy is transferred than with low velocity missiles. The energy liberated by a missile in tissue increases dramatically as the square of the velocity (V). Once contact is made, the missile is decelerated by the resistance of the tissue. The energy released by deceleration of high-velocity missiles forms initial shock waves in both forward and lateral directions. As a result of the enormous explosive force in a lateral direction, a large space, known as a "temporary cavity," is created that attains its maximum volume within 2 to 4 msec after missile impact. After the cavity reaches its maximum volume, the tissue rebounds, narrowing the cavity. Depending on the tissue, the force creating the "temporary cavity" may cause damage for a major distance surrounding wound tract. With high-velocity missiles, the magnitude of tissue injury is extensive and difficult to ascertain accurately soon after injury. High velocity injury may occur not only with a single bullet penetration but also with some of the newer fragmentation shells that throw out pieces traveling over 1000 meters/sec.

The degree to which tissue combats these disruptive forces varies with the individial tissues. Amato et al. (1974) found that the size of the "temporary cavity" is proportional to the specific gravity of the tissue(s) involved and directly related to the ultimate severity of injury. Following passage of high-velocity missiles through lung parenchyma (specific gravity 0.4 to 0.5), the tissue rapidly absorbs the energy and then recoils to leave an almost imperceptible tract. Larger permanent wounds tracts are encountered in tissues with higher specific gravities (liver— 1.01 to 1.02; muscle— 1.02 to 1.04; bone— 1. 11 or greater).

The mass of the bullet (M) also has an influence on the magnitude of injury. Increase in bullet mass enhances the energy transfer to the tissue proportionally. Tumbling of the missile will further accentuate the discharge of energy to tissue. In an in vitro study of wound ballistics, DeMuth noted that expanding bullets used for sporting purposes create a permanent wound tract much larger than that produced by a standard military bullet. The wound volumes resulting from the expanding bullets may be 40 times that due to the nonexpanding type.

When caring for a victim of a bullet injury, one should question the victim or witnesses regarding the weapon and the circumstances of injury (i.e., muzzle distance from wound, etc.). An attempt should be made to obtain as much information as possible about the firearm. Using these data, the informed physician can determine the plausibility of a wound being caused by a given firearm under given circumstances (Table 6.1). Careful wound measurements and determination of the wounding mechanism may spare the investigating physician much embarrassment.

Electrical Energy Electricity is another source of energy that the surgeon has learned to use constructively in operating. An electrical current is a flow of electrons which collides with the stationary nonconductive particles in their path. These collisions cause vibration of the particles within the material, as a result of which the material becomes hot. This process transforms electrical energy into thermal injury.

The magnitude of resistance to electron flow varies widely in tissues. The high resistance of skin and low resistance of muscle to electron flow are cases in point. The control and localization of this heating effect of electrical current comprises the fundamental basis for electrosurgery.

Electrical power is usually generated with a continuously reversing direction of electrical pressure (voltage). The pressure in the line first pushes and then pulls electrons (AC). The frequency of the current in hertz (Hz), or cycles per second, is the time in which the complete cycle of positive and negative pressure occurs. The usual wall outlet provides a current with 120 reversals of the direction of flow occurring each second. Passage of 60 cycles of alternating current through a patient is extremely dangerous since it can induce ventricular fibrillation as well as muscle contractions. Late nineteenth century studies established that involuntary spasmodic contractions of muscle in response to a low-frequency electrical stimulus subside as the frequency of the applied alternating current increases. At frequencies greater than 10,000 Hz, no muscle response is noted. In addition, high-frequency current can flow along paths that virtually block the 60-cycle current. The frequency of the current generated in electrosurgery is 250,000 to 2,000,000 Hz. Heretofore, research in electrosurgery has focused predominantly on electronic technology with only theoretical clinical application. In the future, comprehensive research investigations must be undertaken to relate these modern technologic advances to clinical performance.

The ability of high-frequency current to damage tissue depends on its concentration or density. As the current density increases, its heating effect becomes more pronounced. The size of the active monopolar electrode is deliberately kept small so that concentrated heating will occur at its point of contact with tissue. The ground, or return electrode, must have a large area of contact to ensure low current density and low tissue heating (Fig. 6.6A). The distribution of the current can be even more precisely controlled by making the active electrode bipolar rather than monopolar (Fig. 6.6B). The use of bipolar electrodes, usually in the form of forceps, delineates the tissue through which the current will pass. Bipolar electrodes contain two electrodes and contact the tissue at two points; current flows into the tissue through one arm of the forceps and back out through the other. The entire current is confined to the small area between the two ends of the forceps.

When undamped high-frequency currents are passed through tissue, the active electrode functions as a bloodless knife. The cells at the edges of the resultant wound literally disintegrate. Away from the plane of cutting, one can see elon-

378

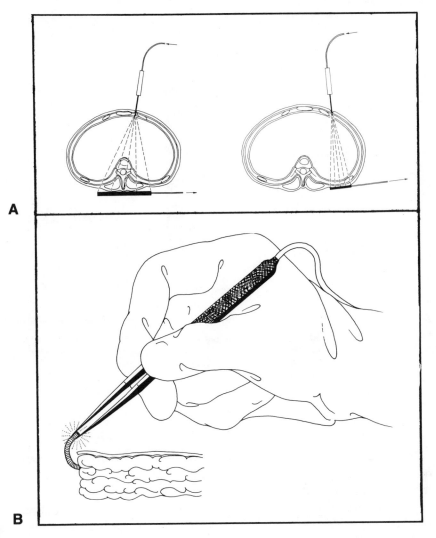

Figure 6.6 **A.** Distribution of current between the active monopolar electrode and the ground electrode. Current is concentrated at the monopolar electrode to produce either cutting or coagulating. Following contact, the current is dispersed at the return (ground) electrode. **B.** Current flow is more concentrated and discrete in the bipolar cautery forceps shown below.

gated tissue cells as well as histologic evidence of a mild thermal injury. Blood vessels at the wound edge are usually thrombosed, accounting for the hemostatic effect of the high frequency current. This type of tissue damage is also associated with an increased susceptibility of the wound to infection. The

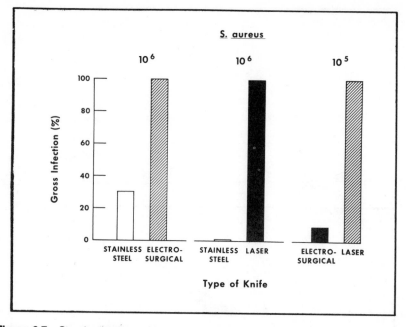

Figure 6.7 Standardized wounds made by either a stainless steel, electrosurgical, or laser knife were contaminated with a specified dose of S. aureus. Four days later, the incidence of gross infection was significantly greater in wounds made by the bloodless knives than those made by the stainless steel scalpel.

wound made by electrosurgery in experimental studies is approximately three times more susceptible to infection than wounds made with the stainless steel scalpel (Fig. 6.7). In a prospective clinical study by Cruse and Foord (1973), the use of electrosurgery almost doubled the infection rates of surgical wounds. *The increased susceptibility of such wounds to infection mitigates against the use of electrosurgery for cutting skin and subcutaneous tissue.*

In massive excisional surgery (e.g., large soft-tissue tumors, debridement of third-degree burns), the threat of blood loss frequently outweighs the potential problems of subsequent infection. In burn wound excisions, Levine and his associates (1975) reported that the operative blood loss during electrosurgical excision was approximately 50 percent less than that encountered during scalpel excision. The operative time was cut in half by eliminating the additional time required to obtain hemostasis after the scalpel was used.

380

When the oscillations are damped, the current accomplishes hemostasis without cutting (Fig. 6.8). This type of current causes a rapid dehydration of cells, and the affected tissue is fused into a structureless homogenous mass with a hyalinized appearance. The vessels within the tissue thrombose. We prefer pinpoint electrosurgical coagulation over suture ligation for small bleeding vessels, but the power should be kept to the absolute minimum needed for vessel thrombosis.

The technique of electrocoagulation has considerable influence on the magnitude of injury. The use of *bipolar coagulation* is a *more precise* method of hemostasis that limits the tissue injury encountered with the more traditional monopolar coagulation. Ferguson (1971) has noted that an equivalent current passed through a monopolar electrode caused approximately three times as much necrosis of the surrounding tissue as the use of bipolar coagulation.

Bleeding from the cut ends of vessels over 2 mm in diameter can rarely be controlled by electrocoagulation. In such cases, hemostasis can be achieved easily with a suture ligature of nonreactive material. The intact vessel should be isolated over a

Figure 6.8 Schematic representation of damped (top) and undamped (bottom) electrical currents. Undamped high-frequency current acts as a bloodless knife while damped current exhibits a hemostatic effect without cutting.

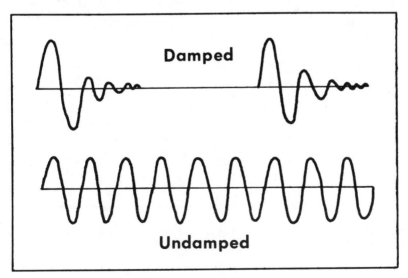

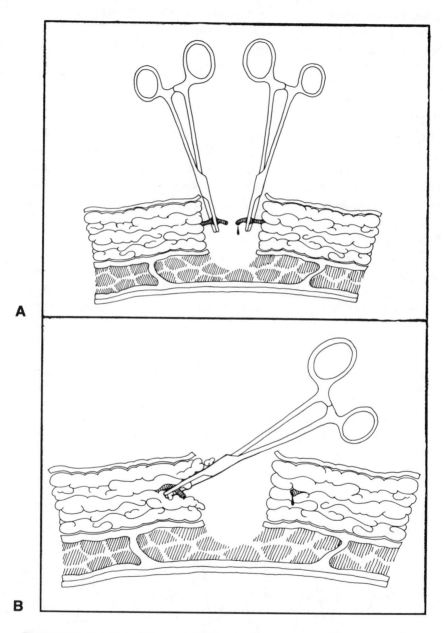

Figure 6.9 Clamping of the vessel before its division (A) results in considerably less tissue injury than does clamping the divided retracted bleeding vessel (B).

short length and clamped with small hemostats applied contiguously. Subsequently, the vessel is divided between the ligatures (Fig. 6.9A). When it can be used, this technique is preferred over cutting the vessel first and then clamping the retracted vessel along with the contiguous blood-stained tissue (Fig. 6.9B). In the latter case Ferguson reported that the amount of strangulated tissue was about five times as much as with the vessel-isolating technique. Furthermore, surgeons should never resort to hot (150 F or 55 C) wet sponges for hemostasis. (This is the point at which a "warm" object begins to feel hot to the hand. Rubber gloves increase the time necessary to feel the heat.) In experimental studies reported by McDowell (1959) this treatment resulted in a hyperthermic injury to tissue that potentiated the development of infection.

When the mechanism and source of electrical energy are not controlled during its application to the human body, the consequences can be disastrous. Accidental acute electrical injury is a result of the transformation of electricity into heat in tissue. Accidental electrical injuries differ from electrosurgical wounds only in the relative frequency, voltage, and distribution of the current delivered to the tissues.

Radiant Energy   As a result of recent scientific advances, surgeons can now employ energy from light as a scalpel. This is one of the many forms of radiant, or electromagnetic, energy. Such energy consists of photons that are both waves and particles. Once it is absorbed by tissue, radiant energy is converted into heat that rapidly increases the temperature of a small volume of tissue. This precise thermal injury results in a relatively bloodless division of tissue. The concept of light as a source of energy is realized in lasers. Light waves emitted from lasers are coherent, and are so nearly parallel that they can travel for miles in a straight line without spreading apart or converging. This coherent light provides tremendous pulses of power that do not diminish over great distances.

This energy source is now being used by some surgeons to cut tissue. Lasers used in surgery get their energy from rotation and vibration of electrons in the CO_2 molecule with a resultant emission of light having a wavelength of 10.6μ. These infrared waves are then directed along an articulated arm, and into a handpiece by means of mirrors located in precision rotary joints. A lens in the handpiece focuses the energy to a point less than 1 mm in diameter. This high concentration of energy at the focal point allows the beam to cut through skin and soft tissue. Despite this technologic advance, laser surgery is limited in usefulness by the cumbersome design of the surgical arm as well as an insufficient level of power. When maneuverability is required, laser surgery is difficult and time consuming.

The hemostatic effect of the laser scalpel makes it especially suitable for massive surgical excisions. In a clinical series of 26 patients subjected to burn wound excision, Levine et al. reported that the blood loss encountered by scalpel excisions was nearly 3.3 times greater than the blood loss following laser surgery. Electrosurgical excision had 1.67 times the blood loss of laser excision. The superior hemostatic effect of the laser over that of electrosurgery is associated with increased damage to the tissue defenses. Experimental wounds made by a laser are approximately tenfold more susceptible to infection than those made by electrosurgery (Fig. 6.7). *This infection-potentiating effect of the laser scalpel mitigates against its use for incisional surgery.* Fortunately, the tissue damage resulting from electrosurgery or the laser does not interfere with the "take" of either autografts or homografts on wound beds with low bacterial counts ($<10^6$ bacteria/g of tissue).

Contaminants of Wounds

Bacteria　Every wound is contaminated to some degree by bacteria. Management of wounds must therefore be considered a practical exercise in bacteriology. There is a key distinction between a wound that is contaminated and one that is infected. Wound contamination refers only to the presence of bacteria, while infection denotes the classical responses to the pathogen. Immediately after bacterial inoculation of a soft-tissue wound, no significant inflammatory response can be detected. At this time, a skilled surgeon can convert a contaminated wound (10^6–10^7) into a clean wound that can be closed safely. In the infected wound, however, primary closure cannot be accomplished without a high risk of failure.

A critical number of bacteria appears to be necessary to elicit infection in soft-tissue wounds. The infective dose of aerobic or facultative bacteria in wounds in healthy tissue is 10^6 bacteria or

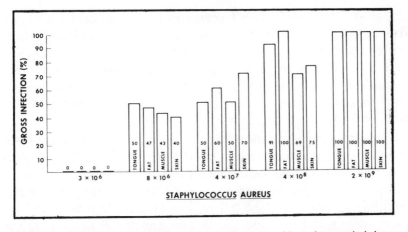

Figure 6.10 Soft tissues in experimental animals were subjected to graded doses of inocula. Four days later, all soft tissue exhibited a remarkable resistance to infection by large numbers of bacteria (3,000,000). In addition, the ability of the different soft tissues to resist infection was roughly comparable.

greater. When aerobic bacterial counts are below this level, the wounds will heal consistently without infection. This remarkable resistance to infection has been identified in all soft tissue tested. In the guinea pig, the ability of tongue, fat, muscle, and skin to resist infection was comparable. Infection in these tissues was only encountered after an inoculation of bacteria numbering greater than 3×10^6 (Fig. 6.10).

Interestingly, the type of obligate aerobic bacteria or facultative species contaminating the wound surface plays a lesser role in the development of infection than does the number of bacteria. For most obligate aerobes or facultative bacteria, infection develops when the number of gram-positive or gram-negative bacteria is 10^6 or greater. The aerobic organisms whose infective dose is 10- to 100-fold greater than 10^6 organisms is the exception rather than the rule. The insignificant role of bacterial virulence of facultative species and obligate aerobes in the development of experimental soft-tissue infection appears to contradict the results of epidemiologic studies of clinical wound infections. In these reports, one specific strain of bacteria is observed to elicit human disease more frequently than another type and is regarded as more virulent. This virulence may be based on ecologic advantages possessed by one microorganism and may not reflect species differences in the host-parasite rela-

385

tionship. The virulence of obligate anaerobic bacteria in soft tissue is dependent on the presence of either aerobic organisms which consume oxygen or compromised host defenses. These anaerobes can then survive and produce tissue injury. When anaerobic organisms are injected into the soft tissue wounds of the uncompromised host (in the absence of dead tissue or foreign body), infection is not encountered.

This important relationship between bacterial counts and clinical wound infection has been a stimulus for the development of quantitative tissue bacteriologic techniques. Measurements are initiated by excising a 2×1 cm sample of tissue that weighs approximately 0.5 g. The biopsy sample is weighed and then suspended in a measured amount of 0.9 percent saline. The tissue can be diced with a knife, but homogenization, using a sterile rotor knife blade is simpler. The homogenate is examined microscopically and quantitative cultures are done for aerobic and anaerobic bacteria. Microscopic examination measures the viable and dead bacteria in the suspension. Results are available to the surgeon within 20 minutes, time enough to influence the surgical decision.

This rapid slide technique gives an accurate and reliable measurement when the specimen contains greater than 2.5×10^5 organisms per g of tissue. Lesser numbers of bacteria are not detectable on microscopic examination. Fortunately, such low levels have little clinical significance. The use of the direct microscopic examination does not replace quantitative serial dilution and plating techniques. These latter techniques are always performed concomitantly with the rapid slide technique since they allow speciation and antibiotic sensitivity testing of the pathogen.

Quantitative bacteriology, consisting of both rapid slide technique as well as serial dilution and plating, is now used routinely by surgeons in our medical center to predict the safety of wound closure (both primary and delayed primary), to determine graft bed receptivity, and to diagnose the onset of burn wound sepsis.

An infective dose of bacteria may be derived from the wounding instrument or from the victim himself. The role of commensal bacteria in the development of infection is a debated issue. Ecologic studies in humans are badly needed. Neglect of this scientific subject has left large gaps in our knowl-

386

edge. Experimentation has focused more on killing the possibly inconsequential numbers of commensal bacteria rather than documenting their role in infection. Obsession with the destruction of bacteria at any cost has disturbing ecologic penalties. The presence of resistant strains of bacteria as a consequence of the use of antimicrobial agents is an illustration.

In the healthy individual, commensal bacteria are localized almost exclusively on the skin and mucous membranes that line all of those cavities and canals of the body that connect with the exterior. These membranes are effective barriers against bacterial invasion.

Microflora of Skin   Different regions of skin contain varied numbers of microorganisms. Differences between regions are more in number than in kind. The predominant organisms encountered on the skin are staphylococci and diphtheroids. These aerobic organisms greatly outnumber strict anaerobes, except in the sebum-rich area, where *Corynebacterium acnes* is prevalent. Gram-negative organisms are scarce on the human skin, residing mainly in the intertriginous regions where they are still out-numbered by the gram-positive bacteria.

Over most of the body surface, bacterial density is quite low, not in millions per cm^2, but more often a few thousand or less. Normally, the organisms are quite sparse on the palms and dorsa of the hands, numbering in the hundreds per cm^2. The majority of organisms (10,000 to 100,000) on the hands reside beneath the distal end of the nail plate, or adjacent to the proximal or lateral nail folds. These recesses frustrate our efforts to disinfect the hands of the surgical team, which are the leading vector of pathogenic bacteria in both the operating surgeon and the surgical nurse. Small numbers of bacteria (400 to 11,000/cm^2) are found on the forearm, a level comparable to that found on thigh, abdominal, or interscapular skin. The hairy axilla, scalp, and perineal regions harbor millions of bacteria.

In most anatomic regions, bacterial colonization is limited to the horny layer of skin that is composed of a sloughing mass of dead cells, full of cracks that harbor bacteria. Beneath this horny layer the stratum corneum, composed of tightly packed cells, provides an effective barrier against bacterial invasion.

The horny layer of pilosebaceous appendages that line the infundibulum of the hair follicle forms a receptacle for bacteria.

However, bacteria rarely descend deeper than the entrance of the sebaceous duct. Similarly, the depths of apocrine glands and sweat glands are devoid of bacteria. Since these organisms reside less than 250μ beneath the surface, they are within reach of topically applied antiseptic agents. *Consequently topical antisepsis can achieve sterility, or near-sterility, in most skin areas of the body.*

Resident bacteria have been identified in unique follicles found in areas that are susceptible to acne: the face, presternum, and upper back. This follicle has been called a sebaceous follicle since the piliary apparatus is a rudimentary structure. Large numbers of gram-positive organisms, mainly *Corynebacterium acnes*, occupy its lumen and are not susceptible to disinfection by topical treatment.

Bacteria applied to the skin disappear rapidly, often in minutes. This apparent "self-disinfecting" property of skin is really a manifestation of desiccation. This same precipitous decline in bacterial count can be observed on inanimate objects such as glass. In contrast, skin hydration encourages bacterial growth. When an occlusive covering is applied to the surface of the skin, a dramatic increase in bacteria is noted. This proliferation may have important clinical implications when wound epidermization is incomplete. *During this time, heavily contaminated skin under occlusive tapes or drapes may be a potential source of infection.*

Microflora of Mucous Membranes   Anaerobes are the predominant organism colonizing the surface of most mucous membranes. The vast majority of investigations of the endogenous microflora of mucous membranes have provided qualitative rather than quantitative data. The relatively few quantitative studies required varied and complex media, extensive identification procedures, special environmental conditions, and fastidious technique. The diverse microflora of some regions, 100 to 300 bacterial strains, defies complete speciation.

RESPIRATORY SYSTEM   Relatively few organisms are recovered from the membranes lining the respiratory passages. The principal habitat of bacteria within the nose is the nasal vestibule, the slightly expanded portion of the nasal cavity beneath the ala. This vestibule is lined by skin and contains some hairs and

388

sebaceous glands, in contrast to the remainder of the nasal cavity which is covered by mucous membrane. Small numbers of facultative aerobes and strict anaerobes are found on the surface of the vestibule. The mucous membrane portion of the nose is often devoid of culturable bacteria. The paranasal sinuses that communicate with the nasal passages are also usually sterile.

The trachea and bronchi in a healthy person are contaminated by few bacteria ($<100/cm^2$). The anatomic relationship of the nasopharynx to the lower airway and the contamination of air which is breathed preclude sterility. However, the self-cleaning action of the respiratory system maintains the tracheobronchial tree relatively free of bacteria.

DIGESTIVE SYSTEM Throughout the human alimentary tract, the types and numbers of bacteria vary considerably. The oral cavity serves as a microbial incubator that supports the growth of facultative species and obligate anaerobes. Concentrations of bacteria within the oral cavity vary widely at different anatomic sites. The pharynx, tongue, buccal mucosa, tooth surfaces, and gingival sulci each have a distinct microflora. The largest numbers of organisms are encountered in the gingival crevices and in plaque on the teeth. The debris removed from the crevices and the plaque on teeth is composed primarily of bacteria in the range of 10^{11} per gram wet weight.

The composite of microorganisms inhabiting the gingival pocket is different from that found in plaque. Plaque contains many facultative streptococci, neisseria, and lactobacilli, while gingival material is composed of large numbers of anaerobic streptococci, Veillonella, *Bacteroides melaninogenicus*, fusobacteria, and spirochetes. The salivary microbial population represents that which has been dislodged from all the oral surfaces consequent to the rinsing of these surfaces by saliva (10^6 bacteria/ml).

Several factors tend to alter the numbers and types of bacteria in the oral cavity; and oral hygiene is one of the most important factors. Good oral hygiene may be defined as a combination of regular and proper use of a toothbrush, periodic removal of calculus and dental plaque by the dentist, and such orthodontic measures as the individual's dentition requires. Under such conditions, the total number of microorganisms in the oral cavity decreases and is predominantly composed of microorganisms tolerant of oxygen. Neglect of oral hygiene results in an increase of the total microbial flora with an anaerobic and putrefactive character. This increase is probably due to an accumulation of food and debris in the gingival sulci and to an increased plaque formation.

The density of the oral microflora changes temporarily during the day. One responsible factor is the flow of saliva which is greater under the stimuli of the waking hours than during the sleeping hours. In contrast, aptyalism, or suppression of salivary secretion, results in an increase in the total microbial population, probably because of the undue accumulation of food debris and the loss of mediating factors inherent in the saliva. The complete loss of teeth will result in a decrease in the total number of oral bacteria in comparison to those with normal dentition or complete dentures.

Most of the oral microflora ingested are destroyed by gastric acid and possibly other factors associated with the mucosa. The stomach is sterile in most fasting individuals. In patients with gastric achlorhydria, bacteria colonization of the stomach with approximately 10^7 organisms per gram of gastric juice is encountered. In normal subjects, the upper small intestine is also virtually free from bacteria except after a meal. Following meals, bacteria number 10^4 or less per ml and usually colonize in the upper bowel (duodenum, jejunum, or upper ileum). This sparse microflora consists mainly of gram-positive organisms that are acid-resistant, i.e., streptococci, aerobic lactobacilli, and fungi. A resident coliform flora has not been demonstrated in this region in normal individuals.

This same microflora without coliforms has been identified in the distal portion of the ileum in one-third of normal individuals. However, the majority of healthy adults exhibit a striking change in the microflora in this area with the appearance of gram-negative microorganisms such as aerobic coliform and anaerobic bacteroides. The concentration of bacteria in the distal portion of the ileum in these people ranges from 10^5 to 10^8 organisms per ml.

The list of diseases associated with heavy contamination of the small bowel is increasing. Bacterial overgrowth appears to be a nonspecific finding in a variety of conditions or illnesses. In patients with induced hypochlorhydria secondary to an

390

ulcer procedure, or primary achlorhydria, an elevated bacterial concentration is encountered in the jejunum. Operative procedures that produce an excessively long afferent loop or denervated segment of bowel provide a fertile area for overgrowth of intestinal bacteria. Elevated bacterial counts are also associated with steatorrhea, diverticula, strictures, and regional enteritis.

Across the ileocecal valve, the numerical proportion of anaerobic bacteria to facultative bacteria increases. In the colon, obligate anaerobes outnumber facultative species such as coliforms by 1,000 to 10,000 to 1. The anerobic organisms—bacteroides, clostridia, and lactobacilli—become the major constituent of luxuriant microbial flora occurring in a concentration of 10^9 for the contents of the intraabdominal colon and 10^{11} per g for the passed feces. Approximately 20 to 30 percent of the wet weight of stool is a solid mass of bacteria, nearly all anaerobes. According to current estimates, the colon harbors more than 200 to 400 distinctive bacterial species. Within a normal individual, the colonic flora is relatively stable so that minimal changes are detectable following periodic stool sampling. In clinical intraabdominal infection following colonic perforation, only a fraction of the normal colonic microflora (an average of five types) is recovered from the site of infection. The factors that account for the survival of these organisms from the infected wound is not completely understood.

Mechanical cleansing of the colon removes gross stool and facilitates the surgical procedure. After only mechanical cleansing, however, the residual contents show the same concentration of both aerobic and anaerobic microorganisms as is found in stool. Many investigators have demonstrated that the addition of antibiotics to the mechanical preparation suppresses the fecal bacteria. This reduction in bacterial count has been associated with a reduced wound infection rate in patients undergoing colonic surgery, as has been confirmed in double-blind, prospective human studies of colonic operations. (For details, see the section on wound healing in the gastrointestinal tract.)

UROGENITAL SYSTEM The urogenital tract in the normal individual is devoid of bacteria except in the vagina, proximal endocervical canal, and the proximal urethra. The vaginal microflora of the premenopausal woman is relatively simple; being composed of an average of five to eight bacterial species that are subject to frequent change. The vaginal microflora includes anaerobic bacteria and aerobic species in concentrations of 10^8 to 10^9. These bacterial counts remain relatively stable until the last premenstrual week at which time the aerobic bacterial counts decrease 100 fold. Anaerobes outnumber aerobic species by 5 to 1. Bacteroides sp., eubacteria, anaerobic lactobacilli, peptococci, and peptostreptococci are the major constituents of the anaerobic microflora. *Bacteroides fragilis* is seldom found in the vaginal flora, although it is frequently identified as the pathogen in infections of the upper female genital tract. In such cases, the source of this organism may be the bowel.

The predominant aerobic bacteria are corynebacteria, *Staphylococcus albus*, lactobacilli, and nonhemolytic streptococci which tolerate the low vaginal pH which is hormonally controlled. *E. coli* is encountered rarely (10 percent) in the vaginal vestibule. When noted, it is recovered in small numbers for short periods of time. These same organisms found in the vagina are also observed in the urethra, but the colony counts are considerably lower ($< 10^3$). High concentrations of vaginal bacteria are present in healthy women until menopause, at which time a sparse microflora and alkaline secretions return.

Diptheroids, *S. albus*, and streptococci (including enterococci) comprise the bulk of the urethral flora of the normal adult male and are encountered in small numbers, usually 1,000 bacteria/ml of urine. Gram-negative enteric bacteria are rare. Thousands of gram-negative bacteria can reside under the uncircumcised foreskin, even though it is easily retractable and visibly clean. Stamey indicates that these foreskin bacteria can be a major source of confusion in localizing the site of infection in the lower urinary tract.

SUMMARY Some regions of the healthy human body contain enough organisms to cause infection. Such heavily contaminated sites include the hairy scalp, axillary and perineal skin, foreskin, nails, mouth, ileum, colon, and vagina. When planning for surgical procedures in these sites, preoperative suppression of the microbiota is essential. Strict adherence to aseptic technique is mandatory to minimize the spread of the endogenous contaminants. In the remaining regions, the microbiota of the healthy individual are usually sparse. However, damage to the host's defenses can change these bacteriologic deserts into teeming jungles of pathogens. The host's defenses can be impaired by a large number of factors, one of which is a foreign body.

Foreign Bodies Foreign bodies in traumatic soft-tissue wounds consist mainly of soil and its contaminants. In missile injuries, clothing and missile fragments are also encountered. Until recently, interest in soil as a wound contaminant has stemmed primarily from the military surgeon's concern over its microorganisms that elicit disease in man. Prophylaxis and management of tetanus and gas gangrene and diseases caused by the soil microflora, have been the subject of many chapters in the history of military surgery. Although it has been recognized for centuries that severe bacterial infection often develops in dirty wounds, there has been little knowledge of the role of nonviable soil components in this infection process.

Soil has four major components: inorganic minerals, organic matter, water, and air. The major component of most soils is inorganic minerals. Typically, the organic content of soils ranges from 1 to 7 percent and is restricted primarily to topsoils. Environmental conditions in swamps, bogs, and marshes encourage the production of soil with as much as 98 percent organic content. This organic component is chemically very reactive as evidenced by its high cation exchange capacity.

The mineral, or inorganic, components of soil vary in size and composition and can be classified according to their particle size (Table 6.2). The coarser components of soil are stone, gravel, and sand. The diameter of the individual stone and

Table 6.2 Three Major Ion Classes of Inorganic Soil Particles

Soil Separate	Visible Using	Size Diameter Limits (mm)
Sand	Naked eye	0.02–2.0
Silt	Microscope	0.002–0.02
Clay	Electron microscope	<0.002

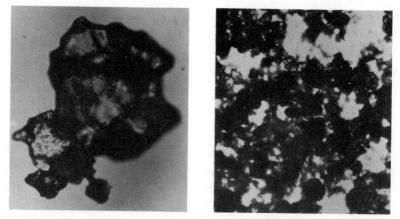

A   B

Figure 6.11 The IPF in inorganic soil reside in the clay fraction which cannot be detected by a light microscope. The larger particles (silt, sand) in inorganic soil are relatively innocuous to the local tissue defenses. **A.** Cecil sand grain–quartz (80×). **B.** Cecil silt (100×).

gravel particles is usually greater than 2 mm. Sand grains vary in size from 0.02 to 2.00 mm and may be rounded or irregular. (Fig. 6.11). These fractions of soil with a large particle size have a relatively small surface area and low level of chemical reactivity. Silt particles, smaller in size than sand, tend to be irregular and diverse in size and shape and are best visualized by a light microscope. There surface area and chemical reactivity are three to four times greater than that of sand.

The smallest inorganic particle in soil is clay, which is not detected by a light microscope. Due to their small size and crystalline structure, clay particles expose a large external surface. In addition, expanding clay minerals have large internal surfaces as well which add to their chemical reactivity and to their ability to damage tissue defenses.

Sterilized samples of topsoil and subsoil, consisting mainly of inorganic matter, potentiate infections. Only 100 bacteria are necessary to elicit purulent discharge from wounds contaminated by 5 mg of either sterile topsoil or subsoil. The fractions that exhibit the greatest capacity to potentiate infection are the clay and organic components. Clay carries a negative charge. Likewise, the organic particle is a highly charged anion that is

394

surrounded by adsorbed cations. Large quantities of cations are dumped into the wound as a result of the addition of these soil infection-potentiating fractions (IPF).

As a result of this cation exchange, the host's defenses are damaged. Soil IPF directly impair leukocytes' ability to ingest and kill bacteria. Soil IPFs also have considerable impact on nonspecific immune mechanisms. Exposure of fresh serum to IPFs eliminates its bactericidal activity without damaging serum opsonins. We have found no way to neutralize the effects of soil IPFs in the wound. Therefore, therapeutic measures should be directed at removing the soil from the wound.

TECHNICAL FACTORS

The surgeon makes judgments that frequently tip the balance in favor of either infection or healing *per primam*. Clinical and experimental studies have provided evidence of the influence of some surgical decisions on the fate of the wound. Based upon them, we can make some specific recommendations.

Local Anesthesia

Local anesthesia ensures the patient's comfort and aids in wound management. *Cleaning of bacteria, soil, and other debris from traumatic injuries, and surgical debridement of infected wounds, cannot be accomplished without anesthesia.*

The ideal anesthetic agent should have rapid onset of action locally with few or no adverse systemic effects. It should not impair the wound's ability to resist infection. This is particularly important in traumatic wounds contaminated with moderate numbers of bacteria. Any further inhibition of tissue defenses will predispose the wound to infection. The effect of the local anesthetic agent on the viability of microorganisms is another important consideration. In infected wounds, an antimicrobial agent may kill the cultured pathogen and interfere with its identification.

Lidocaine hydrochloride is the most commonly employed local anesthetic agent. Loss of sensation occurs within five minutes and lasts for 97 to 156 minutes. This agent displays no antimicrobial activity, and does not damage the local wound defenses. The clinical usefulness of lidocaine can be enhanced by adding the hemostatic agent, epinephrine. Epinephrine is a potent vasoconstrictor that overcomes the vasodilatory effects of lidocaine. The reduction in blood flow induced by epinephrine limits the clearance of the anesthetic agent from the tissue, thus prolonging the duration of anesthesia. As a result, the toxic dose of lidocaine solutions containing epinephrine for local wound infiltration (7 mg/kg, not to exceed 500 mg total) is considerably higher than for the same anesthetic solution without epinephrine (4.5 mg/kg, not to exceed 300 mg). However, the beneficial effect of epinephrine must be weighed against its serious side effects of hypertension, cardiac arrhythmias, and cerebral hemorrhage. Another disturbing side effect of epinephrine is its damage to the local wound defenses. This powerful

Figure 6.12 Soft tissues in experimental animals were subjected to *S. aureus* suspended in either 0.9 percent saline or an aqueous solution of epinephrine. In concentrations of either 1:30,000 (3.3 μg) or 1:100,000 (1μg), epinephrine potentiated the development of infection in soft tissues.

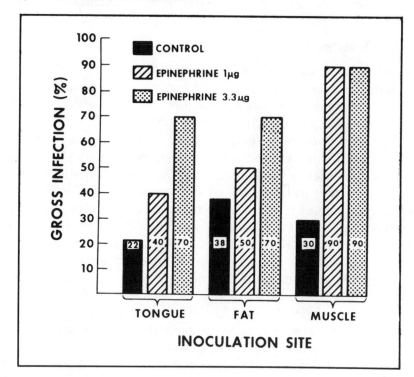

local vasoconstrictor potentiates infection proportional to its concentration (Fig. 6.12).

This damage to tissue defenses mitigates against the use of epinephrine in potentially heavily contaminated wounds like those encountered in traumatic injuries. In these cases, we employ 1 percent lidocaine without epinephrine. The agent is injected through a No. 27 guage needle either through the skin at the wound periphery or preferably as a regional nerve block. Injections through the cut edge of the wound may be less painful than through needles inserted into the adjacent skin but serve to disseminate bacteria throughout uninvolved tissue around the contaminated wound and, in theory, should be avoided. In clean straight lacerations in children, the reduced pain associated with injections into the wound outweighs the risk of infection.

Hair Removal

Although its origins are obscure, shaving has become a routine part of preoperative preparation. However, preoperative shaving has been challenged in recent studies.

In a prospective clinical study, Seropian and Reynolds reported that the infection rate of surgical patients after razor preparation was 5.6 percent as compared to 0.6 percent after a depilatory. These findings agree with those reported by Cruse and Foord. In a five-year prospective study of 23,649 surgical wounds, the infection rate was 2.3 percent in the patients who were shaved. The incidence of infection fell to 0.9 percent in the patients who were not shaved or clipped.

The increased incidence of infection following razor preparation is probably related to the trauma inflicted by the razor. A razor used to shave the skin of surgical patients consists of a blade held in a fixed geometry by the razor head. The exposure of the blade with respect to the razor head is the most important determinant of the blade's performance (Fig. 6.13). If the blade is recessed, the blade will cut the hairs considerably above their infundibula. Extension of the blade beyond the razor head will cut the hair close to the skin. Using the terminology of the advertising media, this is a "close shave." The exposure of the surgical prep razor blade (0.0087 in) is so great

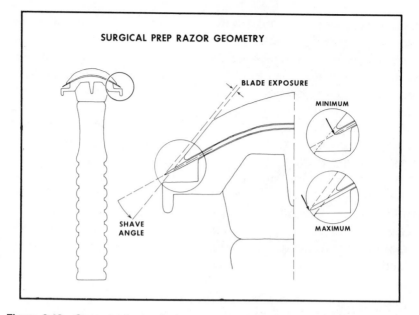

Figure 6.13 Geometry for surgical prep razors. If the blade exposure is minimal, the blade will cut the hairs above their infundibula. The infundibulum of the hair follicle is transected when the blade is exposed maximally beyond the razor head.

that the infundibulum of the hair follicle is transected. As a result of the shave, the wounded hair follicles provide access and substrate for bacteria. Inoculation of shaved skin results in dermatitis. In contrast, skin shaved with a recessed blade is refractory to bacterial contamination.

On the basis of these findings, *hair removal should be employed only when it is anticipated that hair will interfere with performance of the procedure.* In these cases, clipping the hair with scissors or shaving the skin with a razor containing a recessed blade is recommended.

Antisepsis

A wound which has been irrigated with solutions of carbolic acid, corrosive sublimate, or other disinfectant labors under the disadvantage of a more or less extensive area of superficial necrosis.

William S. Halsted, 1890–1891

There is still confusion and misunderstanding of the definition of the term *antisepsis.* The literal translation from Greek is

398

"against putrefaction." In present usage, *antisepsis* refers to the use of antimicrobial chemicals on human tissue, while "disinfection" applies to the employment of these agents on inanimate objects. Surgical scrub solutions contain an antiseptic agent as well as a detergent, or surface active agent. These latter components facilitate removal of surface contaminants by reducing the surface tension between them and the tissue or skin surface.

The clinical efficacy of an antiseptic agent can be evaluated by several parameters. First, the effect of storage on the agent's antimicrobial activity must be appreciated. If it is rapidly inactivated during storage, the antiseptic agent must be freshly prepared prior to use. Second, the agent's spectrum of activity must be understood. Ideally, it must exhibit antimicrobial activity against a broad spectrum of organisms. If the agent is active only against gram-positive organisms, topical treatment of contaminated tissue may result in a potentially harmful shift of the normal flora. The widespread use of antimicrobials acting only against gram-positive organisms is associated with a tremendous increase in gram-negative infections in hospitals. Third, the duration of antimicrobial activity subsequent to contact with living tissues must be recognized. Ideally, the agent should be fast-acting and substantive. A substantive effect is due to the retention of the agent by binding to a tissue (e.g., *stratum corneum*) after rinsing. Bound antiseptic agent limits the proliferation of the residual bacteria. Fourth, the degree to which the agent damages the host, both locally and systemically, must also be known.* Finally, the influence of the vehicle or carrier (i.e., surfactant or detergent) on the performance of the antiseptic agent is important. Inactivation of cationic surface active agents by anionic surface agents is a case in point.

Not all antiseptic agents are used for the same purpose, nor should the requirements for their effectiveness be identical. Specific definitions for the antimicrobial product categories were established in a report by the Advisory Review Panel on over-the-counter (OTC) antimicrobial drug products for repeated daily human use. This report, submitted to the Food and Drug Commission on July 24, 1974, provides detailed in-

*Paracelsus (1493–1541) wrote: "All things are poisons, for there is nothing without poisonous qualities. It is only the dose which makes a thing a poison."

formation regarding patient preoperative skin preparations, surgical hand scrubs, and surgical wound cleansers.

Skin Wound Cleansers   A product in this category is designed to remove bacterial and other contaminants from superficial wounds by its cleansing activity. Such a product may or may not contain an antimicrobial agent. While cleansing the wound, the agent must not damage the tissues or their systemic defenses, or deter healing.

Dilute solutions (1:750) of quaternary ammonium salts ("quats") satisfy many of these requirements. These compounds are cationic surface active agents which are, basically, organically substituted ammonium compounds. "Quats" and other surface antibacterials have been shown to affect cell membrane potential, the consequences of which are clinically apparent at higher concentrations than those recommended for clinical use. Their spectrum of antimicrobial activity is limited. Gram-positive microorganisms are generally more susceptible to these compounds than gram-negative bacteria. The gram-negative pseudomonas species are usually resistant to "quats" and even proliferate in the stored antimicrobial solution, accounting for occasional serious outbreaks of gram-negative infection.

In contrast, the commercially available surgical scrub solutions containing iodophors and hexachlorophene are not safe for use in surgical wounds. These solutions contain toxic anionic detergents that damage the tissue defenses and potentiate the development of infection. Contaminated experimental wounds subjected to a topical treatment with these scrub solutions developed more infections than wounds subjected to 0.9 percent saline. Until this observation was made, detergents and surfactants in surgical scrub solutions were considered by many scientists to be innocuous ingredients.

Pluronic polyol F-68, a nonionic surfactant, is an excellent substitute for those toxic detergents. This surfactant is a member of a family of surfactants, which are made of a series of block copolymers that consist of a water-soluble polyoxyethylene group at both ends of a water-insoluble polyoxypropylene chain. Pluronic polyol F-68, with a molecular weight of 8,350 and ethylene oxide content of 80 percent is safe for human use. The successful use of this polyol as an emulsifying

400

agent for fat emulsions administered intravenously in human subjects lends support to this contention. Similarly, concentrated solutions containing as much as 40 percent Pluronic polyol F-68, when applied topically to open wounds, do not impair resistance to infection. The effect of this surfactant on bacterial viability is also negligible. While Pluronic polyol F-68 does not exhibit any intrinsic antibacterial activity, it will form stable soluble complexes with elemental iodine that possesses antimicrobial capability.

Patient Preoperative Skin Preparation The "ideal" agent for preoperative skin disinfection must be a safe, fast acting, broad spectrum antimicrobial preparation which significantly reduces the number of microorganisms on intact skin, usually following a single application. The most commonly employed antimicrobial agents for wound cleansing are iodophors. These compounds are composed of complexes of iodine that are more stable than iodine in aqueous solution. Iodine is recognized to be a broad spectrum anti-microbial with activity against fungi and viruses as well as gram-positive and gram-negative bacteria.

There are three general preparations of iodine presently in clinical use: (1) solubilized inorganic elemental iodine, such as tincture of iodine, (2) iodine complexed with various surfactant compounds, and (3) iodine complexed with different nonsurfactant compounds like polyvinylpyrrolidone (PVP). In tincture of iodine, all of the iodine is in the free form and is available for instantaneous reaction with both bacteria and other proteinaceous or carbohydrate material. If the iodine solution does not eliminate all the bacteria within these first few seconds, no further significant bacterial kill will be observed since there is no residual activity. This instantaneous availability of iodine accounts for the skin irritation occasionally encountered following topical treatment with this solution. The local toxic manifestation of tincture of iodine necessitates that its use be limited to painting the operative site. It should be restricted from use on open wounds.

The availability of free iodine can be limited by complexing it with either a surfactant, such as a Pluronic polyol, or a protein like PVP. The iodine in these complexes is in dynamic equilibrium between a "complexed" form and a "free" form. Highly

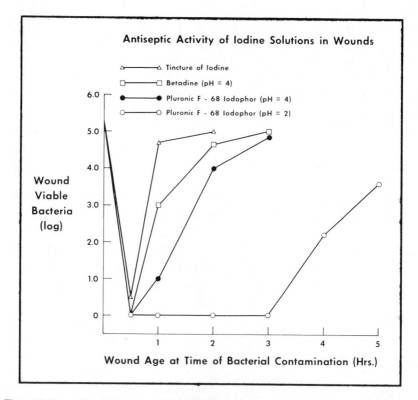

Figure 6.14 Antiseptic activity of iodine solutions in wounds. Standardized experimental wounds were subjected to a topical treatment with different antiseptic agents. At specified times after treatment, the wounds were subjected to repetitive bacterial challenges after which the wound was recultured. The tincture and aqueous iodine solutions were inactivated within 60 minutes, thus losing their antibacterial activity. The antiseptic activity of Pluronic polyol F-68 iodophor persisted the longest.

complexed iodine compounds are very stable, do not stain, have no odor, and are considerably less irritating to tissues than tincture of iodine. Although the level of free iodine is low, it is still highly effective in killing bacteria.

After contact with the wound, such complexes release iodine slowly, resulting in prolonged activity (Fig. 6. 14). Iodine release occurs only when the steady state level of free iodine is depleted by the reaction with the contaminating substance. The parameters of greatest importance to this reaction are concentration of surfactant, amount of iodine, concentration of iodide, and pH of the final solution.

In developing a highly complexed iodophor, the selection of

the protein, or surfactant, to solubilize the iodine is critical. For use in human subjects, Pluronic polyol F-68 has many distinct advantages. Long-term toxicity studies have indicated that it is safe. When it complexes with iodine, the chemical structure of Pluronic polyol F-68 appears to be unchanged since the reaction is easily reversible. In contrast, a significant portion of the PVP binds irreversibly to iodine. PVP reacts with iodine to form carbon-iodine bonds and iodide. The exact nature and toxicity of this new polymeric compound(s) have not been determined.

PVP has had other applications in clinical medicine. German experience at the Russian front in World War II established the effectiveness of PVP in the treatment of shock. About this time it was demonstrated that 35 to 49 percent of the PVP was retained indefinitely in the body after intravenous infusion. This finding stimulated study of the deleterious effects associated with the storage phenomenon.

Numerous clinical reports have noted the formation of cutaneous lesions after the administration of PVP. Although the lesions are not precancerous, they do result in considerable cosmetic deformity. The cutaneous storage phenomenon encountered after the systemic administration of PVP reflects the kidney's inability to excrete molecular weight fractions of PVP greater than 40,000 daltons. Since some of the commercially available PVP iodophors, like Betadine, *do* contain molecular weight fractions greater than 40,000, it would seem prudent to restrict their use to the surface of intact skin. Furthermore, topical application of this iodophor over a large surface area may result in a substantial elevation of serum iodide which is associated with renal failure, metabolic acidosis, and elevation of serum glutamic oxaloacetic transaminase. It is conceivable that those large iodide loads could be, at least in part, responsible for these abnormalities.

Despite of these potential toxic manifestations of PVP-I complexes, many surgeons have continued to apply these agents to contaminated wounds with surprisingly good results. Gilmore and his colleagues have made well controlled studies of the efficacy of PVP-I powders in the treatment of contaminated wounds. In a series of 451 consecutive cases of appendicectomy, topical PVP-I treatment reduced the wound infection rate and was found to be superior to an antiseptic spray.

These beneficial effects of PVP-I in the treatment of contaminated wounds was later reported by Stokes in a prospective randomized study of abdominal surgical patients.

Surgical Hand Scrubs

Rubber gloves must, of course, be worn by all concerned in the operation.
William S. Halsted, 1913

Handwashing before and after contact with a patient is mandatory. Washing one's hands with any of a wide variety of agents, including tap water, removes large numbers of bacteria and successfully reduces the bacterial count. Handwashing prior to donning sterile gloves should be performed with an antiseptic agent that limits the proliferation of bacteria under the occlusive gloves.

The degree to which bacteria proliferate beneath gloves is related in part to the condition of the skin. The microflora of skin afflicted with dermatitis is considerably greater than that of normal skin without inflammation. This elevated skin bacterial count becomes a threat to the patient once the surgeon's glove is punctured. It is certainly prudent to restrict members of the operating team from donning surgical gloves until their dermatitis disappears. Frequently, abstinence from washing their hands with irritating surgical scrub solutions will be the most rapid remedy for the skin condition.

The use of surgical antiseptics on the physician's examining fingers dates back to Semmelweis in 1861. He decreased the incidence of puerpural fever in the obstetric ward by ordering hand washing in chlorinated lime before examining patients. Lister later degermed his hands as well as the operative site and instruments in a 1:20 solution of carbolic acid. Until the 1950s tincture of green soap followed by an alcohol rinse was employed.

Recently, several new antiseptic-detergent solutions have been advocated for surgical hand washes. The antiseptic agents in these new scrub solutions include hexachlorophene, iodophor, and chlorhexidine. For hexachlorophene (3 percent), the potential threat of toxicity seems to outweigh its potential benefits. Surgical scrubs of hands and forearms of adults, five times a day, with a 3 percent hexachlorophene preparation leave levels of 0.5 mg/ml or higher in selected individuals after

404

10 days. Since these levels are considered potentially toxic, the use of hexachlorophene should be limited.

Fortunately, other solutions appear to be safe for human use as surgical hand scrubs. Following hand wash with iodophor or chlorhexidine solutions, the bacterial counts of the skin are suppressed and the buildup of microbial counts under the glove is limited. However, the superiority of one scrub solution over another is difficult to ascertain from the few comprehensive clinical studies completed to date.

Surgical Debridement

Debridment has been considered by many surgeons to be the most important single factor in the management of the contaminated wound. This time-honored technique has two notable benefits. First, it removes tissue heavily contaminated by bacteria and soil IPFs, protecting the patient from invasive infection. Second, it removes permanently devitalized tissues.

All devitalized soft tissue that is left in a wound damages its defenses and encourages the development of infection. The capacities of devitalized fat, muscle, and skin to enhance bacterial infection are about equal. The infection-potentiating effect of damaged skin is further enhanced by exposing it to a dry thermal injury. This observation is consistent with the experimental findings of Algower and Schoenberger who identified a toxin in skin subjected to dry heat. This toxin appears to be generated by a polymeric dehydration of a substance(s) naturally occurring in the skin.

There are at least three mechanisms by which devitalized soft tissue enhances infection. First, *it acts as a culture medium promoting bacterial growth.* Second, *it inhibits leukocyte migration, phagocytosis,* and *subsequent bacterial kill.* Third, *the anaerobic environment within devitalized tissue must also limit leukocyte function.* (At low oxygen tension, the killing of certain bacteria by leukocytes is markedly impaired.)

While the need for debridement of devitalized tissue is undisputed, identification of the exact limits of devitalized tissue in wounds remains a challenging problem, especially in muscle. Determination of the viability of muscle is often difficult, even for the most experienced surgeon. Some surgeons judge viability of muscle at operation primarily by its contractility;

some place greater emphasis on the ability of muscle to bleed; while others judge the condition of muscle on its color and consistency. *There is sufficient clinical evidence to show that muscle is viable if it contracts after being stimulated.* Color is of doubtful value in determining the viability of muscle. These clinical indicators of muscle viability are most accurate when the wound is examined four to five days after the initial operation.

The viability of skin is considerably easier to judge than that of muscle. At 24 hours after injury, a sharp line of demarcation is often apparent between the devitalized and viable skin. In fresh skin wounds in which this demarcation is not precise, the distribution of an intravenously injected fluorescein dye within the tissues may prove helpful. Early staining of the injured tissue by fluorescein is evidence of tissue viability. At times, active bleeding from the distal dermal margin may be present and indicates viability.

In some anatomic sites, like the trunk, debridement is best accomplished by more complete excision of the skin and deep tissues. In these areas, the soft tissue may be free of critical tissues such as nerves or tendons that perform important physical functions. In these regions, heavily contaminated wounds with serpiginous defects can be converted into clean wounds by generous tissue excisions.

The adequacy of debridement may be monitored by forcibly packing the wound with gauze (Fig. 6.15A) or by coloring the wound surface with a vital dye (Fig. 6.15B). Complete excision of the wound, back to a margin of normal tissue, is judged by dissecting in a plane that will not expose the gauze or the blue dye. Suturing the skin edges of the wound prior to excision may further minimize mechanical spread of the wound contaminants into uninjured tissue.

When a heavily contaminated wound contains specialized tissues, such as nerves or tendons, complete excision often is not feasible. In such cases, high-pressure irrigation, followed by excision of all fragments of tissue that are not clearly viable, is indicated. In a compound wound of the hand, selective debridement of nonviable fascia, tendon, fat, and so on, is tedious but still essential.

A specific exception to the general principle of removing *all* devitalized tissue is made in treating specialized tissues that perform important physical functions, regardless of viability.

406

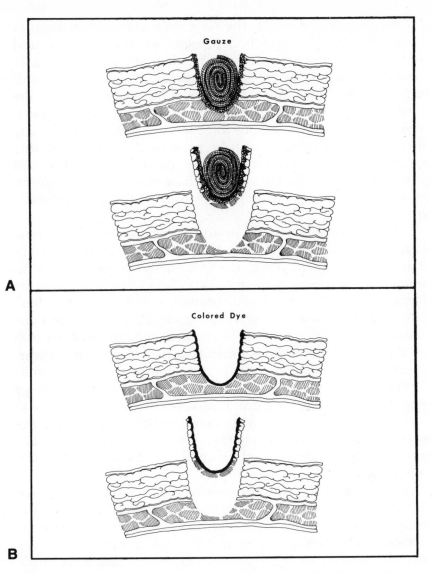

Figure 6.15 Monitoring the adequacy of debridement by forcibly packing the wound with gauze (A) or by coloring the wound surface with a vital dye (B).

Tissues like dura, fascia, and tendon may survive as free grafts without living cells if immediately covered by healthy pedicle flaps. Cells from the wound may then invade the graft as part of the healing process. If these tissues can be rendered surgically clean, they should be left in the wound.

Following debridement, the surgeon's ultimate selection of wound closure technique is dependent on the level of wound contamination and the amount of residual devitalized tissue. In wounds contacted by gross pus or feces, an infective dose of bacteria will often remain on the wound surface despite the most aggressive wound cleaning. If primary closure of such wounds is attempted, serious infection will usually follow. The development of infection can be prevented by subjecting the wounds to *delayed* primary closure. As the wound heals, it gains increased resistance to infection permitting closure on or after the fourth postwounding day without subsequent infection.

For high velocity missile injuries, the magnitude of tissue damage is extensive and difficult to ascertain accurately soon after injury. In these cases, the wound should be explored to remove foreign bodies, to rule out the presence of vascular damage, and to relieve closed compartment pressure that may follow edema or slow bleeding into a muscle compartment enclosed by unyielding fascia. The removal of devitalized tissue is advisable, but in practice is difficult as its definition is unclear. Open wound management is the method of choice with subsequent additional debridement as dictated by the appearance of the wound. An open wound gains considerable resistance to infection on or after the fourth postwounding day. By then, the wound usually contains less than 10^6 bacteria per g of tissue and if it is free of devitalized tissue, delayed primary closure is indicated.

Civilian traumatic wounds resulting from impact injuries or low velocity missiles usually contain devitalized tissue that is easily recognizable by the experienced surgeon. *Debridement, cleansing, and antiobiotic treatment will usually convert these wounds into clean wounds which are amenable to primary closure* by either direct approximation of the wound edges, or by coverage with a flap or graft. There is minimal risk of infection, and significant reduction in the morbidity that results from the use of any method of delayed wound closure.

Mechanical Cleansing

Commonly, surgeons mechanically rid the wound of adherent bacteria and other adherent particulate matter. Mechanical forces must exceed the adhesiveness of the contaminants. The two basic methods employed to cleanse wounds are hydraulic force and direct contact.

In irrigation, the hydraulic pressure of the irrigating stream dislodges the contaminant. The fluid pressure acting on a particle is caused by momentum transfer when the fluid hits the particle's front surface. Following impact, the fluid flows around the particle moving it in the direction of the stream.

The total force component exerted on the particle by the moving stream is defined as "drag." The total drag due to the fluid pressure and stress is expressed by the following equation:

$$\text{Drag} = CA\rho \frac{V^2}{2}$$

where C is an experimentally derived drag coefficient dependent in part on the configuration of the particle; A is the projected area of the particle on a plane perpendicular to flow; ρ is the density of the fluid; and V is the relative velocity of the fluid with respect to the particle.

The magnitude of the hydraulic force is a function of its relative velocity as well as of the configuration of the particle. When subjected to the same irrigating stream, particles with a smaller surface area will experience *less* force than particles with a similar configuration but with a greater surface area. Consequently, it takes significantly smaller hydraulic forces to rid the wound of large foreign bodies than it does to remove bacteria.

The hydraulic force exerted on the particle will increase as the velocity of the irrigating stream is raised. The simplest and most practical methods of raising the velocity are to increase the pressure within the irrigating syringe and to enlarge the internal diameter of the orifice. The maximum pressure varies with the size of the syringe. Small syringes (5, 12 ml) are clinically impractical since delivery of large volumes of fluid would require an extended irrigation time. Therefore, the preferred method is to use a larger bore needle which generates a significantly greater pressure at a surface than fluid delivered through a small bore needle.

The pressure exerted by fluid delivered through a 19 gauge needle by a 35 ml syringe under hand pressure is 8 psi. Irrigation pressure of this magnitude or higher has been classified "high pressure" while irrigation pressure below this level, as with a bulb syringe, has been designated as "low pressure." These definitions have important clinical implications. High pressure irrigation successfully cleanses the wound of small particulate matter, bacteria, and soil. As a result of this cleansing, the infection rate of experimentally contaminated wounds is reduced (Fig. 6. 16). In contrast, low pressure syringe irrigation, even with large volumes of fluid, has negligible capability to remove small particles and has little measurable therapeutic effect except in wounds containing large particulate matter.

Despite the advantage of high pressure irrigation, several theoretical objections have been raised against the routine use of this technique. One commonly expressed concern is that foreign bodies on the surface of the wound may be disseminated more deeply into the wound as a result of high pressure irrigation. On the basis of recent experimental studies, this fear appears to be unrealized. Consequent to high pressure irrigation, the bacteria remain at the surface of the wound even though the irrigant solution may disseminate deeply into the tissues. The tissue penetration of a high pressure irrigating stream is predominantly in a lateral direction similar to that encountered with a jet parenteral injection.

However, concern that high pressure irrigation can damage tissue defenses appears to be justified. Pulsatile or syringe irrigation results in trauma to the tissues that makes the wound more susceptible to experimental infection. This finding serves to remind the surgeon that high pressure irrigation should not be performed indiscriminately, but should be reserved for special use in heavily contaminated wounds. In such wounds, the benefits of this cleansing technique outweigh its consequences, frequently resulting in a marked decrease in the number of bacteria and uncomplicated healing of the wound without clinical infection.

In the clinical setting, high pressure irrigation is accomplished with an inexpensive disposable irrigation assembly consisting of a 19 gauge plastic needle attached to a 35 ml syringe (Fig. 6.17). Sterile electrolyte solution (usually 250 ml of 0.9 percent sodium chloride) is delivered through a one-way valve attached to the syringe barrel via standard intravenous plastic tubing. The tip of the needle, attached to the syringe

410

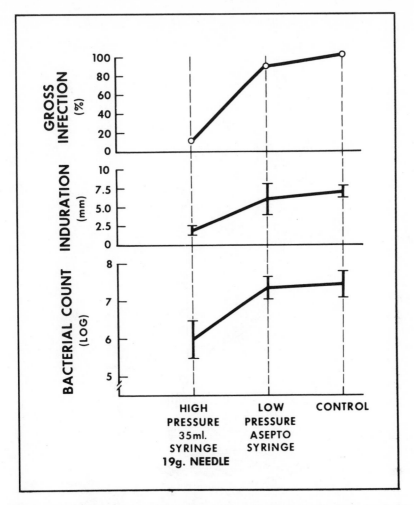

Figure 6.16 Standardized experimental wounds contaminated with similar level of inocula were subjected to either high- or low-pressure irrigation or no treatment prior to closure. Four days later, the inflammatory responses (gross infection, induration) of wounds subjected to high pressure irrigation were significantly less than those of the control wounds or of wounds treated by low pressure irrigation.

filled with saline, is placed perpendicular, and as close as possible, to the surface of the wound; then the surgeon exerts maximal force to the syringe plunger delivering the irrigant to the wound.

Another force often employed by surgeons to cleanse a wound is direct mechanical contact, for example, scrubbing a

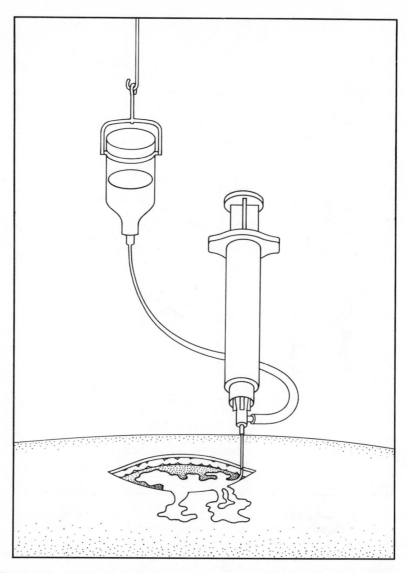

Figure 6.17 High-pressure syringe irrigation assembly. Note that the needle is held as close as possible and perpendicular to the irrigated wound.

dirty wound with a sponge. This technique has proven to be an effective means of removing bacteria from wounds. Unfortunately, despite this benefit, scrubbing the wound with a saline-soaked sponge does not decrease the incidence of infection.

Tissue trauma inflicted by the sponge impairs the wound's

ability to resist infection and allows the residual bacteria to elicit an inflammatory response. The magnitude of the damage to the local tissue resistance is correlated with the porosity of the sponge. Sponges with a low porosity are more abrasive and exert more damage to the wound than do sponges with a higher porosity. The addition of a nontoxic surfactant, such as Pluronic polyol F-68, minimizes tissue damage while maintaining the efficacy of mechanical cleansing. Consequently, use of a surfactant-soaked sponge reduces the incidence of infection in contaminated wounds in experimental animals.

Antibiotics

In laboratory and clinical studies, antibiotic therapy is significantly more effective when the drug is given preoperatively rather than intraoperatively or postoperatively. Delay in antibiotic treatment consistently diminishes its therapeutic merit. When there is an unavoidable delay in administering these drugs, the length of time during which the open wound is exposed plays an important role. As a result of this exposure, a sequence of events occurs that substantially limits the therapeutic value of antibiotics. Insight into the dynamics of these events has been derived from histologic, biochemical, and physiologic measurements that compare primarily closed wounds with open wounds subjected to delayed primary closure.

When any wound is left open, there is a marked increase in vascular permeability. Fluids from the intravascular space extravasate and fill the wound crater. The exudate is rich in a wide variety of proteins, including fibrin. Once outside the vessels, the protein exudate is slowly reabsorbed by the lymphatics, except fibrinogen that partly polymerizes to form fibrin. We believe that the resulting fibrinous coagulum surrounds the bacteria and protects them from contact with any antibiotic that was not already present in the exudate.

The cause of the exaggerated inflammatory response that is seen in exposed wounds has not been defined. However, it may be partly related to environmental conditions. The temperature of the operating theater is usually considerably below the systemic body temperature, encouraging loss of heat from the wound. In addition, evaporation of fluid from the wound surface results in further heat loss and cooling of the tissues.

413

Another consequence of fluid loss from the wound is dessication. Warming the operating theater or covering the wound with wet sponges should reduce these environmental effects.

Paradoxically, the fibrinous wound coagulum that limits the effectiveness of antibiotics may be a crucial positive factor later in the host's defense against infection. The coagulum may serve as a plug in the open mouths of lymphatics preventing dissemination of bacteria and systemic sepsis.

This surface coagulum may be disrupted by a variety of mechanisms. Gentle scrubbing of the surface of the wound with a gauze sponge disturbs the fibrinous cover and allows an antibiotic to gain intimate contact with the bacteria. Consequently, the therapeutic effectiveness of antibiotics is measurably enhanced by this treatment if there is a blood level of antibiotic present at the time of scrubbing.

Enzymatic digestion is a less traumatic and more selective means of disrupting the coagulum. The in vitro fibrinolytic capacity of certain enzymes provides an accurate measure of their ability to potentiate antimicrobial activity. Travase (a proteolytic enzyme produced by *Bacillus subtilis,* the most potent fibrinolytic agent in vitro) is the most effective enzymatic adjunct to antibiotic treatment. Hydrolysis of the protein coagulum can be accomplished within 30 minutes by the topical application of an appropriate aqueous solution of this proteolytic enzyme. Such a brief exposure does not damage either the wound's defenses or its healing capacity.

Finally, the bacterial count of the wound can influence the outcome of antibiotic treatment. When the wound is contaminated by exceedingly large numbers of organisms (greater than 10^9), infection will develop despite antibiotic treatment (Fig. 6.18). This circumstance is encountered when the wound surface is contacted by either pus or feces. In such clinical situations, primary closure of the wound should be avoided. Delayed primary closure should be considered only on or after the fourth day postwounding, at which time the wound will have gained considerable resistance to infection.

The indications for antibiotic treatment of a traumatic wound will depend on the mechanism(s) of injury, the wound's inflammatory response, and the total bacterial count. The mechanism of injury in most traumatic wounds is a shear force secondary to a knife or a piece of glass. Fortunately, these

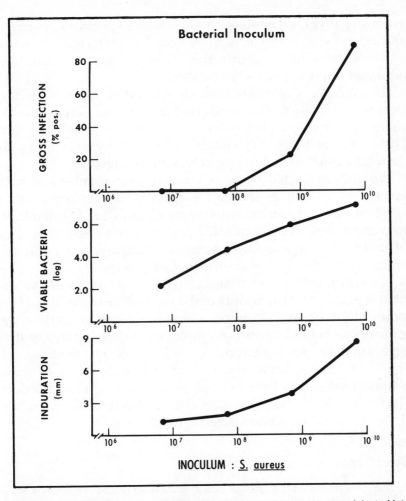

Figure 6.18 Graded doses of a penicillin-sensitive strain of *S. aureus* were injected into the dermis of experimental animals. Immediately after inoculation each animal received an intraperitoneal injection of benzylpenicillin (1,000,000 u). Four days later, the inflammatory responses of the wounds and their bacterial counts were measured. The therapeutic value of antibiotic treatment decreased as the dose of inocula increased.

wounds exhibit a remarkable resistance to infection. One million bacteria or greater are needed to elicit infection. This high level of contamination is rare in shear wounds and such high counts can be detected easily by rapid slide quantitative bacterial counts. Since these wounds are usually contaminated by mixtures of facultative organisms (both gram-positive and gram-negative), an antibiotic with a broad spectrum of activity should be employed if a high count is detected. In shear wounds containing subinfective doses of bacteria, antibiotic administration is not recommended.

An antibiotic is often indicated for penetrating wounds resulting from impact injuries. The weakened local tissue defenses make them susceptible to infection by a relatively small inoculum (10^4 or 10^5 bacteria). Systemically administered antibiotics can penetrate traumatized tissue, at least at its edges.

Wounds contacted by feces contain large numbers of strict anaerobes as well as facultative species. In such cases, both clindamycin and kanamycin may be administered systemically to combat these contaminants. Clindamycin is selected because of its effectiveness against anaerobes; kanamycin is chosen to eliminate the facultative gram-negative species.

For treatment of soft-tissue abscesses, selection of the antibiotic is aided by the results of the rapid slide technique. If the gram stain of the homogenate reveals gram-positive organisms, a cephalosporin is employed. When gram-negative organisms are encountered, an aminoglycoside is chosen. *It must be reiterated that a delay even of an hour or two in antibiotic treatment will greatly limit its therapeutic potential.* When the decision is made to initiate a preventive antibiotic regimen, the drug(s) should be administered immediately.

Dead Space

To drain or obliterate with the greatest care all of the dead spaces of a wound is still an almost universally accepted precept of surgery; and surgeons have a wholesome fear of the presence of blood in wounds.

William S. Halsted, 1890

As Halsted pointed out, since preantiseptic times surgeons have had a great fear of blood in wounds. It was believed that the most feared and dangerous wound diseases arose from the decomposition of blood. Throughout that era, surgeons used various techniques in an effort to free the wound of blood. Insertion of drainage tubes into wounds to allow egress of blood was common practice for securing primary healing. Kocher advocated secondary suture of the surgical wound without drainage tubes after the initial operation. In 1884 Neuber and Kuster recommended complete obliteration of dead space by buried sutures as a means of minimizing the accumulation of blood in the wound.

There were other surgeons, however, who cast doubt on the magnitude of the dangers of blood in the wound. In 1886 Schede commented:

It has required but a short experience with antiseptic surgery to enable us with astonishment to recognize that even very large blood clots in open wounds do not necessarily undergo destruction and decomposition, that they do not necessarily give rise to inflammation and accidental diseases, but that they can take on changes which one may designate as "organization of the blood clot" and which can compare with the conversion of the thrombus in ligated blood vessels.

Other similar observations led to a reevaluation of the thesis on which obliteration of dead space in surgical wounds was based. Halsted indicated that dead space closure of wounds with sutures could even have dangerous consequences. He remarked that "the buried sutures employed to obliterate the dead spaces necessarily enfeeble the circulation and impair the vitality of tissues which otherwise might be able to dispose of large quantities of microorganisms."

Armed with these beliefs, Halsted treated the wounds of 122 patients without drainage and without obliteration of blood clot. "There were no deaths. Of the clean wounds, two suppurated primarily." Halsted believed that this technique of surgical wound management had the advantages that "Tissue defects are beautifully repaired . . ." and that "obliteration sutures are dispensed with."

The importance of obliteration of dead space as a determinant of infection has been examined more recently by Condie and Ferguson in an experimental study. Bilateral transverse wounds were made through the abdominal wall in dogs. Each wound was contaminated with a measured dose of staphylococci. After contamination, wounds in one group were closed in four layers with a running 5-0 nylon suture. No attempt was made to obliterate dead space *between layers*. In the other group of wounds, seven layers were sutured so as to obliterate all potential dead space. Of the 12 wounds subjected to four-layer closure, 11 were infected. When the dead space was obliterated, only three of the 12 wounds exhibited infection. Condie and Ferguson concluded that obliteration of po-

417

tential dead space by suture reduces infection in abdominal wounds.

The benefits of dead space closure by suture were not realized by Ferguson in a clinical study. He noted that significant trauma and necrosis were practically unavoidable when suturing the subcutaneous tissue seen in more obese humans. For that reason, he avoided suture closure of the subcutaneous layer in a series of 268 surgical patients. In only five of these patients did wound infection subsequently develop; this incidence of infection did not differ significantly from that in another group of surgical patients in whom the deep tissues were approximated by sutures. Ferguson commented that "this observation therefore modifies our original conclusion that infection is prevented by suturing all layers in order to minimize potential dead space."

Recent studies performed in our laboratory assessed the potential clinical value of closing dead space with sutures. As expected, the importance of dead space in potentiating infection was clearly identified. Experimentally contaminated wounds containing dead space secondary to tissue loss had a higher infection rate than did those wounds with no dead space when both groups were subjected to the same level of bacterial contamination (Fig. 6. 19A).

However, suture closure of dead space in contaminated wounds containing tissue defects did not alter the results favorably, even when the least reactive sutures were used (Fig. 6.19B). In these cases, the presence of the suture material appeared to potentiate the development of infection (Fig. 6.19C). The harmful effects of suture closure of dead space in experimental animals were also noted in surgical incisions not involving muscle (Fig. 6.19D). Obliteration of the potential space between the cut edges of adipose tissue by sutures potentiated the incidence of infection.

These studies, combined with clinical observations, form the basis for the recommendation that *suture closure of dead space should be avoided in contaminated wounds*. Although dead spaces in wounds should definitely be avoided, the collapse of such spaces should be achieved by physiologic methods such as relaxing incisions, rotation of distal flaps, and splinting dressings that exert gentle surface pressure. The closure of dead space by sutures produces localized areas of wound ischemia and ne-

418

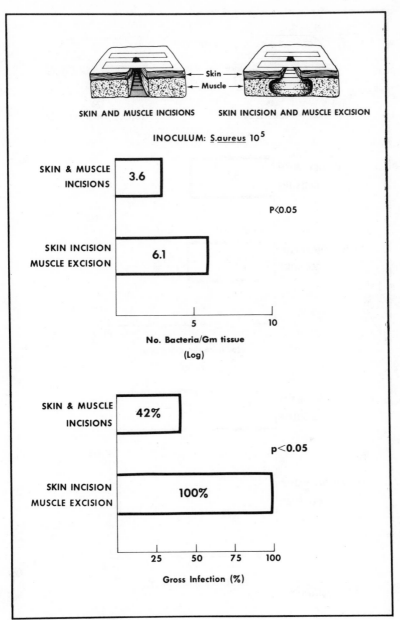

SKIN AND MUSCLE INCISIONS   SKIN INCISION AND MUSCLE EXCISION

INOCULUM: S.aureus 10^5

A

Figure 6.19 A In experimental contaminated wounds, dead space was created by excising muscle adjacent to the wound edge. Four days later, the incidence of infection and the number of viable bacteria were significantly greater in wounds containing dead space than in wounds without muscle excision.

419

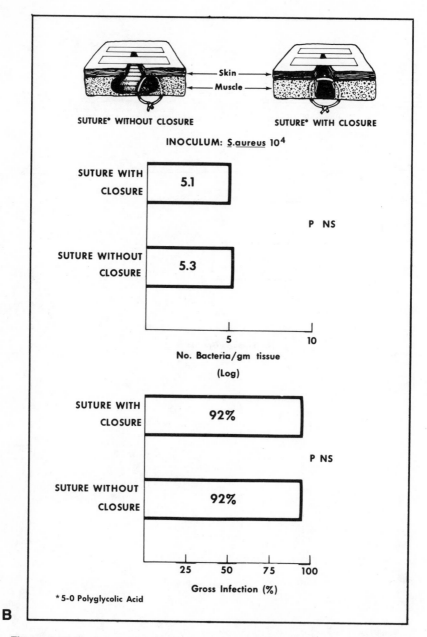

SUTURE° WITHOUT CLOSURE   SUTURE° WITH CLOSURE

INOCULUM: S.aureus 10^4

Figure 6.19 B Suture closure of the excised dead space does not eliminate the infection-potentiating effect of dead space. The infection rate of wounds and their viable bacteria following suture close of dead space was comparable to that of wounds without dead space closure but containing the same quantity of suture.

420

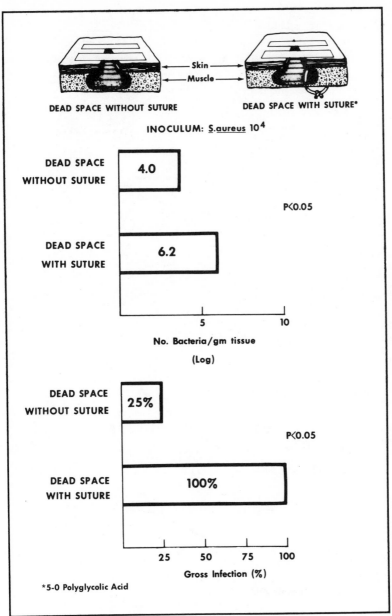

DEAD SPACE WITHOUT SUTURE

DEAD SPACE WITH SUTURE*

INOCULUM: <u>S.aureus</u> 10^4

DEAD SPACE WITHOUT SUTURE — **4.0**

DEAD SPACE WITH SUTURE — **6.2**

$P<0.05$

No. Bacteria/gm tissue
(Log)

DEAD SPACE WITHOUT SUTURE — **25%**

DEAD SPACE WITH SUTURE — **100%**

$P<0.05$

Gross Infection (%)

*5-0 Polyglycolic Acid

C

Figure 6.19 C   The incidence of infection and level of bacterial contamination in wounds following suture closure of dead space was higher than that in wounds without dead space closure.

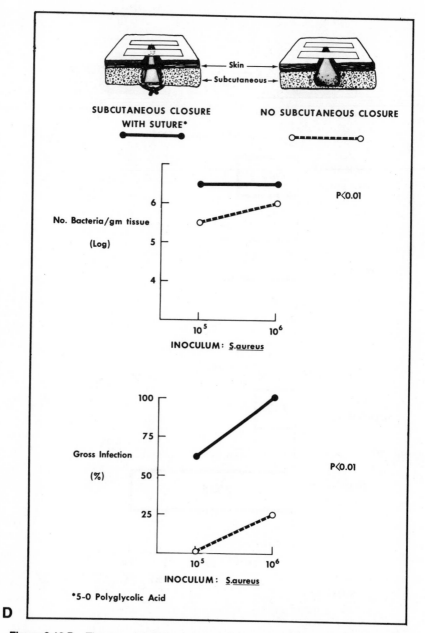

Figure 6.19 D The gross infection rate and the number of bacteria in taped skin wounds subjected to suture closure of subcutaneous tissue were higher than that in wounds without suture closure.

crosis; and the presence of additional suture material adds further danger of wound complication.

Wound Closure

The surgeon's ultimate goal is to restore the physical integrity and function of injured or diseased tissue. While this accomplishment could best be achieved by regeneration, wound restoration usually results from synthesis of scar tissue. This is usually a benign process, but excessive fibrous tissue synthesis can be detrimental to the host itself. By having a detailed knowledge of the biology of wound healing and bacteriology, the surgeon may be able to control scarring in part, and can achieve wound closure with minimal deformity and dysfunction.

The technique of wound closure selected depends largely on the type of wound. In wounds with no tissue loss, primary closure can usually be accomplished. For wounds with associated tissue loss, grafts or flaps are often required to close the defect. The timing of the closure is also critical. A decision must be made as to whether the closure should be immediate or delayed.

The decision to close wounds primarily or to delay closure is based on principles and practices of military surgeons over the centuries. Primary closure of infected or heavily contaminated wounds results in the development of purulent discharge, wound dehiscence, and eventually sepsis. The term *infected* wound refers to a wound that exhibits the classic signs of inflammation as a result of heavy bacterial contamination. Heavy contamination will usually frustrate even the most skilled surgeon's effort to convert the wound into a clean wound that can be closed primarily with safety. Surgical wounds contacted by pus are cases in point. Management of such wounds can best be accomplished by leaving them open until delayed closure can be undertaken without risk of subsequent infection.

The fundamental basis for delayed primary closure is that the healing open wound gradually gains sufficient resistance to infection to permit an uncomplicated closure. The reparative process of open wounds which is associated with this resistance to infection is characterized by the development of capillary buds and young, fibrous tissue which, in their fully de-

423

veloped form, are referred to as a granulation tissue. The resistance of the granulating open wound to infection has been recognized by many, but the exact mechanism of this resistance has not been defined.

The surgical experiences of World War I with management of contaminated wounds established the superiority of delayed over primary closure in the prevention of infection. Surgical experiences of World War II, as well as the Korean and Vietnam conflicts, confirmed the correctness of Surgeon General Kirk's directive in April 1943 in which he advocated delayed primary closure of the combat wound.

The validity of delayed closure following primary debridement of contaminated wounds is strongly reaffirmed in the report (November 1966) of Surgeon General Heaton and his associates. In a group of patients with contaminated battle wounds in Vietnam, Heaton reported an astoundingly low 2.58 percent incidence of massive infection. Using an experimental model, we have confirmed the superiority of delayed closure in the treatment of contaminated wounds. Furthermore, the results of our study suggest that the optimal time for closure of the contaminated open wound is on or after the fourth post-wounding day (Figure 6.20).

DuMortier examined the infectibility of sutured operative incisions during various phases of healing. Utilizing a pathogenic strain of *S. aureus*, an inoculum of bacteria was implanted upon the surface of sutured wounds at different time intervals after wounding. In wounds receiving the inoculum only six hours after wounding, less extensive infection developed. The incidence and severity of infection decreased progressively with time. By the fifth day after operation, the healing closed wound was not susceptible to infection by inoculation, demonstrating a resistance to infection that was comparable to that of intact skin. The taped but not sutured wound gains resistance to topical application of bacteria even more rapidly.

The rapidity with which wounds gain resistance to infection is influenced by the duration of time over which the wound is left open. The gain in resistance to infection by topical contamination of wounds subjected to immediate closure is faster than that encountered in wounds left open for one to seven days and undergoing delayed primary closure (Fig. 6.21). This

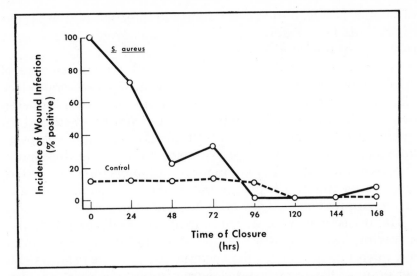

Figure 6.20 Assessment of optimal time for delayed primary closure of contaminated open wounds. Experimental wounds were contaminated with an infective dose of *S. aureus*. Delayed primary closure with tape was accomplished at varying times after contamination. Four or more days after contamination, delayed primary closure was accomplished with negligible infection.

Figure 6.21 In this investigation, the gain in resistance to infection of healing primarily closed wounds was compared to that of healing open wounds. At different times after wounding, the healing wounds received a bacterial challenge with a similar level of inoculum. The healing primarily closed wound displayed a greater resistance to the development of infection than the delayed primarily closed wound.

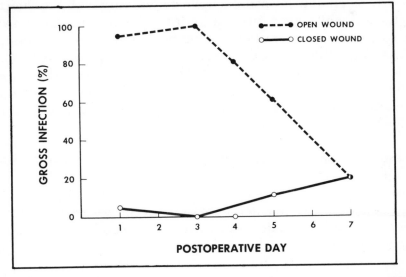

difference between the susceptibility to infection of these types of wounds is probably related to the increased inflammatory response of the open wound.

When wounds are repaired by delayed primary closure of skin and subcutaneous tissue, fine meshed gauze should be placed on the open surface of the tissue and the wound covered by a sterile dressing. The wound should not be disturbed for the first four postoperative days unless the patient develops an unexplained fever. Unnecessary inspection during this period increases the risk of contamination and subsequent infection. On or after the fourth postoperative day, the wound margins can be approximated with minimal risk of infection.

The occasional wound that is destined to develop infection following delayed closure can be identified by using quantitative microbiology. When the bacterial count of the tissue is $<10^5$ per gram of tissue, delayed closure can be accomplished without risk of infection. Wounds containing a higher level are likely to develop infection following delayed closure. Visible shaggy fibrin or pus are frequently seen in these wounds.

Once the decision is made to close the wound, the closure technique must be selected. Ideally, the considerations for the choice of closure method should be based on the biologic interaction of the materials employed and the tissue. The modern surgeon should hold tissue in apposition until the strength of the wound is sufficient to withstand stress.

The technique of closure employed will vary with the clinical situation with which one has to deal. The gaps in our knowledge about the interactions of the biomaterials are staggering. A common theme of the few reportable investigations is that all biomaterials placed within the substance of the wound damage the host defenses and invite infection. On the basis of this information, the merits and shortcomings of several wound closure techniques will be reviewed.

Tissue Adhesives Numerous encouraging experimental and clinical reports have appeared in the literature advocating the use of cyanocrylate tissue adhesives for repair of organs, or as hemostatic agents in emergency or mass combat casualty situations. However, studies performed in our laboratory show that *indications for their use should not include skin closure.* When tissue adhesives are used for bonding skin wounds, the polymer acts as a barrier between the growing edges of the wound. This barrier prevents wound apposition and delays healing. Furthermore, tissue adhesives provide a climate conducive to the development of abscesses. The infection rate in experimentally contaminated wounds closed with a tissue adhesive was significantly higher than in taped wounds. The decreased resistance to infection in wounds containing tissue adhesives was associated with histotoxic reactions in the wounded tissue.

Clips and Staples   Metal clips have been used for closure of skin wounds for many years, primarily for wounds in the head and neck. However, while skin clips have the benefit of speed of application, there are disturbing drawbacks to their use. Harrison and his associates have shown that wounds closed with clips are significantly weaker, have a lower modulus of elasticity, and are able to absorb less energy than similar wounds closed with monofilament nylon sutures in the same animal.

Skin closure can now be accomplished by staples. The major advantage of this closure is speed. Lennihan and Mackereth estimate that stapled wound closure of the incisions in a bilateral vein stripping saves 30 to 35 minutes of time that would be spent suturing. This advantage must be weighed against the demonstrated damaging effect of the staples on local tissue defenses. In recent experimental studies, stapled skin wounds were shown to be considerably more susceptible to infection than taped wounds Fig. 6.22). *This mitigates against the use of staples for closure of contaminated wounds.* We routinely approximate skin grafts to large, clean open wounds using the automatic stapler. The operative time is cut nearly in half by eliminating the additional time required for suture closure.

Sutures

I believe that the obstruction to the circulation produced by sutures and ligatures is often the immediate cause of suppuration in infected wounds . . . .

William S. Halsted, 1890

Sutures remain the most common method of reapproximating the divided edges of tissues. Selection of suture material must be based on the biologic healing properties of the tissues that

427

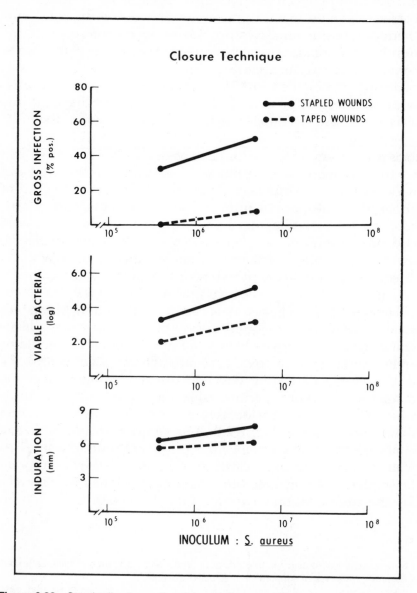

Figure 6.22 Standardized experimental wounds were subjected to graded doses of bacterial inocula prior to closure by either tape or staples. Four days later, the taped wounds displayed considerably more resistance to infection than the stapled wounds.

are to be approximated, the physical and biologic properties of the suture, and the condition of the wound being closed.

Measurements of the in vivo degradation of sutures separate them into two general classes. Sutures that undergo degradation in tissues rapidly, losing their tensile strength within 60 days, can be considered "absorbable" sutures. Those which maintain their tensile strength for longer than 60 days after implantation may be referred to as "nonabsorbable" stutures. This terminology is somewhat misleading since some of the so-called nonabsorbable sutures (e.g., silk, cotton, and nylon) lose their tensile strength rapidly after the second month, and by the sixth month have either disintegrated or are so weak they have little or no effect in reinforcing the tissue.

The absorbable sutures are gut, derived from sheep submucosa or beef serosa, and the synthetics, polyglycolic acid (PGA) and polyglactin (a copolymer of glycolide and lactide). Treatment of gut with chromium salts, a cross-linking agent, prolongs retention of the suture's tensile strength and increases its resistance to absorption by enzymatic action.

The nonabsorbable sutures can be classified according to their origin. Those made from natural fibers are silk, cotton, and linen. Nonabsorbable metallic sutures are usually made from stainless steel alloy. Modern chemistry has developed nonabsorbable synthetic fibers from polyamides (Nylon), polyesters (Dacron), and polyolefins (polyethylene, polypropylene).

Sutures may also be characterized by their physical configuration. Those constructed from one filament are termed monofilament; sutures containing multiple fibers, generally braided, are called multifilament sutures. Both nylon and stainless steel sutures are available in monofilament and multifilament constructions.

The biologic interaction of the suture and the host can be judged, in part, by the degree to which the suture damages the local tissue defenses. There are several mechanisms by which surgical sutures enhance infection. The trauma of inserting a needle is in itself sufficient to cause an inflammatory response. Suturing technique is crucially important. Sutures tied too tightly around the wound edges markedly increase the incidence of infection, even with the least reactive suture (Fig.

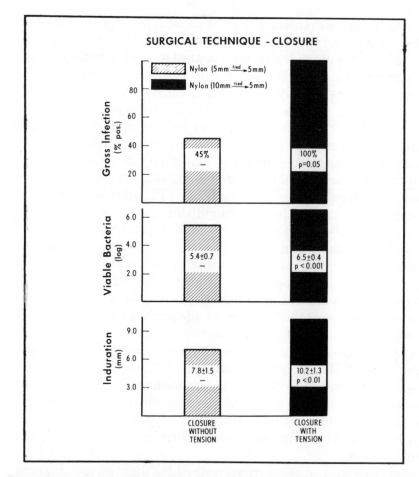

Figure 6.23 Suture closure of one group of contaminated wounds was accomplished with minimal tension on tissues within the suture loop. In these wounds, the exit and entrance of the sutures was 2.5 mm from the wound edge before and after tying the suture. In another group of wounds contaminated with the same level of inoculum, the sutures were tied tightly around the tissues within the suture loop. This was accomplished by passing the suture 5 mm from the wound edge and tying the sutures when the entrance and exit of the sutures were 2.5 mm from the wound edge. The inflammatory responses of sutured wounds closed under tension were significantly higher than those of sutured wounds approximated by sutures tied with minimal tension.

6.23). The mere presence of the suture in the tissue increases susceptibility to infection. The magnitude of this local injury to defenses is related to the quantity of suture within the wound (e.g., diameter [Fig. 6.24A], length [Fig. 6.24B]), and to its chemical composition.

430

In our experimental studies, the incidence of infection in contaminated tissues containing either nylon or polypropylene sutures was lower than with any other nonabsorbable sutures. Among the absorbable sutures, PGA sutures appeared to elicit the least inflammatory response. Postlethwait recently reported that PGA sutures lose tensile strength significantly more rapidly than chromic catgut in the rabbit. After 28 days, PGA exhibited no residual tensile strength while catgut retained substantial strength at this interval. The mechanism of absorption is still unknown but is postulated to be due to the action of the tissue esterases releasing glycolic acid from the suture.

Nylon, although classified as a nonabsorbable suture, is far from being chemically inert. Nylon, in its multifilament form, retains almost no tensile strength after being in tissues for six months. It is Moloney's belief that this degradation in fiber strength may even apply to fine monofilament nylon fibers. The loss of tensile strength is thought to be due to chemical degradation rather than to physical force exerted on the suture. Proteolytic enzymes in the body may aid in the hydrolysis of the suture.

In vitro studies performed in our laboratory indicate that the suspected degradation products of nylon and PGA sutures are potent antibacterial agents. Incubation of S. aureus with varying concentrations of these degradation products results in a marked reduction in the bacterial count. These by-products of nylon and PGA sutures still possess antibacterial activity after being buffered to a pH 7.4. For this reason, it is postulated that the antibacterial activity of the degradation products of nylon and PGA sutures may destroy some of the bacteria associated with the sutures in the wound, thereby minimizing the tissue's reaction to the suture. This hypothesis remains to be confirmed by further experimental studies.

The clinical success of polypropylene sutures in contaminated tissue is related to its biologic inertness. It displays excellent chemical resistance and its tensile strength remains unchanged in tests lasting over two years after implantation in tissue.

Utilizing our experimental model, the physical configuration of a suture was found to play a relatively unimportant role in the development of *early* infection. Although the incidence of

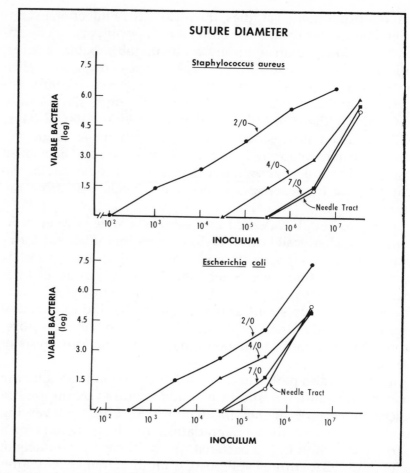

Figure 6.24 Determinants of infection potentiation by suture. The degree to which sutures damaged local tissue's resistance to infection is related to the total quantity of suture within the wound, suture diameter, and length. Graded doses of a specified bacterial inoculum were delivered to tissue containing nylon sutures of varying diameter. Four days

infection in contaminated tissues containing monofilament sutures was lower than in those containing multifilament sutures, these differences were not statistically significant.

Dacron sutures elicited a greater degree of infection in contaminated wounds than did nylon, but less than stainless steel, silk, or cotton sutures. The handling characteristics of untreated Dacron sutures have considerably limited their use in operation. The problems encountered in tying Dacron relate to

432

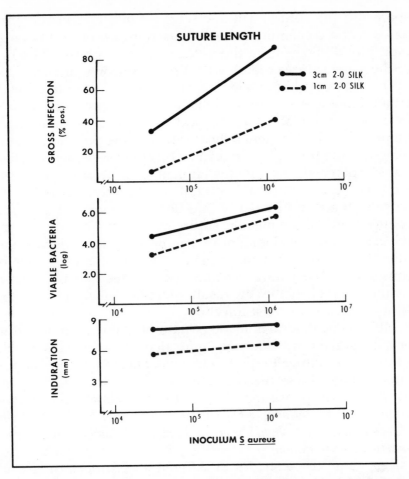

SUTURE LENGTH

after contamination, the magnitude of bacterial proliferation was proportional to the suture diameter. Similarly, the contaminated tissues containing longer suture implants (3 cm) exhibited significantly greater inflammatory responses and bacterial counts than tissues with shorter lengths (1 cm) four days postimplantation.

its high coefficient of friction. When Dacron sutures are tied, excessive friction is encountered between the surfaces of the suture. The multifilament Dacron suture grabs and sticks, and does not slip into place easily. However, coating the surface of Dacron sutures with Teflon or silicone eliminates this excessive friction and allows the suture to slip into place easily. The addition of inert materials to cover the filaments of the Dacron suture did not significantly alter the tissue's inflammatory re-

433

sponse to the suture. The incidence of infection in contaminated tissue containing uncoated Dacron sutures was not significantly different from the inflammatory response of tissues to the same sutures coated with Teflon, silicone, or wax.

The relatively high incidence of infection encountered with either monofilament or multifilament stainless steel sutures may be a result of their chemical or physical configuration. Stainless steel is not generally as inert as pure polymers. Metal may degrade through corrosion or by electrolysis, with a slow transfer of metal ions from the implant to tissue. Both processes are very slow and probably do not significantly alter the resistance of the wound to early infection. However, the physical configuration of the metallic suture may have a more dramatic impact on the development of wound infection. Metallic sutures are so stiff that movement of the host must result in considerable mechanical irritation. It is indeed a small buried weapon. It is likely that the resultant tissue damage impairs the wound's ability to resist infection.

Multifilament sutures made of natural fibers, such as cotton or silk, potentiated infection more than other nonabsorbable sutures. Postlethwait reported that silk and cotton consistently caused more tissue reaction than synthetic sutures. This inflammatory response may impair the tissue's ability to resist infection. *It would appear from these experimental studies that the use of silk and cotton should be avoided in wounds having known gross bacterial contamination.*

Despite all these shades of difference, *even the least reactive suture impairs the wound's local resistance to infection.* (Fig. 6.25). Contaminated tissues containing nylon suture were more often infected than tissue containing no suture but contaminated with the same number of bacteria. A reasonable deduction from these studies is that *sutures should be avoided in contaminated wounds unless they play an essential role in positioning the tissues.* Carpendale and Sereda's observations add factual support to this thesis. In their experimental evaluation of closure techniques in contaminated wounds, Carpendale and Sereda reported 16.7 percent incidence of infections in skin wounds closed with sutures as compared to 0 percent infection rate in taped wounds.

The biomechanical properties of the suture and the healing wound are other important clinical parameters to be considered

434

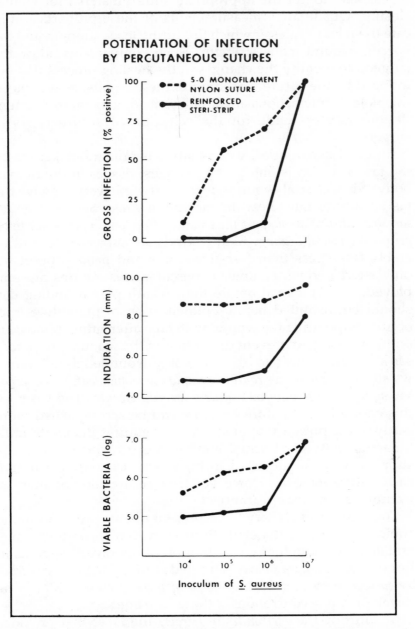

Figure 6.25 Potentiation of infection by percutaneous sutures. Standardized wounds subjected to graded doses of bacterial inocula were closed by either tape or sutures. Four days later, the inflammatory responses of the sutured wounds and their bacterial counts were significantly greater than those of taped wounds.

in the selection of the appropriate suture material for wound closure. Quantitative measurements of these properties indicate the relative rates at which the suture loses strength and the specific wound gains strength. Such comparisons allow the surgeon to identify the changes in the healing process that are induced by the suture. Based upon these results, as well as on the biologic interactions already described, general recommendations can be made for the selection of suture types in surgery.

In soft-tissue injuries, wound stress is primarily taken up by the fascia, which is one of the strongest tissues in the human body. Since fascial wounds regain strength very slowly, the fascial sutures must bear the maximum stress. *Synthetic nonabsorbable sutures can support the wound for prolonged periods of time, permitting fascial healing.* Skin wounds are subjected to considerably less stress than fascial wounds and need support for only short periods of time. If percutaneous sutures are employed, early removal before the seventh postwounding day should be instituted before epithelization of the suture tract occurs. Supporting the wound with tape after suture removal is often necessary to prevent disruption of the wound whose tensile strength is only 5 to 10 percent of unwounded tissue. When we suture the skin, *we routinely employ monofilament, nonabsorbable, synthetic, percutaneous sutures for skin closure.* The basis for this choice is that suture line care can be accomplished more easily in the presence of monofilament sutures than with multifilament sutures. Dermal sutures are occasionally used to support wounds subjected to high skin tensions, permitting early suture removal. However, these sutures do not alter the eventual cosmetic appearance of the scar.

The urinary and biliary tracts present unique problems in the choice of a suture material. Sutures within these tracts may initiate precipitation or crystallization of dissolved elements in urine or bile that are nearly saturated with crystalloids. *Absorbable sutures are used almost routinely in these locations* to limit the development of concretions at the suture line.

In suturing the *gastrointestinal tract*, the layer that provides the strength is the submucosa. Repair of this layer is usually accomplished with interrupted nonabsorbable sutures that do not penetrate the mucosa. This suture line provides support while the healing anastomosis gains sufficient strength to resist disruption. Most surgeons supplement a submucosal suture line with a running absorbable suture in the mucosa for optimal hemostasis. Stapling of the gastrointestinal anastomosis *also* appears to be a *safe* and reliable method of closure. (See chapter on Wound Healing in the Gastrointestinal Tract for details.)

Vascular prostheses and artificial heart valves never become completely incorporated into the tissues. In these cases, sutures must support the prosthesis throughout the patient's lifetime. *Polypropylene and polyester sutures, which maintain their integrity following implantation, are the mandatory choice.*

In vascular surgery, the most serious obstacle to anastomosing blood vessels is thrombosis. As the size of the vessel decreases, the possibility of thrombosis increases. In experimental microsurgical studies, Acland demonstrated that of all injuries to a vessel including intimal damage, the one that produced the greatest amount of thrombosis was the transverse incision closed by a suture. In our laboratory the *magnitude of the thrombosis has been reduced by using monofilament synthetic sutures rather than multifilament sutures.* For large vessels, especially those that are atherosclerotic, we also prefer monofilament synthetic sutures because when they are passed through an atherosclerotic vessel, there is minimal friction, and plaques are less frequently dislodged. Multifilament sutures tend to disrupt plaques providing a nidus for thrombus formation. (See chapter on arterial healing for details.)

The ultimate goal of nerve repair is maximum sensory and motor recovery of the distal denervated part. Surgical technique is a crucial factor in determining the success of nerve repair. Using an operating microscope, fascicles in the divided ends of the nerve must be oriented and repaired using monofilament synthetic sutures swaged to microsurgical needles. *The best results are obtained when end-to-end anastosis is accomplished without tension.* Tension at the suture line invites connective tissue proliferation which presents an obstacle to regenerating axons. (See chapter on peripheral nerve repair for details.)

Tendons transmit muscle action across joints; therefore, tendons must glide without restriction. Following repair of a tendon, adhesions may form between the coapted ends of the tendon and the surrounding tissue. These adhesions may be firm and nonyielding, restricting tendon movement; or loose and filmy, permitting tendon gliding. The nature and degree of adhesions are determined by the mechanism of injury, the associated structures injured, and the individual's healing characteristics. These factors are considerably more important than the suture material employed in the repair. Monofilament steel suture has gained wide acceptance despite its tendency to kink. Monofilament and multifilament synthetic sutures also have their champions. *The superiority of one synthetic suture over another for tendon repair has yet to be proved.* However, the technique used to place the suture is known to be important (see chapter on tendon repair for details.)

Tape Closure   The incidence of infection in contaminated wounds whose edges were approximated by even the least reactive suture was significantly higher than the infection rate of taped wounds subjected to a comparable level of contamination (Fig. 6.25). The superior resistance to infection of taped wounds as compared to sutured wounds indicates that tape closure of contaminated wounds is a significant clinical tool.

The composition of tape, as well as its physical configuration, considerably influence its performance. Selection of a surgical tape is based on adhesiveness, tensile strength, and porosity. Adhesive must be aggressive and provide a firm tape-to-skin bond that resists shear. In the rare case that tapes slip, they usually do so during or immediately after closure. Twenty-four hours later the adhesive bond to the skin is twofold greater than immediately following application.

Surgical closure tape will not adhere to wet skin, even with the most aggressive adhesive. Drying with a gauze sponge often does not completely remove wet exudate, and the residual fluid continues to impair tape adhesion. This problem can be avoided by applying an adhesive adjunct (e.g., tincture of benzoin) prior to tape application. The use of an adhesive adjunct enhances the immediate adhesion of the tape to the skin and prevents tape dislodgement. Inadvertent spillage of the adjunct into the wound damages local resistance to infection. Therefore, the adhesive adjunct is applied (with applicator sticks) in a thin film to the skin at the wound edge.

The tensile strength of a surgical tape must be sufficient to maintain wound approximation during healing. Breakage of nonwoven microporous tape in surgical wounds has been encountered. This weak tape has been strengthened by adding

438

reinforcing rayon filaments to its backing. These additional fibers result in a fourfold increase in tensile strength. In a clinical trial in which the new reinforced microporous tapes were utilized, breakage was not encountered.

Irritation of the skin by tape can be correlated, in part, with tape occlusivity. Tapes that limit moisture vapor transmission lead to an accumulation of fluid underneath the tape promoting tissue maceration and bacterial growth. Microporous tapes allow moisture to be transmitted through the interstices of the tape resulting in a dry skin beneath the tape that is antithetical to the growth of bacteria. Cloth tape is occlusive because of its tightly woven cloth backing and relatively few pores. Transmission of air and moisture vapor is impaired, encouraging bacterial growth. This has important clinical implications, particularly in the early phases of healing when wound epithelization is incomplete. At this time, heavily contaminated skin under the cloth tape may be a potential source of infection.

The ease with which wounds can be closed by tape varies considerably according to the anatomic and biomechanical properties of the wound site. Wounds in skin subjected to minimal static and dynamic tensions are easily approximated by tape. The relatively lax skin of the face and abdomen makes it amenable to wound closure by tapes. In contrast, the taut skin of the extremities, subjected to frequent dynamic joint movements, limits the adherence of tape and the success of closure. The copious secretions from the skin of the axillae, palms, and soles also discourage tape adherence.

Meticulous suture closure of the skin edges of some traumatic wounds approximates skin edges more exactly and gives better eversion of skin margins than tape closure. Undoubtedly, the more accurate approximation of skin edges by skillfully applied suture leads to a more pleasing cosmetic result. The superiority of suture closure becomes most apparent in lacerations resulting from impact injuries. In these cases, closing the wound is often like putting together a jigsaw puzzle and tapes have little practical value.

In the case of lacerations due to sharp wounding instruments, the wound edges can be accurately approximated with tape, a technique that has been used frequently for initial closure, even of facial lacerations, in children. The cosmetic results of such closure have been excellent, and many patients will require no further plastic surgery. One additional bonus of this technique is that the children are spared painful injection of the local anesthetic agent required for suturing. In elective surgery, the sedation will be better; the chance of contamination is reduced; and the blood supply of the damaged tissue is more accurately determined. All of these factors lead to a superior esthetic result with less emotional trauma to the child, and only a single visit to the operating room will be required.

The surgeon's choice of closure technique must also be influenced by the degree of bacterial contamination in the wound. The majority of clean lacerations or avulsions will heal without infection regardless of the closure technique. However, in the contaminated wound, in which a viscus has been opened, the choice of closure technique is critical. Tape closure of these wounds can be undertaken with less risk of infection than with suture closure. The benefit of tape closure in this group of patients has been reiterated by Conolly et al. In their study, the incidence of gross infection in taped wounds was significantly less (about half) than in sutured wounds.

Subcutaneous sutures should be avoided even in elective abdominal incisions, since they act as foreign bodies, impairing the wound's ability to resist infection. Contrary to the usual expectation, tape closure, without a dermal suture, is more easily accomplished in obese patients. The force necessary to approximate wound edges appears less than that in thin patients. In addition, the thick cut edge of adipose tissue tends to evert the skin, facilitating tape closure. In thin patients, supplemental interrupted subcuticular sutures may facilitate tape closure since they take the tension off the wound edge.

Primary closure of the skin and adipose tissue is *never* indicated in heavily contaminated wounds. In such wounds, contacted by pus or known infected fluid during the course of surgery, the number of bacteria deposited exceeds the infective dose, and primary closure will inevitably be followed by infection. In place of primary closure, delayed primary closure by tapes should be employed.

Drainage

A drain invariably produces some necrosis of tissue with which it comes in contact, and enfeebles the power of resistance of these tissues toward organisms. But given necrotic tissue plus infection a drain becomes almost indispensable.

William S. Halsted, 1898

Use of surgical drainage in a clinical setting requires a delicate weighing of potential benefits and harmful effects. The advantages and consequences of wound drainage are detailed in a comprehensive review by Golden et al.

The obvious beneficial effect of drainage is the ability to evacuate potentially harmful collections of certain fluids, such as pus, blood, bile, gastric and pancreatic juices from wounds or body cavities. Pus within a wound or body cavity exerts many deleterious effects on the host and should be removed whenever a localized collection can be drained. Sterile collections of blood per se are not major irritants to tissues, but hemoglobin enhances bacterial virulence. Animal studies with dogs and rats performed by Davis and Yull have demonstrated that an intraperitoneal injection of E. coli (10^8–10^{11} organisms) was not lethal. If, however, hemoglobin at concentrations of 4 g% or greater was added to the inoculum, approximately 70 percent of the animals died within 24 hours. The precise mechanism by which hemoglobin enhances infection is unknown. Red blood cells also enhance subcutaneous infection in experimental animals. Krizek and Davis found that when red blood cells were injected into the same subcutaneous tissue site as E. coli, a serious and often fatal infection occurred, whereas the injection of bacteria alone proved relatively innocuous.

There is also no doubt that collections of bile, gastric juice, or pancreatic juice are harmful. In a recent report, Cohn et al. reviewed the pathophysiology of bile peritonitis. Leakage of sterile bile into the peritoneal cavity causes a generalized exudation of protein-rich fluid. Gallbladder bile is considerably more irritating than hepatic bile, presumably because it is more concentrated. Rewbridge and Hrdina demonstrated that the inflamed and injured intestinal wall permits transmigration of enteric and clostridial organisms that grow rapidly in the bile-laden fluid. The presence of bacteria severely potentiates the damaging effects of the bile, leading to a virulent peritonitis. Extravasated bile should always be removed from the peritoneal cavity.

In instances where no definite localized collection of fluid exists, *drainage must be considered prophylactic, and its potentially harmful effects become more important.* Drains act as retrograde conduits through which skin contaminants gain entrance into the wound. Cerise et al. performed a splenectomy in rabbits and inoculated the skin around the drain tract with type 6 streptococcus, taking care not to inoculate the drain. Twenty percent of the animals had positive intraperitoneal cultures at 24 hours, and 56 percent at 72 hours, compared to a positive culture rate of only 5 percent in undrained animals.

Nora and his colleagues performed laparotomies in dogs and inserted Penrose drains separately into the splenic fossa and in Morison's pouch. Gross intraabdominal infection was detected in nine out of the ten dogs with drains in the splenic fossa. Positive cultures were noted in 90 percent of the dogs in which drains had been placed, whether or not purposeful bacterial inoculation of the splenic fossa drain had been performed. Neither gross infection nor positive bacterial cultures were evident in undrained control dogs. In a clinical study, the same investigators detected skin contaminants on the intraabdominal portion of drainage tubes in 17 of 50 patients who had intraabdominal procedures. *Staphylococcus epidermidis*, a skin contaminant, was found in 14 of the 17 cases. Of the 17 patients with positive cultures, 12 had minimal egress of fluid from the drain tract, and neither the gastrointestinal tract nor genitourinary tract had been opened at operation. Morris showed significantly less infection when closed suction was used in 53 randomized patients undergoing radical mastectomy as compared to the use of standard Penrose drainage, indicating that retrograde contamination might be minimized by the use of a closed system. Closed suction drainage minimizes postoperative infections. Cruse and Foord (August, 1973) in a prospective study of 1,540 patients undergoing cholecystectomy found the following percentage of infections: no drainage (2.9 percent), stab drain (1.8 percent), drain through the wound (9.9 percent), and closed wound suction drain (0 percent). Meticulous postoperative aseptic care of the skin at the drain exit also has much to do with low infection rates.

The air vent within a sump tube provides another potential conduit for organisms. Baker and Borchardt demonstrated that the degree of contamination is proportional to the degree of suction applied. When continuous suction is employed at 10 psi, airborne contamination occurs. Lowering the vacuum pressure attached to suction eliminates this airborne contamination. Plugging the vents with cotton or gauze, or use of a synthetic air filter, provides the same benefit.

442

The presence of drains impairs the resistance of tissues to infection. In an experimental study by Magee et al., placement of drains within experimental wounds exposed to subinfective inoculations of bacteria greatly enhanced the rate of wound infection compared to undrained controls (Fig. 6.26A). Both Silastic and Penrose drains dramatically enhanced the infection rate of soft-tissue wounds in guinea pigs. The rate of infection when the drain was brought out through the wound was similar to the rate when the drain lay entirely within the wound, suggesting a deleterious effect of the drain per se (Fig. 6.26B).

Studies of the impairment of wound healing in the presence of drains have been performed with intestinal anastomoses. Berliner and his associates performed proximal and distal intestinal anastomoses in dogs, draining one anastomosis in each dog. Three of the 20 nondrained anastomoses leaked, compared to 11 of 20 drained anastomoses and, of these, anastomotic disruption proved fatal in four cases.

Manz and his colleagues confirmed the damaging effects of drains on colonic anastomoses in dogs. Of 20 dogs with Penrose drainage at their anastomoses, nine died of anastomotic disruption and peritonitis, and the remainder had extensive adhesions as well as varying degrees of stricture formation. All dogs with drainage had evidence of bacterial contamination at the site of the anastomosis at the necropsy, while the control dogs had only filmy adhesions and no stricture formation. Though the exact mechanism of this effect is unknown, it is obvious that drains are foreign bodies and that they do prevent the collapse of normal tissue against the anastomosis. The drain may also act as a retrograde conduit for bacteria that then contaminate the dead space caused by the drain at the anastomotic site, thereby predisposing to infection and leakage. (See chapter on wound healing in the gastrointestinal tract for further details.)

Dressing

Prevention of wound contamination is considered to be the major purpose of the surgical dressing. The length of time that dressings should cover the surgical wound is based on our knowledge of the period during which the wound is susceptible to bacterial penetration. Warren reports that the wound

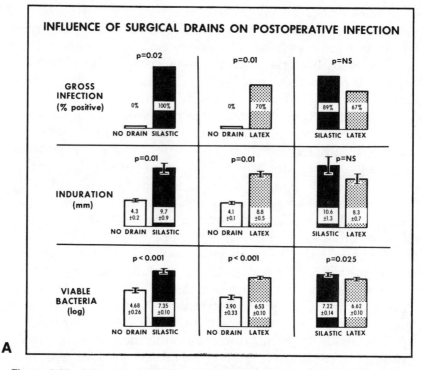

Figure 6.26 Influence of surgical drains on postoperative infection. Experimental wounds were contaminated with subinfective doses of *S. aureus*. **A.** Prior to closure, drains were placed in the wounds and allowed to exit between the wound edges. In contralateral wounds, closure was accomplished without drains. Four days later, the inflammatory responses and bacterial counts of wounds containing drains were significantly greater than those without drains.

edges seal rapidly with a coagulum, thereby eliminating the need for dressings on primarily closed wounds. Other surgeons recommend that the first surgical dressing remain undisturbed until the sutures are ready for removal to prevent the introduction of surface contamination into the wound.

Experimental studies performed in our laboratory demonstrate that, as they heal, sutured wounds become increasingly resistant to the development of infection following surface contamination. Swabbing the surface of the wound with either *S. aureus* or *E. coli* during the first 48 hours after closure did result in localized gross infections. Such surface contamination on the third postoperative day did not produce gross infection in any sutured wound. This susceptibility to infection of the sutured wound during the early postoperative period confirms the ap-

444

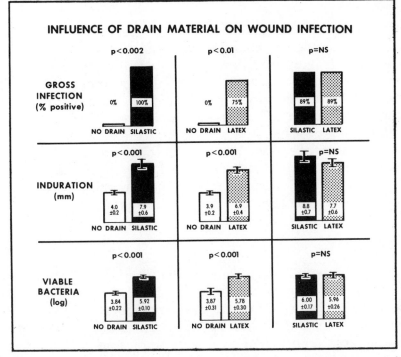

Figure 6.26 (cont.) **B.** The deleterious effect of drains was related to the presence of the foreign body. When drain material was placed entirely within a closed wound, its inflammatory response and bacterial count remained significantly higher than a wound closed without a drain.

parent value of dressings to protect the fresh incision from surface contamination.

Our experiments clearly indicate that *wounds closed with tape have a greater capacity to resist infection than do sutured wounds.* Immediate surface contamination with S. *aureus* did not elicit an infection in any taped wounds. Only one of 14 taped wounds developed gross infection after contamination with *E. coli* immediately after closure. Surface contamination with this same organism two or more hours after closure did not result in infection in any taped wounds. This resistance to infection of taped wounds after surface contamination reduces the need for protective dressings during the postoperative period in wounds free of sutures. In a real sense, the skin suture has the objectionable features of a small drain.

Immobilization

Immobilization of the site of injury is of great value in the care of the contaminated wound. When the site of any injury is immobilized, lymphatic flow is reduced, thereby minimizing the spread of the wound microflora. Furthermore, immobilized tissue demonstrates superior resistance to the growth of bacteria than nonimmobilized tissue.

Whenever possible, the site of injury should be elevated above the patient's heart. Elevation of the injured site limits the accumulation of fluid in the wound interstitial spaces. The wound with little edema proceeds more rapidly to complete rehabilitation than does the markedly edematous wound.

EPILOGUE

We have come full circle from the first chapter. We started by reviewing our knowledge of the reparative process. Details of that process predicted that surgical technique would be a vital determinant of the quality and rate of healing. This chapter summarizes the results of numerous studies on technique and its effects on repair and resistance to infection.

If the reader has found that some of his technical preferences are not featured, it is possible that scientific proof of their efficacy is lacking. However, in practice we must often do as we think best, even without scientific proof that we are correct. To a major extent, surgical technique is still art and craft. On the other hand, the reader may have found information which is contradictory to techniques he employs. We can only say that these are the facts as they have emerged from many laboratories and operating theaters and gleaned from objective studies wherever possible.

We must draw the inevitable conclusion that the surgeon's technique is often more important than his materials. The worst surgeon can defeat the best suture materials, while the technically accomplished surgeon can usually succeed with inferior ones. The objective is, of course, to equip technically accomplished surgeons with the best materials and the best methods.

As surgeons, we must be able to soften the memories of our failures. We tend to reinforce our decisions by recalling our successes. This psychological process, which protects our mental health, should not result in perpetuating suboptimal techniques. In this era of rapid technological advance, we must be prepared to change as the opportunities to improve our techniques arise and the benefits of new techniques are scientifically documented.

The closer the surgeon can approach ideal technique, the wider will be his surgical horizons—horizons that are now limited by infection and failure of repair. The best the surgeon can do under present circumstances is minimize his potential for damaging and infecting tissue. The difference between the currently "acceptable" 4% clean wound infection rate and the 1% rate which is possible may seem small, but it may also be the difference between success and failure—life or death—to three patients in every hundred.

BIBLIOGRAPHY

Mechanical Energy

Amato JJ, Billy LJ, Lawson NS, Rich, NM: High velocity missile injury: An experimental study of the retentive forces of tissue. Am J Surg 127: 454–458, 1974

Cardany CR, Rodeheaver GT, Thacker J, Edgerton MT, Edlich RF: The crush injury: A high risk wound. J Am Coll Emerg Phys 5: 965–970, 1976

Charters, AC III, Charters, AC: Wounding mechanisms of very high velocity projectiles. J Trauma 16: 464–469, 1976

DeMuth WE Jr: Bullet velocity and design as determinants of wounding capability: An experimental study. J Trauma 6: 222–232, 1966

DeMuth WE Jr: The mechanism of shotgun wounds. J Trauma. 11: 219–229, 1971

Jacobs HB: Skin knife-deep knife: The ritual and practice of skin incisions. Ann Surg 179: 102–104, 1974

Electrical and Radiant Energies

Cruse PJE, Foord R: A five-year prospective study of 23,649 surgical wounds. Arch Surg 107: 206–210, 1973

Ferguson DJ: Advances in the management of surgical wounds. Surg Clin North Am 51: 49–59, 1971

Hunt JL, Mason AD, Masterson TS, Pruitt BA Jr: The pathophysiology of acute electric injuries. J Trauma 16: 335–340, 1976

Levine NS, Peterson HD, Salisbury RE, Pruitt BA Jr: Laser, scalpel, electrosurgical and tangential excisions of third degree burns. A preliminary report. Plast Reconstr Surg 56: 286–296, 1975

447

McDowell AJ: Wound infections resulting from the use of hot wet sponges. Surgery 23: 168–174, 1959

Madden JE, Edlich RF, Custer JR, et al.: Studies in the management of the contaminated wound. IV. Resistance to infection of surgical wounds made by knife, electrosurgery, and laser. Am J Surg 119: 206–210, 1970

Antisepsis

Custer J, Edlich RF, Prusak M, et al.: Studies in the management of the contaminated wound. V. An assessment of the effectiveness of pHisoHex and Betadine surgical scrub solutions. Am J Surg 121:572, 1971

Edlich RF, Schmolka IR, Prusak MP, Edgerton MT: The molecular basis for the toxicity of surfactants in surgical wounds. 1. EO:PO block polymers. J Surg Res 14:277, 1973

Gilmore OJA, Martin TDM: Aetiology and prevention of wound infection in appendicectomy. Br J Surg 61:281, 1974

Lavelle KJ, Doedens DJ, Kleit SA, Forney RB: Iodine absorption in burn patients treated topically with Povidone-Iodine. Clin Pharmacol Ther 17:355, 1975

O.T.C topical antimicrobial products and drug and cosmetic products. Fed Reg 39:33107, 1978. Note: The best single reference to all topics under this title.

Rodeheaver GT, Turnbull V, Edgerton MT, Kurtz L, Edlich RF: Pharmocokinetics of a new skin wound cleanser. Am J Surg 132:67–74, 1976

Rogers DE: The current problem of staphylococcal infections. Ann Intern Med 45:748, 1956

Sprunt K, Redman W, Leidy G: Antibacterial effectiveness of routine hand washing. Pediatrics. 52:264, 1973

Stokes EJ, Howard E, Peters JL, et al.: Comparison of antibiotic and antiseptic prophylaxis of wound infection in acute abdominal surgery. World J Surg 1:777, 1977

Walter CW, Kundsin RB: The bacteriologic study of surgical gloves from 250 operations. Surg Gynecol Obstet 129:949, 1969

Debridement

Altemeier WA, Furste WE: Studies in the virulence of *Clostridium welchii*. Surgery 25:12, 1949

Fildes P: Tetanus VI. The conditions under which tetanus spores germinate *in vivo*. Br J Exp Pathol 8:387, 1928

Friedrich PL: Die aseptische versorgung frisher wunder, unter mitteilung bon theirversuchen uber die auskeimungszeit von infectionserregern in frischer wunder. Arch Klin Chir 57:288, 1898

Jones RC, Shires GT: Principles in the management of wounds. In Schwartz, SI (ed): Principles of Surgery. New York, McGraw-Hill, 1974, p. 204

Mandell GL: Bactericidal activity of aerobic and anaerobic polymorphonuclear neutrophils. Infect Immun 9:337, 1974

448

Mendelson JA, Glover JL: Sphere and shell fragment wounds of soft tissues: experimental study. J Trauma 7:889, 1967

Myers MB: Prediction and prevention of skin sloughs in radical cancer surgery. Pacif Med Surg 75:315, 1967

Peacock EE, VanWinkle, Jr. W: Repair of skin wounds. In Surgery and Biology of Wound Repair. Philadelphia, Saunders, 1970, p. 71. Note: required reading for all surgeons.

Scully RE, Artz CP, Sako Y: The criteria for determining the viability of muscle in war wounds. In Battle Wounds, Vol 3, Surgical Research Team, Washington, D.C., Army Medical Service Graduate School.

Bacteria

Bacchetta CA, Magee W, Rodeheaver G, Edgerton MT, Edlich RF: Biology of infections of split thickness skin grafts. Am J Surg 130:63, 1975

Duke WF, Robson MC, Krizek TJ: Civilian wounds, their bacterial flora and rate of infection. Surg Forum 23: 518, 1972

Edlich RF, Rodeheaver GT, Spengler M, Hiebert J, Edgerton MT: Practical bacteriologic monitoring of the burn wound. Clin Plast Surg 4:561, 1977

Marshall KA, Edgerton MT, Rodeheaver GT, Magee CM, Edlich RF: Quantitative microbiology: its application to hand injuries. Am J Surg 131:730, 1976

Robson MC, Krizek TJ: Predicting skin graft survival. J Trauma 13:213, 1973

Robson MC, Lea CE, Dalton JB, Heggers JP: Quantitative bacteriology and delayed wound closure. Surg Forum 19:501, 1968

Roettinger W, Edgerton MT, Kurtz LD, Prusak M, Edlich RF: Role of inoculation site as a determinant of infection. Am J Surg 126:354, 1973

Indigenous Microflora

Klingman AM: The bacteriology of normal skin. In Maibach HI, Hildick-Smith G (eds): Skin Bacteria and Their Role in Infection. New York, McGraw-Hill, 1965, pp. 13–31. Note: A comprehensive and concise review of the subject.

Marples RR: The effect of hydration on the bacterial flora of the skin. In Maibach HI, Hildrick-Smith G (eds): Skin Bacteria and Their Role in Infection. New York, McGraw-Hill, 1965, pp. 33–41.

Pecora DV, Landis RE, Martin E: Location of cutaneous microorganisms. Surgery 64:1114, 1968

Respiratory System

Bjorkwall T: Bacteriological examination in maxillary sinusitis. Acta Otolaryngol 83 (Suppl. 83):1, 1950

Rosebury T: Distribution and Development of the Microbiota of Man. In Microorganism Indigenous to Man. New York, McGraw-Hill, 1962, pp.

310–350. Note: An exhaustive review of the subject. Although it is old, it remains an excellent resource.

Watson ED, Hoffman NJ, Simmers RW, Rosebury T: Aerobic and anaerobic bacterial counts of nasal washings: Presence of organisms resembling *Corynebacterium acnes*. J Bacteriol 83:144–148, 1962

Digestive System

Drasar BS, Shiner M, McLeod GM: Studies on the intestinal flora. I. The bacterial flora of the gastrointestinal tract in healthy and achlorhydric persons. Gastroenterology. 56: 71, 1969

Gorbach SL: Intestinal microflora. Gastroenterology. 60: 1110, 1971

Moore WEC, Holdeman LV: Human fecal flora: The normal flora of 20 Japanese-Hawaiians. Appl Microbiol 27:961, 1974. Note: A classic microbiologic study.

Nichols RL, Broido P, Condon RE, Gorbach SL, Nyhus LM: Effect of preoperative neomycin-erythromycin intestinal preparation on the incidence of infectious complications following colon surgery. Ann Surg 178:453, 1973

Nolte WA: Oral ecology. In Oral Microbiology. St. Louis, Mosby, 1973, pp. 3–44

Urogenital System

Bartleh JG, Onderdonk AB, Drude E, et al.: Quantitative bacteriology of the vaginal flora. J Infect Dis 136:271, 1977

Stamey TA: Urinary Infections. Baltimore, Williams & Wilkins, 1974, pp. 87, 204

Foreign Bodies

Haury BB, Rodeheaver GT, Pettry D, Edgerton MT, Edlich RF: Inhibition of nonspecific defenses by soil infection potentiating factors. Surg Gynecol Obstet 144:19, 1977

Rodeheaver G, Pettry D, Turnbull V, Edgerton MT, Edlich RF: Identification of the wound infection—potentiating factors in soil. Am J Surg 128:8, 1974

Local Anesthesia

Albert J, Lofstrom B: Effects of epinephrine in solutions of local anesthetic agents. Acta Anaesthesiol Scand (suppl) 16:71, 1965

Covino BG: Comparative clinical pharmacology of local anesthetic agents. Anesthesiology 35:158, 1971

Stevenson TR, Rodeheaver GT, Golden GT, et al.: Damage to tissue defenses by vasoconstrictors. J Am Coll Emerg Phys 4:532, 1975

Hair Removal

Cruse PJE, Foord R: A five-year prospective study of 23,649 surgical wounds. Arch Surg 107:206, 1973

Seropian R, Reynolds BM: Wound infections after preoperative depilatory versus razor preparation. Am J Surg 121:251, 1971

Mechanical Cleansing

Madden JC, Edlich RF, Schauerhamer R, et al.: Application of principles of fluid dynamics to surgical wound irrigation. Curr Top Surg Res 3:85, 1971

Rodeheaver GT, Pettry D, Thacker JG, Edgerton MT, Edlich RF: Wound cleansing by high pressure irrigation. Surg Gynecol Obstet 141:357, 1975

Rodeheaver GT, Smith SL, Thacker JG, Edgerton MT, Edlich RF: Mechanical cleansing of contaminated wounds with a surfactant. Am J Surg 129:241, 1975

Stevenson TR, Thacker JG, Rodeheaver GT, et al.: Cleansing the traumatic wound by high pressure syringe irrigation. J Am Coll Emerg Phys 5:17, 1976

Wheeler CB, Rodeheaver GT, Thacker JG, Edgerton MT, Edlich RF: Side-effects of high pressure irrigation. Surg Gynecol Obstet 143:775, 1976

Antibiotics

Edlich RF, Smith QT, Edgerton MT: Resistance of the surgical wound to antimicrobial prophylaxis and its mechanisms of development. Am J Surg 126:583, 1973

Rodeheaver GT, Edgerton MT, Elliot MB, Kurtz LD, Edlich RF: Proteolytic enzymes as adjuncts to antibiotic prophylaxis of surgical wounds. Am J Surg 127:564, 1974

Rodeheaver GT, Marsh D, Edgerton MT, Edlich RF: Proteolytic enzymes as adjuncts to antimicrobial prophylaxis of contaminated wounds. Am J Surg 129:537, 1975.

Dead Space

Condie JD, Ferguson DJ: Experimental wound infections: contamination versus surgical technique. Surgery 50:367, 1961

DeHoll D, Rodeheaver G, Edgerton MT, Edlich RF: Potentiation of infection by suture closure of dead space. Am J Surg 127:716, 1974

Ferguson DJ: Clinical application of experimental relations between technique and wound infection. Surgery 63:377, 1968

Halsted WS: The treatment of wounds with especial reference to the value of blood clot in the management of dead space. Johns Hopkins Hosp Rep 2:255, 1890–1891

Kocher T: Uber die einfachsten mittel zur erzielung einer wundheilung durch verklebung ohne drainrohen. Volkmann's Sammlung klin Vortrage. 224, 1882

451

Kuster E: Uber die anwendung versenkter nahte. Arch Klin Chir 31:126, 1884

Neuber G: Vorschlage zur beseitigun der drainage fur alle frischen wunden. Mitth Chir Klin zu Kiel 1:27, 1884

Schede M: Uber die heilung von wunden unter der feuchten blutscharf. Utsch Med Wochenschr 12:389, 1886

Wound Closure

Acland R: Thrombus formation in microvascular surgery: An experimental study of the effects of surgical trauma. Surgery 73:766, 1973

Afanassief N: Ueber die bedeutung des granulationsgewebes bei der infection von wunden mit pathogene mikroorganismen. Beitr Path Anat 22:11, 1897

Alexander JW, Altemeier WA: Penicillin prophylaxis of experimental staphylococcal wound infections. Surg Gynecol Obstet 120:243, 1965

Alexander JW, Kaplan JZ, Altemeier WA: Role of suture materials in the development of wound infection. Ann Surg 165:192, 1967

Billroth T: Beobactungs-studien uber wundfieber und accidentelle wundkrankheiten. Arch Klin Chir 6:372, 1865

Carpendale MTF, Sereda W: The role of percutaneous suture in surgical wound infection. Surgery 58:672, 1965

Douglas DM: Tensile strength of sutures. II. Loss when implanted in living tissue. Lancet 2:499, 1949

DuMortier JJ: The resistance of healing wounds to infection. Surg Gynecol Obstet 56:762, 1927

Edlich RF, Panek PH, Rodeheaver GT, et al.: Physical and chemical configuration of sutures in the development of surgical infection. Ann Surg 177:679, 1973

Edlich RF, Rodeheaver GT, Kuphal J, et al.: Technique of closure: Contaminated wounds. J Am Coll Emerg Phys 3:375, 1974

Edlich RF, Thul J, Prusak M, Madden J, Wangensteen OH: Studies in the management of the contaminated wound. VIII. Assessment of tissue adhesives for repair of contaminated tissue. Am J Surg 122:394, 1971

Edlich RF, Tsung MS, Rogers W, Rogers P, Wangensteen OH: Studies in the management of the contaminated wound. I. Technique of closure of such wounds together with a note on a reproducible model. J Surg Res 8:585, 1968

Halley CRL, Chesney AM, Dresel I: On the behavior of granulating wounds of the rabbit to various types of infection. Bull Johns Hopkins Hosp 41:191, 1927

Conolly WB, Hunt TK, Zederfeldt B, Cafferata HT, Dunphy JE: Clinical comparison of surgical wounds closed by suture and adhesive tapes. Am J Surg 117:318, 1969

Harrison ID, Williams DF, Cuschieri A: The effect of metal clips on the tensile properties of healing skin wounds. Br J Surg 62:945, 1975

Harrison JH, Adler RH: Nylon as a vascular prosthesis in experimental animals with tensile strength studies. Surg Gynecol Obstet 103:613, 1956

Heaton LD, Hughes CW, Rosegay H: Military surgical practices of the United States Army in Viet Nam. Cur Probl Surg 19, 1966

452

Herrmann JB: Tensile strength and knot security of surgical suture materials. Am J Surg 37:209, 1971

Kirk N: U.S. War Department. Army Service Forces. Office of the Surgeon General. Circular Letter No. 91, April 26, 1943

Lennihan R Jr, Mackereth MA: A comparison of staples and nylon closure in varicose vein surgery. Vasc Surg 9:200, 1975

Moloney GE: The effect of human tissues on the tensile strength of implanted nylon sutures. Br J Surg 48:528, 1961

Noetzel W: Ueber die infection granulirender wunden. Arch Klin Chir, 55:543, 1897

Postlethwait, RW: Long-term comparative study of non-absorbable sutures. Ann Surg 171:892, 1970

Postlethwait RW: Polyglycolic acid surgical suture. Arch Surg 101:489, 1970

Schimmelbusch C: Die aufnahme bakterielle keime von frischen und blutenden wunden. Deutsche Med Wchnschr 20:575, 1894

Terzis J, Faibisoff B, Williams B: The nerve gap: Suture under tension vs. graft. Plast Reconstr Surg 56:166, 1975

Usher FC, Allen JE, Crosthwait RW, Cogan JE: Polypropylene monofilament. A new biologically inert suture for closing contaminated wounds. JAMA 179:780, 1962

Van Winkle W Jr, Hastings JC: Consideration in the choice of suture materials for various tissues. Surg Gynecol Obstet 135:113, 1972

Weeks PM, Wray RC: Management of Acute Hand Injuries. A Biological Approach. St. Louis, Mosby, 1973

Williams DF: The reactions of tissues to materials. Biomed Eng 6: 152, 1971

Drains

Baker BH, Borchardt KA: Sump drains and airborne bacteria as a cause of wound infections. J Surg Res 17:407, 1974

Berliner SD, Burson LC, Lear, PE: Use and abuse of intraperitoneal drains in colon surgery. Arch Surg 89:686, 1964

Carrel A: Cicatrization of wounds. XII. Factors initiating regeneration. J Exp Med 34:425, 1921

Carrel A, Hartmann A: Cicatrization of wounds, the relation between size of the wound and the rate of cicatrization. J Exp Med 125:965, 1967

Cerise EJ, Pierce WA, Diamond DL: Abdominal drains: Their role as a source of infection following splenectomy. Ann Surg 171:764, 1970

Cohn I Jr, Cotlar AN, Atik M, et al.: Bile peritonitis. Ann Surg 152:827, 1960

Davis JH, Yull AB: A toxic factor in abdominal injury. II. The role of the red cell component. J Trauma 4:84, 1964

Golden G, Chandler JG, Fox J, Edgerton MT, Edlich RF: Surgical drainage: Collective review. Submitted to Surg Gynecol Obstet.

Halsted WS: Concerning drainage and drainage tubes. Trans Am Surg Assoc 16:103, 1898

Howard JM, Singh LM: Peritoneal fluid pH after perforation of peptic ulcers: The myth of "acid-peritonitis." Arch Surg 87:483, 1963

Krizek TJ, Davis JH: The role of red cell in subcutaneous infection. J Trauma 5:85, 1965

Magee C, Rodeheaver GT, Golden G, et al.: Potentiation of wound infection by surgical drains. Am J Surg 131:547, 1976

Manz CW, Latendresse C, Sako Y: The detrimental effects of drains on colonic anastomoses: An experimental study. Dis Colon Rectum 13:17, 1970

Morris AM: A controlled trial of closed wound suction. Br J Surg 60:357, 1973

Nora PF, Vanecko RM, Bransfield JJ: Prophylactic abdominal drains. Arch Surg 105:173, 1972

Rewbridge AG, Hrdina LS: The etiological role of bacteria in bile peritonitis. An experimental study in dogs. Proc Soc Exp Biol Med 27:528, 1929–1930

Smith M, Enguist IF: A quantitative study of impaired healing resulting from infection. Surg Gynecol Obstet 125:965, 1967

Thal A, Perry JF, Jr, Egner W: A clinical and morphologic study of forty-two cases of fetal auto pancreatitis. Surg Gynecol Obstet 105:191, 1957

Dressings

Fomon S: The Surgery of Injury and Plastic Repair. Baltimore, Williams & Wilkins, 1939, p. 495

Reid R: Complications of the wounding. In Maingot R (ed): The Management of Abdominal Operations, 2nd ed, Vol 1. New York, Macmillan, 1957, p 289

Schauerhamer RA, Edlich RE, Panek P, et al.: Studies in the management of the contaminated wound. VII. Susceptibility of surgical wounds to postoperative surface contamination. Am J Surg 122:74, 1971

Warren R: Surgery. Philadelphia, Saunders, 1963, p 43

7

WOUND MANAGEMENT IN SELECTED TISSUES

Peripheral Nerve Repair
    Lynn D. Ketchum
Vascular Repair
    Wesley S. Moore
    James M. Malone
Tendon Healing
    Lynn D. Ketchum
Fracture and Cartilage Repair
    R. Bruce Heppenstall
Burns
    Thomas K. Hunt
Wound Healing in the Gastrointestinal Tract
    Clifford W. Deveney
    J. Englebert Dunphy

Introduction

In this section, we present discussions of repair in certain important tissues of the body. As seen in previous chapters repair is a relatively nonspecific process designed primarily to restore anatomic continuity of disrupted tissues. Repair generally accomplishes the task of restoration of the physical integrity of tissues, but restoration of biologic function is frequently much less satisfactory. In the area of restoration of biologic function, the skill and knowledge of the surgeon can play a particularly important role. A thorough understanding of the fundamental principles of the healing process is essential for the most successful results. For instance, tendon injuries, particularly in the hand, are difficult to manage because the repair process may prevent continued function; but a firm grasp of the basic principles of management of this type of injury can offer the skilled surgeon the best chance for a functional result. Much the same applies to nerve injuries, vascular injuries, and to the repair of visceral and bony tissues. In every case, the surgeon must avoid letting the repair process impair function, but at the same time he must guide it to restoration of anatomical continuity.

The surgeon's mechanical skills can be employed with maximum effectiveness only if he has the knowldge and understanding of the fundamental principles of the repair process on which he so totally relies. With this knowledge and with skilled judgment applied to each individual patient, the young surgeon can soon achieve mastery of even the most difficult problems in wound management. We hope that we have contributed to this goal.

Peripheral Nerve Repair
Lynn D. Ketchum

THE HEALING PROCESS

In the healing of a transected tendon, we hope that not only will the divided tendon ends heal with sufficient tensile strength to transmit a significant force, but will perform the specialized function of gliding. Similarly, surgeons expect that a healing nerve develop sufficient tensile strength to resist separation when it is stretched, that it glide, as the joints it traverses are flexed and extended, and that it develop the highly specialized function of transmitting numerous electrical impulses simultaneously in two directions.

Nerve injuries include simple compression, crushing, stretching, and transection. Though the end result of these four mechanisms is alteration and/or cessation of neural transmission, the prognosis of each is significantly different. To understand how various forms of nerve injury affect function, a brief review of the anatomy of a typical mixed peripheral nerve is helpful (Fig. 7. 1). A peripheral nerve consists of numerous axons that are extensions of nerve cells in the spinal cord. Axons are insulated by myelin, which is in essence a Schwann cell, cushioned by mesenchymal tissue and nourished by an intrinsic and extrinsic vascular supply. Each nerve has an outer layer of connective tissue known as the epineurium. Encased

459

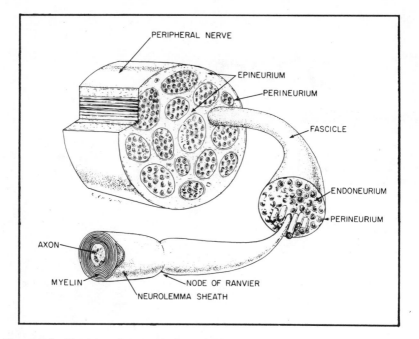

Figure 7.1   The internal anatomy of a peripheral nerve, demonstrating the epineurium, perineurium, and endoneurium with multiple axons being found within a single fascicle, each fascicle being covered by perineurium

by the epineurium are numerous bundles of nerve fibers called fascicles or funiculi, each in turn encased by a multilayered connective tissue membrane called perineurium. Each layer of perineurium is covered with a basement membrane. The perineurium functions as a diffusion barrier to numerous substances including proteins to help maintain an environment similar to the central nervous system within the endoneurial space which is within the perineurium.

Each fascicle contains many nerve fibers. These fibers are separated from each other by a loose tissue lattice of collagen fibrils, fibroblasts, and capillaries, called the endoneurium.

Peripheral nerve fibers are differentiated into myelinated and unmyelinated types. Each myelinated axon is surrounded by a series of Schwann cells, each forming a myelin sheath for a regular length of axon known as the internodal length. The diameter of the nerve fiber correlates with its axon sheath thickness and internodal length. The junctional area interposed

460

between two Schwann cells, known as the node of Ranvier (Fig. 7.1), occurs at approximately 1 mm intervals along myelinated fibers. In the case of unmyelinated axons, several axons are ensheathed by a chain of Schwann cells distributed at intervals along the length of the fiber. Thus at any level there is one Schwann cell for several axons. A thin extracellular coat or basal lamina surrounds both myelinated and unmyelinated fibers and serves as a conduit. This structure, known as the endoneurial or Schwann tube, provides the critical framework that guides regenerating fibers to their peripheral terminations during reinnervation. Furthermore, the action potentials are conducted differentially in the two types of fibers. In the unmyelinated fibers, the spread of current is continuous and conduction appears to be a uniform process; whereas in the myelinated fibers conduction is discontinuous, saltatory (leaping), and the impulse skips from one node of Ranvier to the next because the insulating nature of the myelin sheath allows current to pass through the membrane only at the nodes. This factor brings about a considerable increase in the conduction velocity of myelinated fibers. The conduction velocity is proportional to the diameter of the underlying fibers and greater internodal distance, and can range from 100 meters per second to less than 2 meters per second.

In a mixed peripheral nerve, there are both motor and sensory fibers. Efferent (motor) fibers innervate extrafusal (skeletal) muscle fibers. They are divided into those having a diameter of 9 to 17 MU, which are responsible for muscle contraction, and smaller fibers, known as fusimotor or gamma fibers, which have a diameter of 3 to 8 MU and innervate the intrafusal fibers of the muscle spindle, a proprioception receptor. Efferent fibers of the autonomic nervous system are the smallest motor fibers, mostly unmyelinated and conduct at a velocity of less than 2 meters per second.

Afferent fibers are both myelinated and unmyelinated and have cell bodies in the dorsal root ganglia. It has been demonstrated that large myelinated sensory fibers (group A-beta fibers) can be subdivided by their response to mechanical stimuli into quickly adapting and slowly adapting fibers. The quickly adapting fibers can be further subdivided into a group of maximally responsive to 30 cps vibratory stimuli and a group maximally responsible to 256 cps. Clinically the slowly adapting

461

fibers are interpreted as those mediating the perception of a constant touch stimulus (as Von Frey or Weber). The quickly adapting fibers perceive not only vibration, but moving touch stimuli (such as any object, e.g., a pencil eraser moving across a fingertip). This phenomenon is important because there is a pattern of return of sensory perception following nerve recovery with certain types of sensation such as pinprick being perceived first and two point discrimination last. The usefulness of this fact in the sensory reeducation of the patient following peripheral nerve repair will be discussed later.

For normal nerve function, nerve cells must have a continuous and adequate supply of oxygen through the intraneural vascular system. While transection of a nerve results in loss of excitability in its distal part within three to eight days, complete ischemia is followed by rapid deterioration of nerve function within 30 to 90 minutes; however, if blood flow is reestablished, as with release of tourniquet, recovery of nerve function occurs concomitantly.

There are two integrated but functionally independent microvascular systems, extrinsic and intrinsic, providing a blood supply to peripheral nerves. The extrinsic system is composed of segmentally arranged vessels varying in size, which originate from nearby large arteries and veins as well as from smaller adjacent muscular and periosteal vessels. As these vessels approach a large nerve trunk, they run in a mesoneurium and branch distally and proximally (small nerves do not have a mesoneurium). When the local nutrient vessels reach the epineurium, they divide into ascending and descending branches and anastomose with the intraneural intrinsic system, which is composed of epineurial, perineurial, and endoneurial plexuses and their communicating vessels.

The well-developed perineurial plexus has a close relationship with the intrafascicular, endoneurial vascular bed, which extends the whole length of the nerve and consists mainly of capillaries.

Under normal conditions, only part of the intraneural bed is functioning at any one time. Empty capillaries can be seen in the endoneurial space, and they start to function immediately when warm saline is applied or when the nerve is slightly traumatized.

The question of nerve vascularization during mobilization is important clinically. Nerves can be mobilized extensively with minimum histologic, neurophysiologic, or clinical evidence of ischemic damage. Up to 14 cm without transecting it or 7 cm of a transected nerve can be mobilized without impairment. The intraneurial blood supply is impaired when a nerve is elongated by 8 percent and blood flow comes to a standstill when the nerve is elongated by 15 percent.

The epineurial blood vessels normally allow the passage of small amounts of circulating serum proteins across their walls and these proteins can diffuse close to the perineurium but do not pass through this impermeable structure. The endoneurial vessels have unique permeability qualities. When radioactive labeled albumin is injected intravenously, the protein remains in the lumen of these vessels and the tracer does not pass into the extracellular space of the endoneurium. Waksman refers to this as the blood–nerve barrier.

Mast cells may be found along the intraneurial microvessels; they can synthesize, store, and release heparin and biogenic amines, which are thought to cause increased permeability of the vessels. Thus mast cells may play an important role in edema in nerve injury.

NERVE INJURY

Within 70 to 100 hours after nerve transection, normal neuromuscular transmission fails and action potentials no longer conduct. Within a few more days, myelin sheaths begin to break down.

The axon is a cytoplasmic process of the centrally located cell. The cell, itself, reacts to an axonal injury by swelling, which may last several months. Although little change is seen in the proximal part of the axon, the distal part undergoes Wallerian degeneration, the rate of which depends upon the presence and thickness of the myelin sheath. Unmyelinated fibers degenerate most rapidly. Within 24 to 48 hours after injury, the neurofibrils in the axoplasm of the segments degenerate and disappear. The axoplasm of the distal segment appears to increase in optical density and begins to clump, leaving large vacant spaces within the myelin sheath, or in the case of unmyelinated fibers within the enveloping Schwann cell membrane.

About 48 hours after injury, the myelin sheath begins to show characteristic changes, losing its sharp layered appearance and becoming more homogeneous. The Schwann cells respond vigorously to nerve injury, particularly those close to the site of injury. Macrophages, from both intra- and extraneural sources, appear in the first few days and presumably remove degenerated products. Schwann cells proliferate early and the proliferation persists until the late phase of repair. This is the predominant cell type in the distal, densely cellular segment; and these cells have a specific function in guiding regeneration. Endoneurial fibroblasts multiply as well and begin to lay down collagen during the repair process. This collagen is laid down both around and between the regenerating tubules. In the distal segment, the axon tubules tend to collapse and become compressed, and in some cases obliterated as a result of active cellular proliferation and collagen deposition. (Collagen accumulated during reinnervation does not resorb as in cutaneous wounds.)

This process of Wallerian degeneration occurs throughout the entire distal segment beyond the nerve injury and in the proximal segment to the first node of Ranvier. Following an injury, changes also occur in the vascular elements of a nerve. There is an almost immediate exudation of circulating albumin at the site of trauma, and during the following days, the extravascular albumin rapidly spreads distally in the endoneurial space. In addition to these early changes, there is a second wave of increased permeability, which usually peaks about two weeks posttrauma, probably due to formation of immature vessels with special permeability properties.

Following crush, there is abnormal permeability at the site of trauma, starting on the first day and persisting for at least four months. Once inside the endoneurium, protein (albumin) spreads mainly in a distal direction. The permeability of the perineurium distal to the trauma site remains unchanged; however, it was concluded that even localized trauma to a nerve may change the environment of the nerve fibers far away from the primary injury for a long time, due to the diffusion of proteins (albumin) from the tissue surrounding the traumatized region.

REGENERATION

Following injury, changes in the nerve cell occur in preparation for repair. Active protein synthesis begins sometime in the first few weeks after injury in the cell body; then the products of protein synthesis migrate down the axon to the site of repair and beyond into the eventually changed distal segment. In addition to central events, glial cells (the supporting cells of nervous tissue) proliferate in the surroundings of the nerve cell.

At the site of injury, cellular bridge formation is seen in the distal tubules, which basically become columns of Schwann cells surrounded by collagen sheaths. These columns tend to migrate centrally and hook up to the proximal segment, and are best thought of as bridges over which new axons will travel. In the central segment, axons actively form numerous branches that push distally as a result of axon streaming and a measurable increase in axoplasmic pressure. Axons are also guided by a natural affinity that the axon has for the Schwann cell's surface. This phenomenon is called homotropism. Axonal branches enter the distal tubules and tend to crowd the Schwann cell processes to one side. The reentering axons are smaller than normal and many may be present in a single tubule, which may undergo remyelinization gradually as the guidance function of the Schwann cell ceases. Initially, the number of axonal branches reaching the distal segment far exceeds the normal number, up to four times the normal by some estimates. As regeneration proceeds, the axonal population diminishes, and eventually in the healed nerve, fewer than normal axons are present—a form of functional remodeling peculiar to the peripheral nerve.

The distal injured nerve segment or graft does not act as a group of empty tubes conducting the regenerating axons, passively waiting for axonal refilling. Regeneration is an active invasion and displacement process in which the pushing forces of axonal streaming, increased axoplasmic pressure, and central protein synthesis are opposed by distal Schwann cell proliferation, collapsed tubules, and collagen accumulation.

Myelin sheaths first make their appearance on the regenerating axon at about six to seven days. Nodes of Ranvier appear some two weeks later. Myelin continues to be laid down for approximately one year.

The flow of axoplasm into the distal coapted segments does not occur immediately and is impeded by edema, mechanical stress of bringing the nerves together, inflammation, and collagen synthesis. There is a delay of five to six weeks before any evidence of regeneration can be detected.

NERVE REPAIR

Having looked at the process of degeneration and regeneration, what is the best technique of repairing divided nerve for optimum regeneration? Obviously until the ideal tissue cement

Figure 7.2 These drawings depict epineurial and perineurial nerve sutures. **A.** In the epineurial nerve suture, the suture goes through the epineurium and does not touch the fascicle at all. **B.** In contrast, in the perineurial, or interfascicular, nerve suture, the suture goes through the perineurium of each fascicle. In this way, fascicles of similar size in the same area of opposing transected ends of a peripheral nerve are coapted. *(Courtesy of Ethicon, Inc.)*

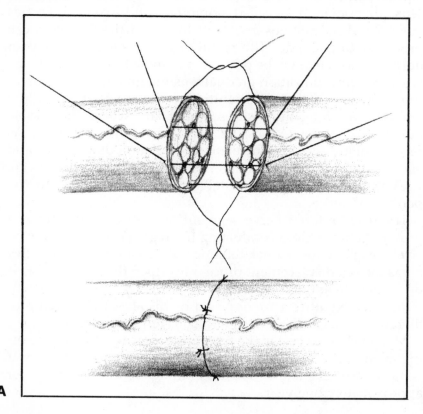

A

is found, the two divided ends must be coapted by sutures. The suture technique, diameter, and composition should be such as to minimize the inflammatory reaction in and around the nerve. The amount of fibroplasia and resultant collagen synthesis is directly related to the inflammatory reaction. One of the two main deterrents to regaining good nerve function is excessive scar tissue obstructing the properly oriented flow of axoplasm. The other is disorientation of axons into the wrong endoneurial tubes, so that either sensory axons enter motor endoneurial tubes, and vice versa, or sensory axons enter sensory endoneurial tubes but different ones than they originally traversed, so that the cerebrum does not interpret correctly the information returned to it by the stimuli of different end-

Figure 7.2   B

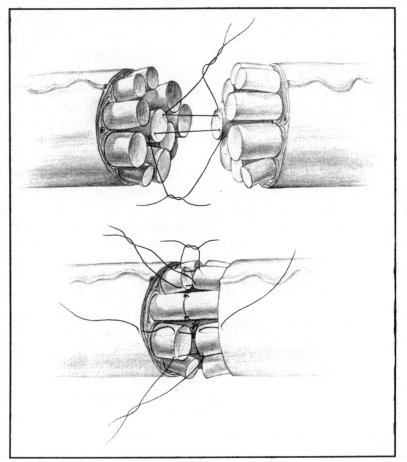

B

organs. If inflammation can be minimized, the regenerating axons retain the ability to cross the fibrous barrier at the area of repair and then to open endoneurial tubes collapsed by cellular proliferation and collagen proliferation.

There are two techniques currently in use for the primary repair of divided nerves: the epineurial and the perineurial, or interfascicular, suture techniques (Fig. 7.2). In the epineurial technique, sutures are placed in the epineurium only, taking care to align blood vessels (external topography) of the proximal and distal segments so that the homotropic process (i.e., the attraction of like tissues to each other) will occur and fascicles will have the best opportunity to reunite with their respective distal counterparts. The topographic orientation is lost after one or two weeks, which is an important reason to repair nerves primarily if the epineurial approach is used. The perineurial approach has the theoretical advantage of directly suturing individual fascicles to like counterparts. The advantage is somewhat theoretical because fascicles are not color coded and many are of similar size, so it is still possible to suture sensory fascicles proximally to motor fascicles distally.

The technique of perineurial repair embodies the ultimate refinements to date in surgical technique, second only to microvascular repair. It is difficult to perform perineurial repair without magnification. It is made easier with a 2x or 4x loupe and greatly facilitated by an operating microscope using a magnification of 8 or 16 power. Instruments designed for microsurgical procedures should be used, as the 8-0 and 9-0 sutures cannot be held by large, clumsy ratcheted needle holders. Suture material should be nonreactive and nonabsorbable, such as nylon. As seen in Figure 7.2B, the needle is placed through the side of a fascicle and then through another fascicle of matching size in the same area of the opposing transected nerve end. In this way every fascicle is sutured, care being taken to minimize handling and crushing. The repair is usually done after hemostasis has been achieved and a tourniquet is usually elevated to maintain a dry field. Following repair, joints are appropriately flexed or extended to minimize tension on the repair. After three weeks, sufficient healing should have occurred to prevent disruption of the nerve. Therefore, gentle motion is begun and progressively increased at weekly intervals.

468

The first significant report of perineurial repairs, published in 1972, generated several good experimental studies of perineurial versus epineurial repair, and a few clinical reports. In one study of 40 repaired median and ulnar nerves monitored by EMG in Rhesus monkeys, significantly improved results were found in the interfascicular repair group. However, in another study comparing the two techniques in cats, there was no statistical difference in repairs evaluated histologically, by muscle weights and by functional results. Yet another experimental study comparing the two techniques found that after epineurial repair of rabbit sciatic nerves, 60 percent of normal myelin production was found in the distal segments compared to 23.8 percent for interfascicular repairs.

Most of the collagen in peripheral nerves is in the perineurium. Morphologic observations suggest that after nerve transection, the endoneurial Schwann cell tubes in the distal nerve segments become progressively constricted by deposition of endoneurial collagen and that this endoneurial fibrosis results in a permanent reduction in the diameter attained by regenerating axons. It is felt by those investigators that dissection, the trauma of suturing, and the suture material per se, potentiate the inflammatory response sufficiently that increased collagen deposition decreases the amount of axonal regeneration.

With this in mind, another investigator injected the area around the nerve repair with the antiinflammatory agent, triamcinolone, and found significantly decreased amounts of collagen both around and in the area of nerve repair without adverse influence on regeneration.

The question of epineurial versus perineurial (interfascicular) repair remains moot and unanswered, though it is obvious that inflammation must be minimized. What answers have come out of these investigations are that there is a limit to the distance a nerve can be mobilized from its external blood supply and the amount of tension that can be placed on the nerve ends to be coapted. As mentioned above, 7 cm is the maximum distance a transected nerve can be mobilized without producing cell death and fibrosis. In addition, tension on the anastomosis leads to poor results because it renders the nerve ischemic followed by the inevitable chain reaction of degeneration and collagenous repair. It has been established that tension leads to fibrosis in the healing of other tissues, and recently it has been found to be perhaps the most formidable offender in nerve repair.

How much is too much tension? In the ideal repair, freshly divided nerve ends are coapted and there is minimal tension. However, severed nerves retract and if a repair is not done primarily, it will be more difficult to bring them together with minimal tension. Furthermore, scar tissue covers the perineurial bundles and nerves will have to be resected to free those bundles. A gap of less than 2.5 cm is the optimum distance to be overcome for good results. Results of experimental studies of nerve repair in which there was mild stretching (4 cm gap) were equivalent to those obtained with a properly fitted nerve graft. With a gap of over 4 cm, considered moderate stretching, results are better when a graft is used without tension.

Nerve grafting has been done for some time but the recent development of suturing a graft under optimal tension, i.e., minimal tension with no redundancy, together with staggering suture lines of the fascicles to minimize circumferential scar contracture, led to results that are significantly better than nerve repairs under moderate tension. The donor site of the graft obviously must not leave a motor or sensory deficit and the sural nerve or lateral antebrachial cutaneous nerve are good donor sources in that regard. Several smaller nerves are preferred over one large nerve, as any large nerve will in all likelihood leave a deficit and the central cells will not survive; multiple small nerve grafts are known as cable grafts and have an improved chance for survival with function.

Following repair, nerve recovery may be monitored by several means to ascertain whether or not regeneration is occurring. The simplest clinical test is the Tinel's sign, where the examiner percusses along the course of the nerve, going from peripheral to central. Where the patient experiences an electric shock of greatest intensity indicates the advancing area of regeneration. The progress of regneration can also be checked using evoked potentials: a recording electrode is placed along the nerve proximal to the repair and the stimulating electrode is placed along the nerve distal to the repair. Stimulation proceeds along the nerve progressively and centrally until an action potential is recorded.

If nerve regeneration does not occur or does so with unsatisfactory results, it is likely that the nerve repair was disrupted for one or more reasons during the healing process, or that sufficient collagen was deposited between nerve ends during healing to prevent penetration of the axons down the distal endoneurial tubes with the formation of a neuroma (Fig. 7.3A,B).

Whether the nerve repair can be salvaged can be determined by surgical exploration. The nerve is first freed of surrounding scar tissue, then the conductivity through the repair is checked at surgery using evoked potentials. A stimulating electrode is placed on the nerve distal to the neuroma and a recording electrode is placed proximal to the neuroma. When the nerve is electrically stimulated distally from the stimulating electrode, the speed and intensity with which it is received by the pickup electrode is recorded. Obviously if no signal is recorded, the nerve is not transmitting electrical impulses. If conduction is slow with diminished amplitude, then there is an obstruction and a decreased number of functioning axons. When conduction is reasonably good, the author merely instills an antiinflammatory agent into the paraneurial tissues to prevent recompression. If conduction is poor, an internal neurolysis can be done by dissecting the fascicles apart using a careful delicate technique under magnification to decompress the individual fascicles; after internal neurolysis, conduction is rechecked. If conduction is reestablished, treat as above; individual fascicles may be checked using a new technique of microelectrophysiologic diagnosis, which will be used with increased frequency in the future. If some of the fascicles do not conduct, individual fascicular grafts can be done. If there is no conduction across the nerve repair, the neuroma should be excised and a nerve graft placed in the gap under minimal tension. Following resection of a neuroma, mobilizing the nerve and repairing it under tension, or with multiple joints flexed, is not recommended. Under these circumstances, the neuroma will probably recur when the joints are extended because of the significant tension that will develop on the nerve anastomosis. Since the area of healing is frequently in a bed of scar, compared to the normal soft, pliable tissue that the nerve originally rested in before injury, the nerve will not glide nor-

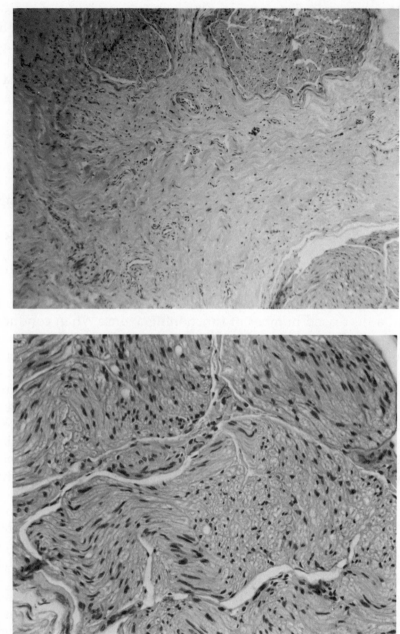

Figure 7.3 **A.** The amount of fibrovascular tissue that is seen in a neuroma. There are only a few fascicles present and the axons are smaller than normal. In this particular case, the nerve repair was stretched accidentally through a fall and the patient developed a neuroma. **B.** Higher power view of one of the fascicles seen in **A.** There is considerable vacuolization and many of the axons are smaller than normal.

mally, which only increases the amount of tension at the site of repair rather than distributing the tension equally throughout the nerve.

What is the expected functional result in the repair of a mixed peripheral nerve such as the median nerve at the wrist? A recent review of the literature revealed that less than 2 percent of such repairs regained normal two point discrimination (3 to 4 mm). Why were there such poor results? A certain percentage of these repairs disrupted and a certain percentage developed a neuroma in continuity; but most of the cases had good axonal penetration with reinnervation of end-organs, though of a decreased magnitude, as tested by nerve conduction velocities. One recent study of 19 patients showed that although up to puberty there is a linear correlation between nerve conduction velocity and two point discrimination, after puberty there is no correlation and that most of the adults studied had moderately good conduction while some had good two point discrimination and others did not with no predictable pattern. In another study, 23 fingertips were biopsied after repair of peripheral nerve injuries, and histologic evidence of end-organ regeneration was correlated with nerve function. The degree and level of the reinnervation did not correlate with clinical testing or subjective impression of the result. This means that although end-organs are reinnervated by regenerating axons, they are almost certainly not the original axons that innervated those end-organs, and the brain cannot unscramble or decode the barrage of the many and varied new messages that it is receiving from these end-organs.

Since the messages are there, the only way to restore function is to reeducate the patient beginning at the first sign of distal sensory recovery. Using pinprick, constant touch, moving touch, and vibration of 30 cps and 256 cps, it has been demonstrated that a typical pattern of sensory recovery occurs prior to the return of two point discrimination.

First to return distally is perception of pinprick, then the perception of 30 cps, either concurrently or just ahead of moving touch, then constant touch, then 256 cps. An example of a reeducation program would be the following: If 30 cps stimulus is perceived at a distal level, but moving touch is perceived only at a more proximal level, the patient can be started on perceiving moving touch stimuli; or if 256 cps stimulus is perceived at some distal level, but constant touch is perceived only at a more proximal level, it is the appropriate time to reeducate the patient on constant touch stimulus appreciation. The 256 cps stimuli does not test for fibers that moderate constant touch, but the fibers for which it does test return distally after the return of those for constant touch. Thus, if the 256 cps stimulus is perceived more distally than constant touch, we assume that the constant touch fibers are regenerated distally, but the patient has not learned to interpret their altered profile.

SUMMARY

Optimal results in the repair of peripheral nerves demand a precise approximation of the severed nerve ends with minimal stimulus of inflammation and fibroplasia, minimal mobilization of the nerves with suture under minimal tension, and careful patient follow-up with reeducation at the appropriate time.

BIBLIOGRAPHY

Almquist E, Eeg-Olofsson O: Sensory-nerve-conduction velocity and two-point discrimination in sutured nerves. J Bone Joint Surg 52-A:791, 1970

Bora FW Jr, Pleasure DE, Didizian NA: A study of nerve regeneration and neuroma formation after nerve suture by various techniques. J Hand Surg 1 (2): 138–43, 1976

Cabaud HE, Rodkey WG, McCarroll HR, Mutz SB, Niebauer JJ: Epineurial and perineurial fascicular nerve repairs: A critical comparison. J Hand Surg 1 (2): 131–37, 1976

Dellon AL, Curtis RM, Edgerton MT: Reeducation of sensation in the hand after nerve injury and repair. Plast Reconstr Surg 53 (3): 297–305, 1974

Grabb WC, Bement SL, Koepke GH, Green RA: Comparison of methods of peripheral nerve suturing in monkeys. Plast Reconstr Surg 46 (1): 31–37, 1970

Jabaley ME, Burns JE, Orcutt BS, Bryant WM: Comparison of histologic and functional recovery after peripheral nerve repair. J Hand Surg 1 (2): 119–30, 1976

Lundborg G: Structure and function of the intraneural microvessels as related to trauma, edema formation, and nerve function. J Bone Joint Surg 57-A (7): 938–48, 1975

Millesi H, Meissl G, Berger A: Further experience with interfascicular grafting of the median, ulnar, and radial neves. J Bone Joint Surg 58-A (2): 209–17, 1976

Orgel MG, Terzis JK: Epineurial vs. perineurial repair. Plast Reconstr Surg 60 (1): 80–9 1, 1977

474

Peacock EE Jr, Van Winkle W Jr: Surgery and Biology of Wound Repair. Philadelphia, Saunders, 1970, p 449

Remensnyder JP: Physiology of nerve healing and nerve grafts. In Symposium on Basic Science in Plastic Surgery, vol 15. St. Louis, Mosby, 1976, p 196

Smith JW: Microsurgery of peripheral nerves. Plast Reconstr Surg 33 (4): 317–29, 1964

Terzis JK, Dykes RW, Hakstian RW: Electrophysiological recordings in peripheral nerve surgery: A review. J Hand Surg 1 (1): 52–66, 1976

Terzis J, Faibisoff B, Williams HB: The nerve gap: suture under tension vs. graft. Plast Reconstr Surg 56 (2): 166–69, 1975

475

VASCULAR REPAIR
Wesley S. Moore
James M. Malone

The study of vascular repair is a relatively new field, which explains why there are minimal data and only limited understanding of the subject. This section summarizes currently available information in two broad categories: repair of autogenous vessels and the healing of prosthetic vascular grafts.

REPAIR OF AUTOGENOUS VASCULAR TISSUE

"Normal" healing of vascular conduits varies with the type of surgical procedure. Thromboendarterectomy, artery-to-vein

476

anastomoses, artery-to-artery anastomoses, and simple arteriotomy with primary closure all stimulate their characteristic patterns of repair.

Blood vessels are composed of three primary histologic layers: the internal layer or intima, the medial layer or muscular coat, and the external fibroaponeurotic or adventitial layer. The intimal surface of vessels is covered by a specialized cell type called the endothelial cell. This "nonwetting" cellular layer seems primarily involved with hemostasis, extravascular water regulation, fibrinolysis of thrombus, and vascular healing following injury. Normal endothelial cell turnover is slow and nonhomogeneous. However, arterial intimal thickening is a common nonspecific response to diverse types of injury. Intimal proliferation may also vary directly with hemodynamic factors, and is, of course, a feature of arteriosclerosis.

The two most important aspects of vascular healing are the reestablishment of a nonwetting endothelial surface and development of a strong elastic/muscular media. Investigation of the mechanism of intimal regeneration has suggested four possible origins of neoendothelial cells: (1) medial smooth muscle cells, which migrate through the wall of the injured vessel, (2) circulating endothelial cells, (3) circulating macrophages and mononuclear cells, and (4) junctional zone, that is, graft/host pannus extension at the anastomosis. The primary origin of new elastic fibers for the subintimal elastic lamina is felt to be from the medial smooth muscle (myointimal) cells.

Normal healing is divided into three phases: substrate, proliferative, and resorptive. This three-phase sequence appears to be inviolable. During the first two to three days fibroblasts appear in the wound and collagen production begins shortly following their appearance. The combination of old and new collagen provides wound strength.

By the fifth or sixth day, new collagen synthesis accelerates and wound strength increases rapidly. This proliferative phase continues for several weeks. New collagen synthesis occurs in combination with lysis of old collagen. The process of wound healing becomes a balance between lysis and synthesis of collagen. Any imbalance in the rates of old collagen lysis and new collagen synthesis results in a failure of wound healing; either anastomotic failure on the one hand, or stricture on the other.

In the resorptive phase, fibroblasts and tissue macrophages

disappear and the excess collagen is removed. During the latter stage of absorption, the amorphous mass of collagen, seen in early wound healing, gradually becomes an interlocking network of collagen fibers.

Unlike other tissues, blood vessels contain a special type of collagen (Type 3) which possesses special properties that allow some elasticity of the collagen tube, enhancing its characteristics as a vascular conduit.

Healing of Thromboendarterectomy Wounds

The animal model that is most commonly used to study healing following thromboendarterectomy is the rabbit or primate aorta. The intima is stripped by a single passage of a Fogarty catheter, providing a standardized reproducible model for study. Immediately following mechanical injury of the normal rabbit aorta, the subintimal and exposed medial surfaces are covered with a coagulum composed of fibrin, platelets, red blood cells, and leukocytes (Fig. 7.4). By 24 hours, junctional zones near the normal endothelium bordering the denuded segment of vessel show early endothelial cellular ingrowth and localized mitosis; however, both the early endothelial cellular ingrowth and the rate of endothelial mitosis may vary with different species studied. In addition, the rate of neoendothelization varies directly with the thickness of the initial platelet-fibrin-red and white cell thrombus; the larger the thrombus, the slower the reendothelization and the thicker the final neointimal layer.

The size of the original thrombus may vary with the degree of medial injury, the species variability of platelet function, the blood flow through the vessel being studied, the turbulence of flow, and the ultrastructure and thrombogenicity of the vascular lining. Variations of the depth of the initial thrombus probably account for the focal variations in the rate of neo- or pseudointimal growth.

At three days, light microscopic evaluation will reveal occasional endothelial cells; subendothelial thickening, inflammation, fracture, and disruption of the internal elastic lamella; medial necrosis with leukocyte infiltration; mitosis of medial smooth muscle cells; and mononuclear adventitial infiltration and no increase in total collagen content (Fig. 7.5).

478

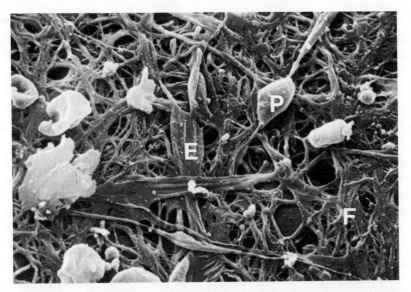

Figure 7.4 Early fibrin deposition on a grossly bare area of endarterectomy. Segments of elastic lamina are visible in the fibrin mesh (F-fibrin, P-platelet, E-elastic lamina) ×4, 375. *(From Moseley HS, Connell JS, Krippaehne WW: Healing of the canine aorta after endarterectomy. Ann Surg 180:331, 1974.)*

Figure 7.5 The arterial wall exhibits large necrotic areas and infiltration with leukocytes in the luminal part. *(From Helin P, Lorenzen I, Garbarsch C, Matthiesen ME: Repair in arterial tissue. Circ Res 29(1):542, 1971.)*

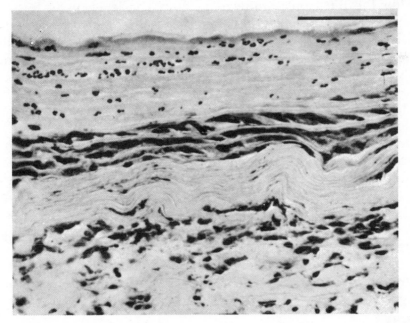

By six to eight days, one can see calcification of the internal elastic lamella, endothelial thickening, and a small increase in the number of neoendothelial cells. The initial leukocyte infiltration varies directly with the extent of the injury, but the decrease in leukocytes correlates with increased endothelial regeneration. Polymorphs and lymphocytes are replaced by monocytes (macrophages). The macrophages may direct collagen production by fibroblasts and serve, with platelets and thrombin, as a cellular coordinator of wound healing. The most probable source of the neoendothelial cells appears to be medial smooth muscle cells. It is of particular interest that platelets do not stick to these "myointimal" cells, that is, the "myointimal" cell is nonwetting.

Vascular permeability, as measured by I^{125} albumin uptake, is increased for 3 to 30 days following intimectomy. Similarly, scanning electron microscopy will show increased permeability of neoendothelial cells to macromolecules. The increase in neoendothelial permeability probably represents increased cellular pinocytosis and an increased gap in the intracellular spacing.

Total collagen content is not increased for the first six days. Chondroitin-4, 6-sulphate, measured by S^{35} sulphate uptake into sulphated glycosaminoglycans, is increased continuously after the third postintimectomy day. The level of hyaluronic acid is elevated during postinjury days 3 to 6 and then gradually decreases to normal by postinjury day 60. All of the changes in collagen content, chondroitin-4, 6-sulphate and hyaluronic acid are subject to wide focal variations which reemphasizes the nonuniformity of neoendothelial growth.

Two weeks following intimectomy, there is increased neoendothelium, irregular subendothelial (myointimal) thickening, new collagen and newly synthesized elastin in the media, and scattered, necrotic, calcified and noncalcified foci of inflammation. Both the calcified and noncalcified inflammatory foci are sites of monocytic proliferation and increased collagen synthesis. At this point, total collagen content exceeds control levels for the first time during the healing process. Adventitial neovascularization is increased.

By 30 days, there is continued neoendothelial and subendothelial (myointimal) thickening, continued collagen production in the myointima, and giant cell infiltration into areas of focal inflammation. By 60 days, calcified inflammatory foci are absorbed. Total collagen content and total chondroitin-4, 6-sulphate levels are elevated compared to control values; however, hyaluronic acid levels have decreased to preintimectomy control levels. There is little elastin present; however, the total eleastin content slowly increases during the succeeding months. Neoendothelial permeability has approached preinjury levels at two months. However, intracellular spacing increases slightly but permanently post-injury, and endothelial resistance to filtration and diffusion of water and solutes is decreased. *In other words, one intimal injury causes chronic alteration of endothelial permeability.*

Normal endothelial cells are spindle shaped and their cellular axes correspond to the direction of blood flow. However, neoendothelial cells are rounded, and initially have a random orientation. With time, the neoendothelial cells tend to flatten and become oriented parallel to the long axis of the vessel.

Healed neointima is usually several cell layers thick, rather than one cell layer thick as is normal; but by six months postintimectomy, the neointima thins to a one or two cell thickness. Failure of cellular thinning at specific foci probably reflects sustained myointimal proliferation. Since smooth muscle cells are stimulated by platelet debris and plasma proteins, the areas of focal myointimal thickening seem to correspond to initial sites of thick fibrin-platelet-red and white cell thrombus.

Elastin formation appears to be related to smooth muscle proliferation. Elastin may not become normally organized for the first six months following intimectomy.

By six months all species studied demonstrate complete healing of the intimectomized surface. As noted, however, the neoendothelial cells are not "normal" in shape, intracellular configuration, or function.

The healing sequence following intimectomy is important to the surgeon performing thromboendarterectomy. Disruption of the middle and outer layers of the arterial media, as when thromboendarterectomy is performed in a plane that is too far from the lumen, is associated with decreased patency and/or increased intimal fibrosis. A similar result may occur if the intimectomy leaves a rough or graded surface against the direction of blood flow. Because of the increased thrombogenicity of the newly intimectomized surface, there may be a place for the use of platelet inhibitors such as aspirin, persantoin, or dextran prior to and following thromboendarterectomy, but the definitive work remains to be done.

Healing of Anastomoses between Arteries and Veins

The early work of Carrel demonstrated the feasibility of using venous autografts in the arterial position. While it is true that degenerative changes including atherosclerosis, dilatation, and aneurysm formation have been observed in venous-arterial autografts, vein grafts are still satisfactory conduits for arterial replacement or bypass. They are the graft choice for many procedures, including coronary artery bypass, femoral-popliteal bypass, and patch angioplasties.

The techniques for preparation, dissection, and harvesting of an autogenous vein for arterial reconstruction are important. Storage of fresh autogenous vein in normal saline causes significant venous endothelial damage. There may be a loss of 40 to 50 percent of venous endothelial cells, as well as damage to cells in the subendothelial layers.

Following implantation of a vein in the arterial tree, 60 to 70 percent of the venous endothelial cells disappear within 48 hours. The areas of denuded venous intima are covered by platelet-fibrin-red and white cell clots. The surviving cells appear normal. Intimal proliferation can be seen near the venous internal elastic lamella. These changes persist for one or two weeks.

In the interval of two to four weeks, neointimal proliferation continues (Fig. 7.6). By four weeks, 80 to 90 percent of the venous graft is reendothelized. However, endothelial cellular orientation is still random and there are focal areas of intimal hyperplasia. Reendothelization is complete by six to eight weeks but with a random orientation of cells.

By 12 weeks, the venous endothelium and arterial endothelium are joined and the segments are now joined. However, areas of focal neointimal hyperplasia and random cellular orientation still persist. During the next three to six months

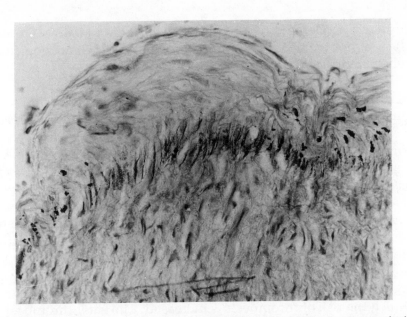

Figure 7.6 Transverse section through area of intimal proliferation in a two-week-old venous graft. *(From Wyatt AP, Taylor GW: Vein grafts: Changes in the endothelium of autogenous free vein grafts used as arterial replacements. Br J Surg 53:943, 1966.)*

fibroblasts progressively infiltrate the vein media and adventitia. The venous internal elastic lamella disappears between six to nine months following implantation.

Close examination of the venous intimal proliferation reveals the nonhomogeneous, almost random cellular distribution. We presume that growth and migration of endothelial cells are inhibited by cell to cell contact (contact inhibition); nevertheless, fibroblasts migrate between the endothelial cells, probably due to their random array and increased spacing. These fibroblasts then undergo extensive mitosis with rapid cellular extension into the subintimal areas. There is some suggestion that this aberrant fibroblastic proliferation occurs only in areas of thickened mural thrombus, much akin to the intimal changes seen during the healing of vessels following thromboendarterectomy. When arterial-venous endothelial healing is complete, this abnormal fibroblastic response stops. The cellular mechanisms governing this process remain unknown; myointimal fibrosis remains a common defect in the healing of vein grafts. Some feel that these sites of myointimal hyperplasia will later undergo accelerated atherosclerotic degeneration. In spite of these abnormalities, vein grafts exhibit normal thrombogenicity when compared to arteries.

Review of the healing of vein to artery anastomoses provides several important bits of information for the clinical surgeon. First of all, *a vein should be handled or manipulated as little as possible during its harvesting. A graft should be left in venous continuity as long as possible. When removed, it should be stored in cold heparinized blood. Vein grafts should never be stored in crystalloid solutions; these media will minimize cell damage but will not prevent it. Second, venous endothelial cells are disrupted by vessel overdistention and high pressure.* Therefore, care should be taken when testing or "dilating" vein grafts with a hand syringe filled with heparinized blood. Last, *healing of the autogenous vein graft approaches completion only after six to eight weeks.* The first two months is a critical time in the life of a reconstruction during which the risk of thrombosis is increased. The early thrombosis rate might be reduced by a period of anticoagulant administration or by the use of antiplatelet drugs until healing or neoendothelization is complete. Once again, proof is lacking.

Healing of Artery-to-Artery Anastomoses and Arteriotomies

The process of primary arterial healing has many similarities to the healing that takes place following intimectomy and arterial-venous anastomosis; however, there are several major differences. Both artery-to-artery anastomoses and arteriotomies approximate and heal similar tissues, so that the reparative process is primarily at the suture line. Freshly cut arterial tissue surfaces are less compromised by injury than their vein graft counterpart. Arteries are thicker than veins and can sustain more trauma during mobilization without incurring endothelial damage. Both artery-to-artery anastomoses and arteriotomies tend to be performed in areas of a relatively "normal" artery, which also leads to better healing characteristics.

Also, the endothelia of artery-to-artery anastomoses and arteriotomies heal by pannus extension (i.e. continuous autogenous endothelial growth across a suture line) rather than by cellular ingrowth from within the conduit wall. Humans are able to extend an endothelial pannus for no more than 6 to 10 mm in either direction from the suture line. Other animals vary.

During the first week following artery-to-artery anastomosis or arteriotomy closure, arterial collagen content, anastomotic strength, and healing times are similar to the healing curves seen for other tissues. There are few mitoses in the first 24 hours, but there is a marked increase by 48 hours. Complete neoendothelization of an arterial anastomosis or arteriotomy is seen by scanning electromicroscopy within 10 days; however, cellular orientation of the endothelium remains random. By 21 days, cellular orientation has returned to normal. Regeneration of the elastic lamina is not as rapid, nor is the end result as close to normal structure.

There is an intense inflammatory reaction around the suture that may last three to four weeks depending on the reactivity of the suture material utilized. The elastic lamella defect, which was most marked during the first week, is repaired by four to six weeks (Fig. 7.7). The origin of new elastic fibers appears to be from medial smooth muscle cells.

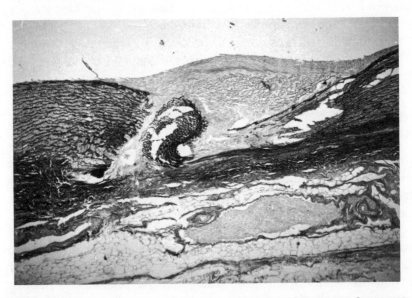

Figure 7.7   Site of artery-to-artery anastomosis five weeks after operation. Suture material is marked by the arrow. There is distortion of the elastic lamina and filling of the "depression" in the aortic wall by endothelial proliferation and new elastin formation. × 50. *(From Tawes RL Jr, Aberdeen E, Berry CL: The growth of an aortic anastomosis: An experimental study in piglets. Surgery 64(6): 1122–1132, 1968.)*

Healed arterial anastomoses remain excessively permeable, which we believe is due to increased intercellular spacing. Primary arterial anastomoses heal faster than either arterial-venous anastomoses or intimectomized vessels. The most important factors associated with disorders of primary arterial healing are the initial tension on the suture line and the type of suture material employed. Active vascular disease within the arterial wall also retards the rate of arterial healing.

There are several important clinical concepts that can be stressed. *First, arterial strength following end-to-end repair or arteriotomy increases in a curve similar to that for most other wounds so that stress on the anastomosis or arteriotomy should be kept at a minimum for at least two weeks. Second, arterial anastomoses and arteriotomies heal much more rapidly than either arterial-venous anastomoses or thrombo-endarterectomized vessels. Third, arterial anastomoses in children constructed with nonabsorbable suture should be interrupted at least once to permit enlargement of vascular diameter. Fourth, tucks taken in the suture line may result in disruption of the laminar flow and can contribute to progressive stenosis of the anastomosis. Finally, the surgeon should employ the most inert suture material available (i.e., braided dacron or monofilament polypropylene) as this incites the least fibrosis at the suture line and permits a more rapid resolution of the suture-induced inflammatory response.* This rapid inflammatory resolution is associated with less disturbance of normal arterial structure.

HEALING OF
ARTERIAL PROSTHESES

Prosthetic grafts, as such, do not heal, but rather they incite a modified foreign body reaction. This response, when controlled, can be used to advantage in order to simulate a "tissue-like" morphologic appearance and function.

Grafts of different materials and structural designs produce variations of the foreign body response that may have significance in both the immediate and long-term function of the prosthesis. This discussion addresses the phases of "healing" common to all cloth prostheses, and cites known differences between currently available grafts. One section is devoted to the two major healing complications associated with prosthetic vascular grafting: anastomotic aneurysm and infection.

486

Fabrication of Prosthetic Vascular Grafts

While many plastic materials have been tried in the vascular system, Dacron and Teflon are the two materials currently identified as the most suitable for prosthetic graft fabrication. Multifilament thread made of either dacron or teflon fibers can be used to either knit or weave a tubular graft. The weaving process essentially eliminates porosity as documented by the inability of the graft to leak fluid through its interstices.

Knitting, on the other hand, provides for porosity, which assumes a major importance in subsequent phases of "healing" and neointimal development. Porosity of a graft is measured by the volume of water that leaks through one square centimeter of cloth per minute at a pressure of 120 mm of mercury. The size of each individual pore, as well as the overall porosity, can be regulated by the fineness (denier) of the thread used for fabrication and by the number of stitches or needles per inch employed in the knitting process. In addition, the knitting process may employ different types of stitches that will improve stability and prevent unraveling of thread edges.

Finally, different surface characteristics can be imparted to the prosthesis; the introduction of elevated loops of yarn imparts a pile or velour surface to either the luminal or adventitial surface of the graft, or both. The use of the velour concept has recently assumed major importance. A final surface modification is the introduction of crimping of the tubular graft either as a series of concentric rings or random pleats in the tube. This is done to provide for some elasticity in the longitudinal axis and also to prevent kinking of the prosthesis during the time of implantation and later as it conforms to body contours.

The Phases of Healing

Phase I Immediately following implantation, fibrin is deposited on the luminal surface of all prosthetic grafts. Red cells, white cells, and platelets become trapped in this fibrin mesh and a coagulum forms on the graft surface. At this stage, the surface is highly thrombogenic but complete thrombosis is usually prevented by the high flow rate within the graft, particularly in larger protheses. As grafts of smaller diameter are employed, the propensity for graft thrombosis increases. The

487

critical diameter below which a high percent of graft thrombosis will occur is 5 mm.

Phase II Over the next few weeks, fibrolasts surround the prosthesis. A collagen matrix, which ultimately becomes a mature fibrous tissue capsule, surrounds the plastic grafts. The interstices of the graft, particularly knitted grafts, are infiltrated by collagen to a degree that is proportionate to the porosity and type of the material. Most prostheses do not develop a firm bond between the perigraft fibrous tissue capsule and the interstitial fibrous tissue that permeates the graft material. A potential and easily dissectible space remains between the graft and the capsule. However, porous dacron grafts tend to have a close apposition of the capsule and the graft in contrast to woven Teflon grafts that stimulate little fibroblastic response and often have a fluid collection between the graft and the poorly developed capsule. The knitted dacron velour prothesis, and in particular the external velour graft, is exceptional in this regard in that a tight transmural fibrous tissue bond develops. Experimental and clinical data suggest that this is a desirable characteristic and signifies a preferable or more advanced state of "healing."

Phase III The final phase of healing represents the metamorphosis of the fibrin lining into a pseudo- or neointima. In this phase the greatest variations occur between grafts of different design, and variations in patient responses are seen. Since most information has been obtained from animal experimentation, the translation to humans is inexact. However, human graft material recovered at various times following graft implantation has helped to validate the patterns documented in animals.

The intimal healing phase varies from essentially no change (from Phase II), to infiltration of the fibrin lining by fibroblasts and maturation into a cellular lining with final covering of a cellular neointima containing cells that closely resemble endothelium when viewed by scanning electron microscopy. Clearly, this more advanced phase of healing is the most desirable course, and grafts that will incite this type of response should be the prostheses of choice.

The grafts that demonstrate the poorest intimal healing are the woven grafts, the knitted grafts of low porosity, and those knitted grafts with many pores but with small pore size (Fig. (Fig. 7.8A). The grafts that appear to have the best intimal healing are the velour prostheses (Fig. 7.8B).

The mechanism of intimal healing is still speculative. Sauvage speaks of the "trellis" theory in which he proposes that fibroblasts advance along the course of the external velour loops in order to gain access to the compacted fibrin layer developing on the luminal surface. There is some evidence that fibrin split products may activate macrophages to stimulate fibroblast accumulation. Once such access is gained, he reasons, the fibroblasts infiltrate the fibrin layer, spreading a collagen matrix and developing into mature, cellular, fibrous tissue.

The origin of endothelial cells on this material or lining is controversial. Four possibilities have been proposed. First, ingrowth from anastomotic ends; a normal reaction following any graft implantation is the ingrowth of a pannus of intima from the host artery, however, this pannus ingrowth is usually limited to about 1 cm from each end. Second, transmural ingrowth with intimal budding of cells that ultimately mature into endothelium. Third, transmural ingrowth of capillaries that provide endothelial cells that spread over the luminal surface (rather similar in concept to regeneration of epithelial cells from skin appendages in second degree burns). Fourth, surface deposition of cells, perhaps even fibroblasts, that have a multiple potential to develop into endothelial cells.

In any event, the manner and completeness with which a graft heals has a major impact on its resistance to subsequent complications, particularly infection and thrombosis. Likewise, the bonding of the neointima, whether it is simply a compacted fibrin layer or a cellular lining, is of particular importance. A pseudointimal lining that is not bonded to the fabric may dislodge and embolize. In contrast, a cellular neointima that is closely bonded to the graft develops characteristics that more closely emulate autogenous artery and presumably functions better, particularly in small grafts with low flow.

The intima of autogenous vessels possess fibrinolytic properties that tend to resist surface thrombus formation, particularly in states of low flow. Measurements of surface thrombogenicity among various prostheses revealed that the most thrombogenic grafts are those that have linings composed of compacted fibrin, and those that are least thrombogenic are the ones that have a cellular neointima.

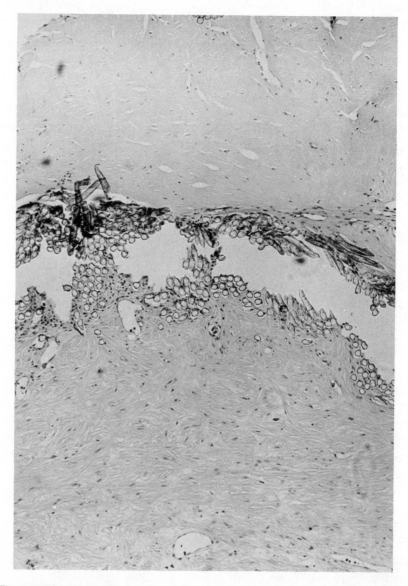

A

Figure 7.8A Microscopic section of ultra lightweight knitted prosthesis three months postimplantation. The prosthesis is lined with compacted fibrin and thrombus. Note the lack of transmural cellular ingrowth. *(From Roon AJ, Moore WS, Goldstone J, Towan H, Campagna G: Comparative surface thrombogenicity of implanted vascular grafts. J Surg Res 22:165–73, 1977.)*

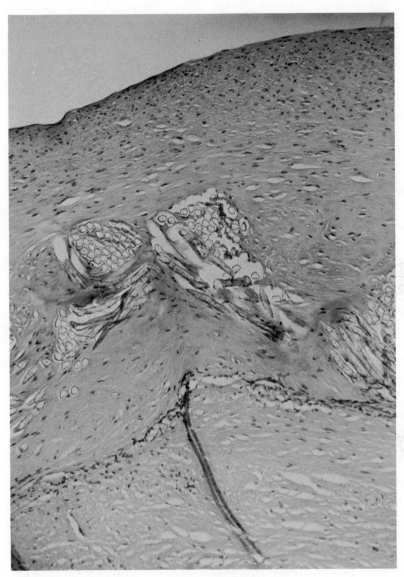

B

Figure 7.8B Microscopic section of velour graft three months postimplantation. Note neointimal lining and high degree of transmural cellular ingrowth. *(From Roon AJ, Moore WS, Goldstone J, Campagna G: Comparative surface thrombogenicity of implanted vascular grafts. J Surg Res 165, 1977.)*

Abnormal Healing of Vascular Prostheses

Anastomotic Aneurysm   The bonding of a prosthetic graft to a host vessel is entirely dependent upon the suture material. This dependency goes beyond the initial time of implantation and extends, in fact, for the life of the patient and the reconstructive procedure. If the suture breaks, pulls out of the host arterial wall, or is absorbed, a separation will occur at the graft-artery interface. Initially, the separation is bridged by the fibrous tissue capsule that surrounds the graft and is contiguous with the periarterial scar. However, since this fibrous tissue capsule lacks elastic tissue, the force exerted from within by arterial pressure causes the bridging capsule to expand and dilate. As dilatation occurs, forces on the arterial wall increase according to the physical principle that the lateral forces in a vessel under pressure are directly proportional to the diameter of that vessel (LaPlace's law). Thus, once an anastomotic aneurysm starts, its rate of expansion will accelerate until it either ruptures or produces a graft thrombosis as a result of impingement on the lumen of the graft.

False aneurysm can be prevented by using a permanent, nonabsorbable suture and by taking deep suture bites, thus incorporating enough host artery to prevent the sutures from pulling through the arterial wall. This is particularly important if the anastomosis of the graft is made to an endarterectomized vessel, since removal of the intima and media leaves the vessel wall in an initially weakened condition.

The early reports of false aneurysms occurred at a time when it was common practice to use silk suture for performing vascular anastomoses. Contrary to popular opinion, silk is an "absorbable" suture. As a biologic product, it is degradable and removed by the host phagocytic response, usually completely within four years from the time of implantation. Therefore, the practice of using silk sutures for arterial-prosthetic graft anastomoses led to a high incidence of anastomotic aneurysm formation. Monofilament polyethylene suture has also been associated with anastomotic disruption since this material tends to degenerate with time and subsequently fractures. The best results with prosthetic graft anastomoses have been obtained with multifilament braided Dacron sutures or with monofilament polypropylene. While polypropylene appears to maintain its integrity, care must be exercised in its use. Grasping the polypropylene suture with a vascular forcep will fracture the suture material and lead to disruption. This tendency represents the major disadvantage of a monofilament suture in that the surgeon and the patient are fully dependent upon a single strand in contrast to the braided suture which has greater inherent margin of safety due to its multifiber construction.

Infection in Vascular Protheses Acute infection in a newly-implanted vascular graft is due to contamination, usually secondary to a break in surgical technique and cannot be attributed to a defect in healing. However, graft infections appearing many months to years following initial implantation may very well be due to a healing deficiency. Experimental work in our laboratory has demonstrated that newly-implanted vascular grafts are susceptible to contamination with blood-borne bacteria.

The raw intimal surface of a prosthetic graft serves as a suitable site for circulating bacteria to settle and establish an infection. This susceptibility persists as long as the luminal surface is uncovered by a cellular neointima. Healing time and healing completeness vary with the type of graft employed. In an experimental study comparing four types of prosthetic graft materials, which included a standard weight knitted Dacron, ultra-lightweight knitted Dacron, expanded Teflon, and external velour Dacron, the velour grafts "healed" faster, had the highest incidence of cellular neointimal completeness, and the lowest incidence of infection following a standard bacteremic challenge. In essence, it develops resistance to infection by blood-borne bacteria more rapidly.

Newer Vascular Prostheses

Newer vascular conduits made of tissue, plastic, and combinations are being developed and tested. Included in this group are the bovine heterograft, the umbilical artery and vein, and compound grafts made by allowing a fibrous tissue to infiltrate a wide mesh fabric suspended on a plastic mandril and implanted in a subcutaneous position for six weeks prior to use as a vascular conduit. Finally, there is a "new breed" of vascular grafts which is neither knitted nor woven but extruded as a

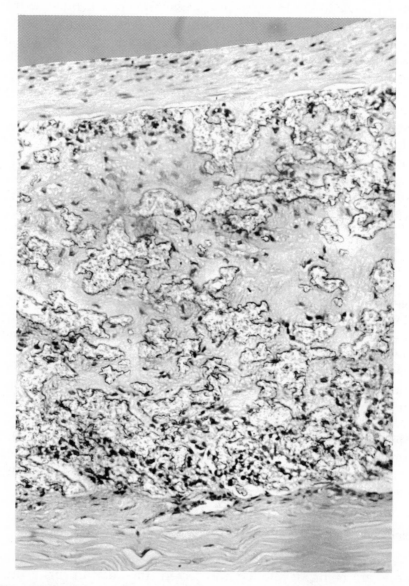

Figure 7.8C Photomicrograph of expanded teflon graft sectioned three months post-implantation. Note the cellular neointimal lining and the very extensive transmural cellular ingrowth. *(From Roon AJ, Moore WS, Goldstone J, Towan H, Campagna G: J Surg Res, 22:168, 1977.)*

porous tube made of air-infiltrated, or expanded Teflon (Gortex® and Impra®). Information concerning the healing characteristics of these new grafts is limited, but new tissue does penetrate Gortex.®.

The bovine heterografts are prepared by subjecting bovine carotid arteries to protein enzymatic digestion which leaves a collagen tube. The collagen tube is then tanned and stored in a liquid sterilizing solution for subsequent implantation. The host reaction to bovine heterograft is minimal. A surrounding fibrous tissue response develops, but there is no fibroblastic infiltration of the graft, nor is there any evidence of an attempt at neointimal formation. While the bovine heterograft is unsatisfactory for arterial reconstruction, it has proved useful as an access for hemodialysis.

The umbilical vein is quite similar to the bovine heterograft in that it is a tanned, nonviable tissue conduit that must be supported by Dacron mesh in order to prevent aneurysmal degeneration.

The principle of the "mandril" graft was an intriguing one in that the final product consisted of a viable fibrous tissue tube supported by a Dacron matrix. Late results, however, have been unsatisfactory in that the fibrous tissue maturation appears to continue following vascular implantation. This has led to stricture and thrombosis of the implant and the anastomosis.

The experience to date with expanded Teflon has been encouraging. This has been particularly important in small vessel replacement. Since the Teflon surface is nonwettable, it has a low surface thrombogenic potential. A thin cellular neointima rapidly develops and the microinterstices of the wall become infiltrated with fibroblasts and capillaries (Fig. 7.8C). So far, it seems less susceptible to separation and embolization of the neointima than conventionally prepared teflon implants.

SUMMARY

The ideal vascular substitute has not yet been developed, but the necessary characteristics are becoming better defined. These include a low thrombogenic potential at the time of implantation and a rapid host cellular response leading to tissue infiltration of the prosthesis, with the ultimate product being soundly incorporated in the host tissue and possessing a complete, thin, cellular neointima that is tightly adherent to the underlying graft.

BIBLIOGRAPHY

Berger K, Sauvage LR, Rao AM, Wood SJ: Healing of arterial prostheses in man: Its incompleteness. Ann Surg 175:118, 1972. This paper describes experience with vascular grafts recovered from patients with respect to intimal healing.

Bradbeer J, Jackson DS, Fletcher WS, Krippaehne WW, Dunphy JE: Biochemical studies of the connective tissue reaction to dacron aortic prostheses. J Surg Res 10:431, 1965. This explores the adventital and intimal reaction around dacron prostheses with respect to the biochemistry of collagen.

Brais MP, Braunwald NS: Tissue acceptance of materials implanted within the circulatory system. Arch Surg 109:351, 1974.

Carrel A: Ultimate result of arotic transplantation. J Exp Med 15:389, 1912. This classic paper describes the utilization of homograft aorta as a vascular transplant.

Clark RA, Stone RD, Leung DYK, et al.: Role of macrophages in wound healing. Surg Forum 27: 16, 1976. This paper explores the relationship between the macrophage, wound healing, and collagen production.

Dardik H, Ibrahim IM, Sprayregen S, Dardik II: Clinical experience with modified human umbilical cord vein for arterial bypass. Surgery 79:618, 1976.

Dent TL, Weber TR, Lindenauer SM, et al.: Cryopreservation of vein grafts. Surg Forum 25:241, 1974.

Eckman CA, Scott HW: Influence of experimental staphylococcic infection on arterial anastomoses and grafts. Bull Soc Int Chir (2): 1960. This paper relates the early experimental experience with the effect of infection on prosthetic grafts comparing the response of homografts with that of Dacron prostheses in the presence of sepsis.

Ejrup B, Hiertonn T, Moberg A: Atheromatous changes in autogenous venous grafts. Functional and anatomical aspects. Case report. Acta Chir Scand 121:211, 1961. This is a case report describing the early atherosclerotic changes seen in an autogenous vein graft.

Faulkner SL, Fisher RD, Conkle DM, Page DL, Bender HW Jr: Effect of blood flow rate on subendothelial proliferation in venous autografts used as arterial substitutes. Circulation (Suppl 1) 51, 52: 1975. This describes the relationship between blood flow and subendothelial changes in venous autograft conduits used as arterial substitutes.

Florey HW, Greer SJ, Poole JCF, et al.: The pseudointima lining fabric of the aorta. Br J Exp Pathol 42:236, 1961. This study, performed in living dogs, used a silver stain fixative to capture endothelial repopulation in vascular graft substitutes.

496

Foster JH, Berzins T, Scott HW: An experimental study of arterial replacement in the presence of bacterial infection. Surg Gynecol Obstet 108:141, 1959.

French JE: Atherosclerosis in relation to the structure and function of the arterial intima with special reference to the endothelium. Int Rev Exp Pathol 5:253, 1965. This paper explores the relationship between endothelial hypertrophy and atherosclerosis as a causative mechanism.

Gaylis H, Corvese WP, Linton RR, Shaw RS: The rate of healing of arterial autografts. Surgery 45:41, 1959.

Glagon S, Ts'ao CH: Restitution of aortic wall after sustaining necrotizing transmural ligation injury: Role of blood cells and artery cells. Am J Pathol 79:7, 1975. This is an experimental study in which a transmural injury of a rabbit aorta was produced by ligature. The origins of the neoendothelial cells were then explored on follow-up.

Griffith CA, Eade GC, Zech RA, et al.: A new technique for compilation arterial grafts. Vinyon "N" cloth support with a long autogenous arterial strip. Surg Gynecol Obstet 101:225, 1955.

Hansen OK, Kraft, Mouritzen C: Biologic and semibiologic vascular grafts. Surg Gynecol Obstet 138:940, 1974.

Harrison JH: Influence of infection on homografts and synthetic (teflon) grafts. Arch Surg 76:67, 1958.

Harrison JH, Davalos PA: Influence of porosity on synthetic grafts. Arch Surg 82:8, 1961. This is an early experimental study exploring the pore size of soft prostheses with regard to capillary and fiber tissue ingrowth.

Helin P, Lorenzen I, Garbars CH, et al.: Repair in arterial tissue: morphological and biochemical changes in the rabbit aorta after a single dilation injury. Circ Res 29:542, 1971. This is an experimental study in which the biochemical changes following intimectomy were explored, as well as documentation of the origin of endothelial cells following the single passage of a Fogarty catheter as a means of producing an intimal injury.

Humphries AW, Hawk WA, DeWolfe VG, et al.: Clinicopathologic observations of the fate of arterial freeze-dried homografts. Surgery 45:59, 1959.

Malone JM, Moore WS, Campagna G, Bean B: Bacteremic infectability of vascular grafts: The influence of pseudointimal integrity and duration of graft function. Surgery 78:211, 1975. This compares the bacteremic infectability of vascular prostheses as a function of graft type and duration of implantation following a single challenge of intravenously introduced bacteria.

Moore WS, Hall AD: Late suture failure in the pathogenesis of anastomotic false aneurysms. Ann Surg 172:1064, 1970. This clinical paper documents the relationship of pseudoaneurysm formation and the use of an absorbable suture, vascular silk.

Moore WS, Hall AD, Allen RE: Tensile strength of arterial prosthetic anastomoses. J Surg Res 13:209, 1972. This experimental paper measures the tensile strength of vascular anastomoses with and without material in order to demonstrate the role of periadventital fibrous tissue response.

Moore WS, Swanson RJ, Campagna G, Bean B: Pseudointimal development and vascular prosthesis' susceptibility to bacteremic infection. Surg

Forum 25:250, 1974. This study documents the relationship between the completeness of neointimal development and the susceptibility to bacteremic infection.

Moore WS, Swanson RJ, Campagna G, Bean B: The use of fresh tissue arterial substitutes in infected fields. J Surg Res 18:229, 1975. This experimental paper demonstrated that autogenous arteries could be successfully implanted in an infected field with the expectation of healing and preservation of arterial function.

Moseley HS, Connell RJ, Krippaehne WW: Healing of the canine aorta after endarterectomy. A scanning electron microscopic study. Ann Surg 180:329, 1974. This experimental study explores the changes in medial and endothelial cells following arterial endarterectomy.

Nomora Y: The ultrastructure of the pseudointima lining synthetic arterial grafts in the canine aorta with specific reference to the origin of the endothelial cells. J Cardiovasc Surg (Torino) 11:282, 1970.

Ochsner JL, DeCamp PT, Leonard GL: Experience with fresh venous allografts as an arterial substitute. Ann Surg 173:933, 1971. This clinical report documented the experience with fresh allograft saphenous vein used as arterial substitutes. It demonstrated that patency was achieved when there was ABO compatibility between donor and recipient.

Perloff LJ, Reckard CR, Rowlands DT, Barker CF: The venous homograft: An immunological question. Surgery 72:961, 1972. This experimental paper demonstrated that allograft veins, used as arterial substitutes, did incite a rejection phenomenon.

Poole JCF, Sabiston DC, Florey HW et al.: Growth of entothelium in arterial prosthetic grafts following endarterectomy. Surg Forum 13:225, 1962.

Poole JCF, Cromwell SN, Bennditt EP: Behavior of smooth muscle cells and formation of extra cellular structures in the reaction of arterial walls to injury. Am J Pathol 62:391, 1971. This experimental paper discusses the origin and function of the viable intimal cell with regard to vascular healing.

Poole JCF, Sabiston DC, Florey HW et al.: Growth of endothelium in arterial Pathol Bact 75:133, 1958.

Ramos JR, Berger K, Mansfield PB, Sauvage LR: Histologic fate and endothelial changes of distended and nondistended vein grafts. Ann Surg 183, 205, 1976. This study documents endothelial disruption, as seen on scanning electron microscopy, following venous distention with excessive pressure.

Reichle FA, Stewart GJ, Essa N: A transmission and scanning electron microscopic study of luminal surfaces in dacron and autogenous vein bypass in man and dog. Surgery 74:945, 1973. This is an experimental study comparing the healing of vascular prostheses and contrasting data with that of autogenous veins using the modalities of electron microscopy.

Roon AJ, Moore WS, Goldstone J, Towan H, Campagna G: Comparative surface thrombogenicity of implanted vascular grafts. J Surg Res 22:165, 1977. This is an experimental study that demonstrated a lowering of thrombogenic potential of the endothelial surfaces of vascular grafts as a function of the completeness of cellular intimal lining.

498

Sauvage LR, Berger K, Wood SJ, Nakagawa Y, Mansfield PB: An external velour surface for porous arterial prostheses. Surgery 70:940, 1971.

Sauvage LR, Berger KE, Wood ST, et al.: Interspecies healing of porous arterial prostheses. Arch Surg 109:698, 1974. This experimental study demonstrated and compared the healing of vascular prostheses in various animal models. It demonstrated that the dog came the closest to the human in healing response.

Schramel RJ, Creech O: Effects of infection and exposure or synthetic arterial prosthesis. Arch Surg 78:271, 1959. This is the earliest experimental paper demonstrating the susceptibility of newly implanted vascular grafts to infection of bacteremic origin.

Schwartz CJ, Caplin BA: Non-homogeneity of aortic endothelial cell turnover. Am J Pathol 70:549, 1973. This experimental study demonstrated that the repopulation of endothelium in healing in a vessel occurs in a random fashion.

Schwartz SM, Stemerman MB, Benditt EP: The aortic intima. II Repair of the aortic lining after mechanical denudation. Am J Pathol 81:15, 1975. This is an excellent review on the origin of endothelial cells in an experimental model.

Smith U, Ryan JW, Michie DD, et al.: Endothelial projections as revealed by scanning electron microscopy. Science 173:925, 1971. This experimental study discusses the biologic function of endothelial microvilli.

Spaet TH, Lejnieks I: Mitotic activity of rabbit blood vessels. Proc Soc Exp Biol Med 125:1197, 1967.

Spaet TH, Stemerman MB, Veith FJ: Intimal injury and regrowth in the rabbit aorta; medial smooth muscle cells as a source of neointima. Circ Res 36:58, 1975. This paper discusses the various sources and origin of the neointimal cell and provides an indepth discussion of the myointimal cell.

Swanson RJ, Moore WS, Campagna G: Effect of time on vascular prostheses susceptibility to infection of bacteremic origin. Surg Forum 24:28, 1973. This is an early report relating the decreasing susceptibility to infection of bacteremic origin as a function of the healing time.

Tilney NL, Boor PJ: Host response to implanted dacron grafts. A comparison between mesh and velour. Arch Surg 110:1469, 1975. This discusses the relationship of graft pore size and fabrication to the rapidity and completeness of tissue healing.

Wesolowski SA, Seaman AR: Growth and differentiation of the endothelial lining of the vascular prosthesis by scanning electromicroscopy. J Abdom Surg 13:219, 1971.

Weyman AK, Plume SK, DeWeese JA: Bovine heterografts and autogenous veins as canine arterial bypass grafts. Arch Surg 110:746, 1975.

Williams GM, ter Haar A, Krajewski C, Parks LC, Roth J: Rejection and repair of endothelium in major vessel transplants. Surgery 78:694, 1975. This is an excellent review article on the endothelial changes that occur following tissue incompatibility.

Tendon Healing
Lynn D. Ketchum

Primary tendon healing, which is defined as the fusion of the two ends of a divided tendon brought into apposition, can occur from both within and without the tendon. For many years it was believed that the tendon was an inert, almost avascular structure, whose cells were so specialized that they were incapable of contributing to the healing process. Healing was then thought to take place solely by ingrowth of both fibroblasts and capillaries from the paratendinous tissues. It is true that a significant, even major part of tendon healing occurs in this manner, but it is important to recognize that intrinsic tendon repair exists, and can be exploited clinically. In most cases, where the distances over which tendons glide is small and where surrounding structures are flexible, whether tendon injuries heal from extrinsic or intrinsic resources is clinically immaterial. However, in some instances, the encouragement of intrinsic repair and discouragement of extrinsic repair has major value for the trauma victim.

Most tendon repair problems are seen in Zone 2 of the hand,

the so-called No Man's Land (Fig. 7.9). In this area the flexor tendons glide in a synovial sheath and have a precarious blood supply. Tendons in other areas are richly endowed with a blood supply and are less intimately encroached upon by unyielding structures. Consequently, healing and restoration of function generally occur uneventfully. Since any significant problems in tendon healing would be encountered in Zone 2 of the hand, the emphasis in this section is on healing in that area.

Figure 7.9 Zones of the hand. *(Courtesy of Ethicon, Inc.)*

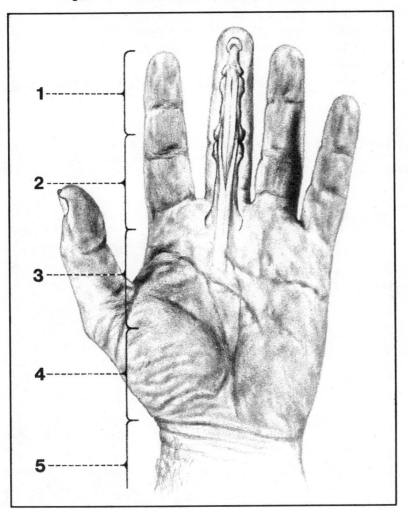

SEQUENCE OF EVENTS IN PRIMARY TENDON HEALING

As with wound healing elsewhere in the body, tendon healing begins with an inflammatory reaction. This process is essentially the same as the advance of the "wound module" as described in the chapter on normal repair. There is an outpouring of fibrin and inflammatory cells proportional to the size of the wound and the amount of trauma. Fibroplasia is influenced by the inflammatory reaction. If there is traumatized, ischemic tissue with foreign material, a greater inflammatory reaction occurs which is a significant stimulus for the formation of excessive reparative tissue (i.e., collagen deposition).

A few fibroblasts appear in the wound by the second day, and the number thereafter increases rapidly (Fig. 7.10). The inflammatory phase is still very evident by the fourth day, and will not decrease until the eighth to tenth day. By day 21 there

Figure 7.10 The wound milieu surrounding a tendon at four days. There are inflammatory cells, fibroblasts, fibrin, and early collagen deposition in the peripheral environment of the tendon.

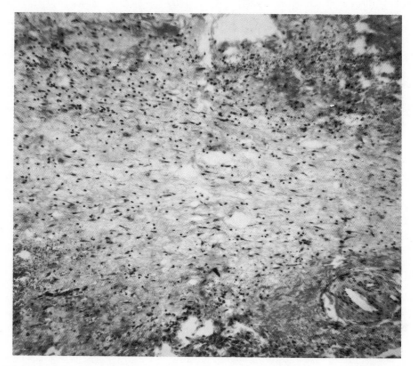

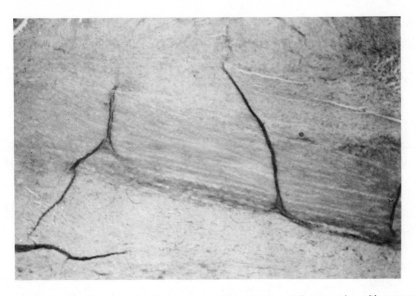

Figure 7.11 The fibrovascular tissue surrounding a tendon at three weeks, with a mass of fibroblasts, collagen, and capillaries.

is a mass of fibrovascular tissue surrounding the tendon (Fig. 7.11). The fibroblasts within the neighboring tendinous tissue are slower to respond. By the fourth day there is an increase in thickness of fibroblasts covering the tendon itself. Fibrovascular tissue migrating from the paratendinous tissues blends in with the epitenon layer of cells covering the tendon to form the tendon callus. By 28 days, most of the fibroblasts and collagen between the tendon stumps are oriented longitudinally. New collagen fibers in the tendon scar remain as small, parallel, longitudinally oriented fibers until the end of the third post-operative month, when there is evidence of early collagen bundle formation. This progresses so that by about four months after the operation, collagen in the scar between the tendon ends is in the form of large bundles identical microscopically to those of the tendon.

The contribution from the paratendinous tissues in the tendon healing process cannot be denied and is certainly an important contributing factor, as are the capillaries from that source, which are important for three reasons: First, they bring in oxygen necessary for cell survival. The oxygen also acts as a co-substrate for the hydroxylation of proline during collagen synthesis. Second, the capillaries deliver inflammatory cells to

503

remove foreign material, such as suture. Third, they bring in the amino acid building blocks for protein synthesis.

Frequently the paratendinous response takes the form of a mass migration of cells with large numbers of inflammatory cells, capillaries, and fibroblasts, and subsequent secretion of collagen firmly uniting not only the tendon ends to each other, but also the tendon to all structures in peripheral contact with it. The healing reaction essentially joins the tendon to its surrounding sources of vascularity and fibroblasts. Through such a process, a tendon heals and develops significant tensile strength; but it all too frequently loses its specialized function of gliding without which it could just as well be left unrepaired. Fortunately, the quantity and quality of these adhesions can be modified somewhat. One of the frontiers of applied surgical research is the modification and control of this "adhesive" reaction.

INTRINSIC TENDON HEALING

The massive reaction of the paratenon overshadows the response of the tendon itself. It was not until the tendon could be isolated from that response that it could be shown that, indeed, the tendon can and does contribute significantly to its own healing. Early attempts to demonstrate an intrinsic healing potential of tendons were rebuffed, but the evidence that has accumulated in the last five years is convincing.

Segments of tendon have been divided, separated from their blood supply, repaired and then placed into an intact tendon sheath bathed only by synovial fluid. The cells of tendons treated in this manner survive, except for those in the center. The epitenon, as well as the endotenon, becomes hyperplastic (Fig. 7.12). The junctures of these tendon repairs, bridged by fibroblasts and collagen, attain significant strength to resist rupture. The fibroblasts in the epitenon and endotenon secrete collagen as seen on scanning electron microscopy. Metabolic studies demonstrate the presence of both anabolic and catabolic processes within tendons. Cells demonstrate an increased uptake of tritiated proline into new collagen in these free tendon segments, indicating that the cells were not just surviving while nourished by synovial fluid but were synthesizing protein. Furthermore, adhesions did not form in these isolated tendon segments.

504

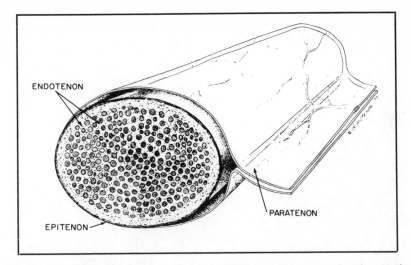

Figure 7.12 A segment of tendon where it is covered by paratenon rather than tendon sheath. Paratenon is a loose, filmy structure, endowed with a rich blood supply which communicates with the tendon itself. The tendon is covered with a thin layer of cells, the epitenon (Figure 7.13A) and the tendon fibers within are supported and separated by the endotenon.

Isolated segments of tendons placed in a synovial compartment survive and metabolize, except for the centralmost cells. On the other hand, tendon segments simply degenerate when isolated from both blood supply and synovial nourishment by envelopment in polyethylene sheets. Although longitudinal strength remains for weeks in such isolated segments, the fibrous bundles in the tendons literally fall apart when subjected to lateral stress; and sutures pull through the bundles with ease, indicating that there is little effective repair by several weeks. At three weeks, there is complete avascularity and collagenous disintegration. A tendon segment totally isolated from nourishment undergoes cell death and collagen lysis.

The epitenon component of tendons has been shown to grow in three directions. This has been studied by isolating tendons in a sheath; i.e., opening the sheath, dividing the tendon in two places, dividing the mesentery to that segment, then closing the sheath (Fig. 7.13 A,B). Under these conditions, the epitenon increases in thickness (centrifugal). Cells of the epitenon move longitudinally down into and across the area of tendon juncture, and grow centripetally down into the tendon itself, whereby it is difficult to distinguish the growth of the

505

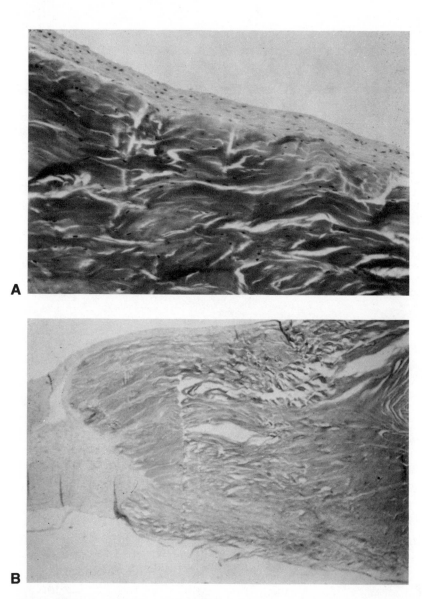

A

B

Figure 7.13 **A.** demonstrates the centrifugal growth of the epitenon. **B.** and **C.** (see facing page) show the epitenon growing longitudinally towards its counterpart on the other side of a divided tendon end, while joining the fibers from the endotenon in the area of the tendinous junction.

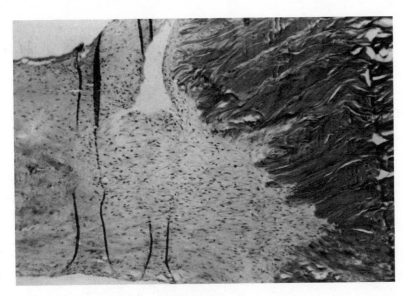

C

Figure 7.13   C

fibroblasts of the endotenon (see Fig. 7.9 C). The endotenon, which also becomes hyperplastic, separates the fiber bundles of the tendon.

BLOOD SUPPLY

The fact that collagen metabolism is an active process all over the body, albeit at a slow rate in the most inert bone, means that collagen within a tendon is being continously secreted and remodeled and that the secreting cells that are present normally, are capable of contributing to the repair process. To survive and function, they must derive nutrition from either synovial fluid or blood supply. Isolation from both leads to cell death and collagen disintegration. Synovial fluid is an important source of nourishment. What happens then, when the synovial sheath is removed surgically except for short segments of pulleys, and the blood supply is interrupted by trauma, surgical dissection (or both) with the tendon consequently apposed to fibro-fatty tissue? In answering that question, it is necessary to examine the blood supply of flexor tendons in Zone 2 and determine the effects of interfering with segments of that blood supply.

The blood supply of normal tendons within a synovial sheath has been shown to be segmental (Fig. 7.14). There is a proximal

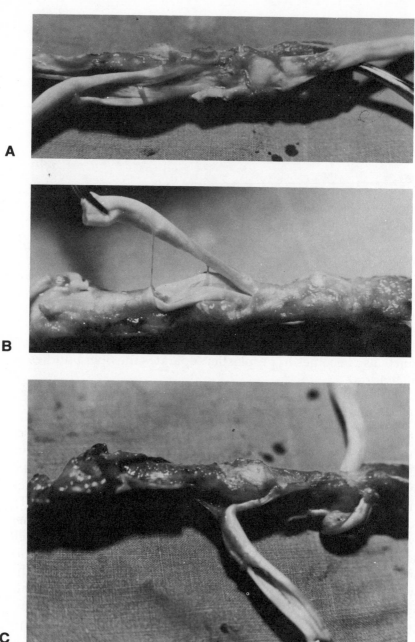

Figure 7.14   A. The chiasma of Camper where the fibers of the flexor superficialis cross over with a hiatus between them through which the flexor profundus tendon passes. **B.** The vinculum longus to the flexor profundus coming through the flexor superficialis tendon at the level of the chiasma of Camper, distal to the pulley at the proximal phalanx. **C.** The flexor superficialis tendon reflected, demonstrating its vinculum breve. The blood vessels run through the vincula.

system originating in the palm that continues distally in a longitudinal direction within the tendon and is in continuation with the synovial folds in the proximal reflection of the tendon sheath. Second, there is an intermediate system originating from the vinculum longus of the flexor profundus tendon and vinculum brevis of the flexor sublimis tendon that are in continuity at the level of the proximal interphalangeal joint. Third, a distal segment originates from the vinculum brevis of the flexor profundus tendon at its insertion. That this segmental distribution is critical has been demonstrated when the tendon is isolated on any one of these three sources of blood supply. Blood does not pass further than that particular segment; that is, if the proximal segment is the sole source of blood supply, then blood does not pass into the middle and distal zones. Thus in a tendon transfer, these two zones would be ischemic and would behave essentially as a tendon graft.

Tissue oxygen supply is one of the factors that affects the tendon healing process. Tendon cells need oxygen and the nutrients found in blood and synovial fluid to survive. If the blood supply is surgically or traumatically divided and the tendon sheath stripped except for small pulley segments, cells will die unless capillaries grow in from surrounding tissues. It has been shown that if small bowel is stripped of its mesentery, *adhesions will form to that segment only in the area of devascularization.* If omentum is wrapped around a bowel segment stripped of mesentery, it will adhere firmly through numerous neovascular attachments. Omentum wrapped around a segment of bowel with intact mesentery will not adhere at all, which suggests that ischemia is a potent stimulus to the formation of adhesions.

It is interesting that early attempts to study tendon healing removed the blood supply to the central third of the flexor profundus tendon because the sublimis tendon was excised, and along with it the vincula. In addition, limbs were immobilized, thus preventing lengthening of any adhesions; tendon sheath was stripped away and suture material, frequently silk, one of the most tissue reactive sutures, was introduced into the tendon. This can hardly be faulted because the same procedures were followed in clinical practice at that time. However, better materials and techniques are now available, with corresponding improvements in laboratory and clinical procedures.

All of the above-mentioned variables have now been studied in isolation and in combination in the repair of divided tendons. Restricting adhesions do not adhere to a partially (80 percent) divided tendon in Zone 2 when the tendon is immobilized, when it is not sutured and the sheath is intact. Nor do they occur when the tendon is sutured if the sheath is intact and the tendon is not immobilized. Nor do they form when the sheath was removed, and the tendon sutured but not immobilized. The experimental conditions causing restrictive adhesions were immobilization of a sutured tendon with an excised sheath.

Why do adhesions occur if the vincula is intact and the middle third of the tendon has an "intact blood supply" in the above-mentioned situation? Two separate studies have shown that the microcirculation of the tendon can be impaired by (1) sutures and (2) tension, alone, or in combination. That this situation can be, in fact, avoided is shown in Figure 7.15. (See also 7.17 B and C). Ischemia then sets up the stimulus for ingrowth of capillaries from surrounding paratendinous tissues to provide nutrition to the tendon cells.

Figure 7.15 The intratendinous blood supply going right up to the juncture of two divided tendon ends which have been coapted. This repair has been made with four simple sutures and tension has been removed from the repair allowing the blood supply to nourish the tendon right out to the severed ends.

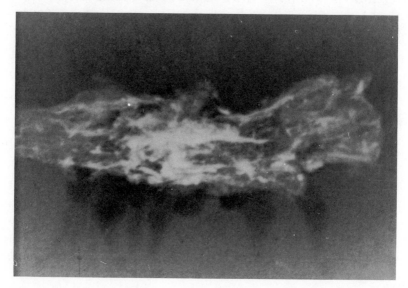

The concept of a "one wound unit body construction" is certainly valid in the situation where the tendon has been divided, sutured, the tendon sheath removed, and the tendon immobilized. This is the concept in which tendon repair is seen as an agglomeration of reactions of surrounding structures participating in the healing of the entire wound. The tendon is only a part of this wound. Fibroblasts migrate in all directions and eventually unite all exposed sturctures in a mass of collagen. In a wound in which the tendon sheath is removed but the tendon and mesotendon are not disturbed, there will be no adhesions to the tendon; and it will remain pearly white. The traumatized tendon, then, is particularly vulnerable to the one wound healing concept described above and must be protected in one of the following ways:

The blood supply must be preserved. Since the vincula longus to the flexor profundus is intimately associated with the vincula brevis of the flexor superficialis, the flexor superficialis should not be disturbed in this region, much less removed. Removal results in significantly increased amounts of scarring and adhesions to the profundus tendon, and also results in loss of stability to the volar side of the proximal interphalangeal joint.

If the vincula longus of the profundus and the vincula brevis of the sublimis are traumatically divided, the stage is set for ischemic tendon with degeneration and excessive scarring. This problem can be avoided if the sheath can be repaired, allowing synovial fluid to bathe the area of repair and serve as a physical barrier to limit the amount of paratendinous tissue migrating to the damaged tendon. Fortunately, tendon sheath can regenerate rapidly. From the evidence at hand it appears that a limited resection of the tendon sheath just sufficient to prevent triggering of the repaired tendons is indicated.

Wherever suture material enters a tendon, fibrovascular tissue will migrate to and into the tendon. Thus, the amount and size of suture material should be minimized. The suture material should be nonreactive, such as polypropylene, nylon, or stainless steel. Furthermore, a nonconstrictive type of suture should be used such as the Mason and Allen, Kessler, or lateral trap technique, particularly in Zone 2 (Fig. 7.16). These techniques minimize damage to the tendon's microcirculation. Since the microcirculation enters from the dorsum, volar

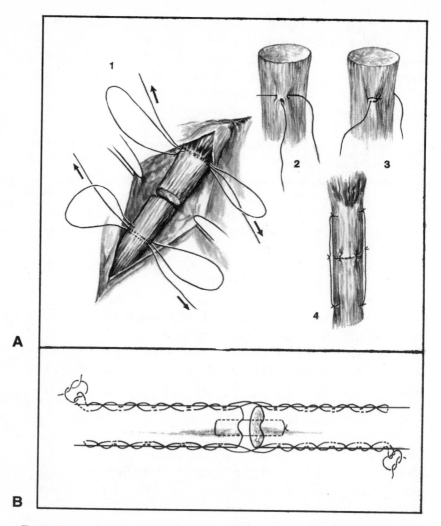

Figure 7.16 **A.** The Mason and Allen suture technique, of which the Kessler is a modification *(Mason, M., and Allen, H.S.: The Rate of Healing of Tendons: An Experimental Study of Tensile Strength, Ann Surg 113:424–459, 1941).* **B.** The lateral trap. These three techniques spare the center of the tendon and tend to prevent strangulation of its microcirculation. *(Ketchum, L.D., Martin, N.L., and Kappel, D.A.: Experimental Evaluation of the Factors Affecting the Tendon Gap and Tendon Strength at the Site of Tendon Repair. Plast Reconstr Surg 59:708, 1977 © 1977 by American Society of Plastic and Reconstructive Surgeons, Inc.)*

placement of sutures is less likely to interfere with the microcirculation. Actually, the technique that interferes least is the placement of four simple sutures of a nonreactive 5-0 material coapting the divided tendon ends. This has the further advantage of requiring less exposure, less sheath resection and less

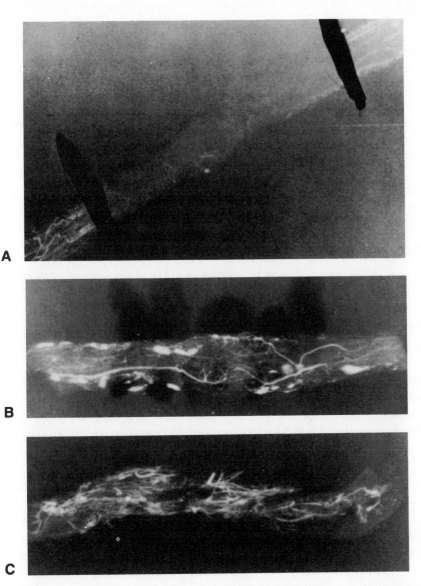

Figure 7.17   **A.** Repair not protected from tension. Normal tension is being exerted on the repair. Note that tendon is avascular for approximately 1 cm on each side of the anastomosis. **B, C.** Repairs protected from tension. These tendons were anastomosed with four simple sutures around the periphery; and all tension was taken off of the repairs. Note the excellent vasculature around the anastomosis at one week postrepair.

trauma from handling of the tendon with forceps. The strength of a repair using this technique is minimal initially and must be treated as such. But at six weeks, the strength of such a repair will not be significantly different from that attained through the use of any other suture technique, demonstrating the importance of the tendon healing process. The ultimate strength is not dependent upon suture technique or suture material. Of utmost importance in this regard is the relaxation of the suture line by flexion of the wrist and metacarpophalangeal joints, thus allowing the microcirculation to function unaffected by tissue tension (Fig. 7.17).

If these measures are not or cannot be taken, placement of a silicone rod to create a new sheath will probably be required in order to achieve a functional repair.

COLLAGEN ORGANIZATION AND REMODELING

In tendons, as in wounds elsewhere in the body, the ultimate strength of the area of repair is produced by the deposition and organization of collagen. A solution of collagen monomer bridges the tendon junction and polymerizes into fibrils. Collagen fibrils at the interface cross-link with each other and with the remaining original collagen of the tendon on each side of the junction. If the abundant deposition of collagen were not counterbalanced by a remodeling process, a tendon callus, or overabundant scar, of such magnitude would develop that the tendon could never function as a gliding structure. By the second day postwounding, collagenase is present in the wound, and somewhere between the fourth and sixth week collagen synthesis and collagen degradation reach an equilibrium. The total collagen content becomes stable, with a corresponding diminution in the number of fibroblasts and amount of ground substance (proteoglycans) required to maintain normal turnover. As collagen metabolism reaches equilibrium, the effects of remodeling can be seen visually and functionally. Fibroblasts and collagen fibers at the tendon interface align themselves parallel to those of the tendon, while the fibroblasts and collagen fibers in the extratendinous milieu remain in a haphazard configuration (Fig. 7.18). This is most likely caused by the effect of stress on the collagen biopolymer. Even though tension on the tendon anastomosis has been reduced by postoperative splinting, there is nevertheless a small amount of tension pro-

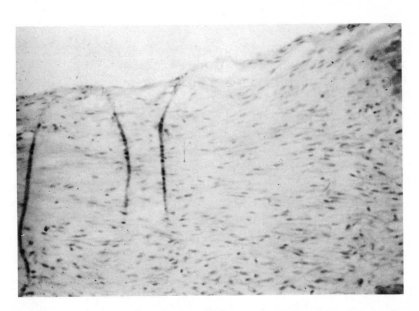

Figure 7.18 A tendon juncture at three weeks, in which the fibroblasts and collagen fibers are lining up parallel to each other and to the tendon fibers.

duced by the attached muscle, which is exerted on the small tendinous portion of the larger wound. We hypothesize that this tension on the cells in that area now separates the one big wound into extratendinous and tendinous divisions. Stress (in the form of tension) on a biopolymer produces a piezoelectric effect, resulting in the development of an electrical potential. An electrical potential has been demonstrated on the surface of intact tendons and is abolished at tendon division. However, the potential is reestablished by one week postrepair. Since collagen molecules have an electrical charge, it is highly probable that their orientation is enhanced by these two phenomena. This organization of collagen fibers leads to an increase in the tensile strength of the area of tendon repair. When active motion of the tendon is initiated at the appropriate time, collagen reorganization continues and tensile strength and resilience accrue.

Early active mobilization (less than three weeks) by contraction of the attached muscle is contraindicated, as demonstrated by the results of every study on primary tendon healing. Early active mobilization does not lead to an increase in tendon gliding. On the contrary, it imposes tension on the suture line with resultant ischemia, tenomalacia, and possible tendon rupture or gap formation between tendon ends. Such a gap must be filled with fibrovascular tissue to heal. There will be a greater stimulus to adhesion formation, and remodeling time will take longer. Repaired tendons mobilized early have a greater initial tendon strength if they stay together, but gliding is not improved and the danger of rupture is great.

Controlled passive mobilization is beneficial, however. While pharmacologic treatment of the healing tendon modifies the amount of fibroplasia, controlled passive mobilization modifies the quality of the adhesions. Controlled passive motion actively elongates adhesions to tendons from paratendinous tissues preventing the spot-welding effect of short adhesions in direct apposition to the tendon. Three to 5 mm of passive tendon gliding, repeated 10 to 12 times and done 2 to 3 times daily is sufficient to achieve the effect. It can be done by gentle external manipulation or by limited active extension, since, during active extension there is reciprocal relaxation of flexor tendons that allows passive extension of a flexor tendon repair. This limited motion, done with the wrist flexed and fingers protected from full extension by rubber band traction, so that a minimum of tension is exerted at the suture line, has only a very temporary effect on the microcirculation within the tendon. This technique is effective both experimentally and clinically in decreasing the tethering effect of adhesions.

Another way of regulating tendon healing and adhesion formation is to modify the inflammatory reaction. If antiinflammatory agents, such as triamcinolone, are instilled in the paratendinous tissues, there will be a dose-dependent modification of inflammation from a slight decrease to the virtual cessation of wound healing (Fig. 7.19). Obviously, the goal of such treatment is to decrease inflammation and subsequent fibroplasia sufficiently to prevent an all-enveloping encasement of scar tissue that restricts gliding, but, at the same time, allow sufficient fibroplasia from without and within the tendon to accomplish adequate healing across the wound.

The strength of the adhesions (as well as the tendon repair) can also be modified by agents such as BAPN (β-amino-proprionitrile*). BAPN has been used experimentally to inter-

---

*See Chapter 2, "Disorders of Repair and Their Management." β-aminoproprionitrile, by preventing cross-linking of adjacent lysines, inhibits formation of intermolecular bonds in collagen, thus rendering the collagen a soft gelatinous mass. It has this effect on paratendinous repair *and* on tendinous collagen as well.

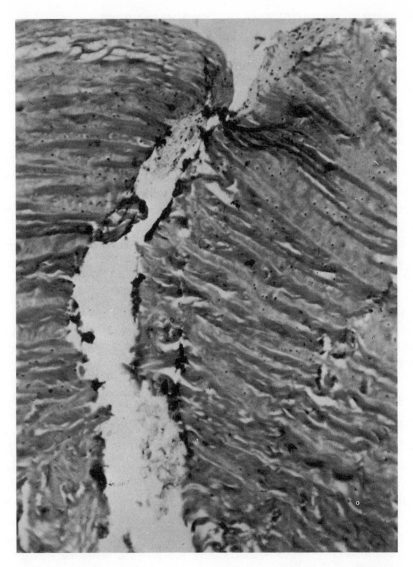

Figure 7.19 Tendon healing stopped by steroids. The reduction in the macrophage population in this three-week-old repair is dramatic with subsequent lack of fibroblasts and collagen.

fere with the cross-linking capability of the collagen molecules, so that the tendon is capable of pulling through the mass of "glue" which surrounds it. Although this method has been used successfully in animals, it has several theoretical disadvantages and is not, as yet, clinically applicable.

517

At first, the repair is weak; it is essentially as strong as the suture material for the first seven to ten days. In fact, at about the fifth to seventh day postrepair, the tendon wound is actually weaker than it was immediately after repair. The tendon collagen becomes soft in the area of repair just as it does in any other soft tissue wound, and its ability to hold sutures is decreased. Why is this? Certain suture techniques, such as the Bunnell (figure-of-eight stitch), commonly used in the repair of flexor tendons, produce a constricting effect on the microcirculation of the tendon in the area of repair. Furthermore, irrespective of suture technique, significant tension on the repair produces the same effect. An avascular segment of tendon undergoes cell death and collagen lysis resulting in a soft, weak tendon.

With time, the strength of the repair increases. Its ultimate functional capacity will depend on several factors: 1) suture technique, 2) the degree and method of mobilization and application of tension to the sutured tendon, 3) antiinflammatory treatment, and 4) preoperative conditions such as joint stiffness involvement of digital nerves, and so on.

Suture Technique

It is a natural inclination to use a suture technique that binds the tendon securely and restricts the shearing effect of suture through it. However, this is a self-defeating maneuver. The more invasive suture techniques provide greater initial strength to the tendon but constrict its microcirculation, predisposing the tendon to both gap and adhesion formation. By the time repair is well established, usually six weeks, tendons sutured with a figure-of-eight, or other invasive techniques, have the same tensile strength as those repaired with just four simple sutures.

Mobilization

Tendon repairs that are totally immobilized are significantly weaker than those that are not totally immobilized. As already mentioned, gliding is not improved by early active mobilization and the threat to gap formation and tendon rupture mitigates against its use. Strength of tendon repairs undergoing early controlled passive mobilization has not been studied. A tendon that is immobilized for three weeks and is then mobilized, triples its tensile strength in just two weeks. The clinical correlate is that if a tendon suture line is effectively protected and a program of timely, progressively increased stress is placed upon it, its strength will improve rapidly.

Antiinflammatory Agents

A tendon injury whose environment has been altered by installation of antiinflammatory agents can be isolated from the paratendinous inflammatory response, and the subsequent fibroplastic events are modified there. Healing proceeds more slowly, but at six weeks there is adequate tensile strength within the tendon, and gliding is significantly better than in untreated tendons.

Associated Injuries

Results of tendon repair are poor when joints are also damaged and when both digital nerves are damaged. In fingers in which only one nerve has been damaged, results of tendon repair are not compromised. The level of injury in Zone 2 is not a determining factor, although it is well recognized that injuries outside of Zone 2, but still in the hand, do much better than those in Zone 2. Injury to tendons in more than one digit is in itself not important, but the condition of each individual digit determines the outcome. Results of tendon repair in patients over 40 years old are not as good as those in younger patients.

The above discussion has focused primarily on the divided flexor tendons within the digital sheath. Because of their vascular vulnerability and proximity to dense unyielding structures, these injuries have traditionally resulted in poor functional recovery. However, even less experienced surgeons can achieve far better functional results with flexor tendons outside of digital sheaths and with extensor tendons. The reason for this is that these are surrounded by a paratenon endowed with a rich blood supply, and they are not in close proximity to dense unyielding structures such as fibro-osseous tunnels.

TENDOLYSIS

The end results of tendon repair can be predicted approximately six months following repair, at which time 90 percent of the functional recovery will have been attained. If there is poor function and dense adhesions limit gliding, a tendolysis, or freeing of the tendon, can be performed. This is a serious undertaking and not one for the inexperienced surgeon. Invariably, tendons that become adherent do so to all surrounding structures, including the tendon sheaths forming the pulleys (Fig. 7.20). Great care must be taken to avoid destroying the pulleys, as this will cause the tendons to bowstring, increasing their moment arms (defined as the perpendicular distance from the tendon to the joint axis) and decreasing the effective excursion that produces a full range of motion at a given joint.

If joint motion in a finger is assumed to be circular, which for practical purposes it is at the distal and proximal interphalangeal joints, then as a tendon pulls a joint through 60 degrees of motion, it has traveled one radian (approximately) of a circle. That distance is equivalent to the distance from the center of the circle (joint) to the tendon. For 90 degrees of motion, the distance traveled will be 1.5 times that for 60 degrees of motion. If a tendon has a moment arm of 2 cm, it will have an excursion of 2 cm for 60 degrees of motion and 3 cm for 90 degrees. If a particular pulley is destroyed and the tendon bowstrings at that point so that its moment arm now becomes 3 cm, then it can only take that joint through 60 degrees of motion.

Second, the blood supply to the tendon may be interrupted over a critical segment of the tendon, making it vulnerable to "spontaneous" rupture. Experimentally it has been shown that tendolysis is indicated in tendon repairs with poor function where sufficient improvement can be obtained to justify this procedure. Clinically, tendolysis has not been useful when only a limited amount of adhesion is present.

If tendolysis is unsuccessful, or if the tendon ruptures following repair or tendolysis, function may be salvaged by the formation of a pseudotendon sheath. This is accomplished by inserting a silicone rod that produces a smooth mesothelial lined bursal canal through which a tendon graft may be passed when the sheath is mature (90 to 120 days usually). This procedure is a subject of secondary tendon repair and will not be discussed here.

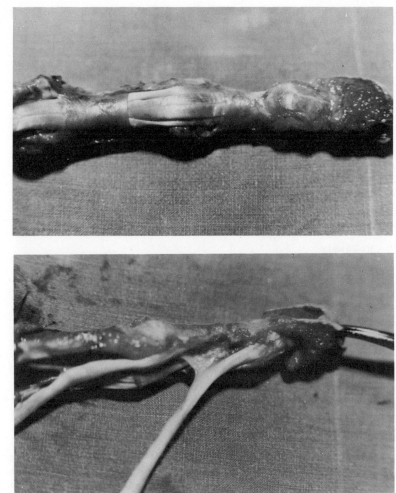

A

B

Figure 7.20   **A.** The close relationship of the flexor superficialis and plexor profundus in the finger. Two pulleys are seen at the level of the middle and proximal phalanx. The integrity of pulley systems in the fingers is essential to the efficiency of tendon gliding. **B.** The pulleys have been removed and the flexor tendons separated from each other. The vinculum breve of the flexor profundus tendon is seen at the level of the distal interphalangeal joint.

SUMMARY

The problem of tendon injury, especially in the hand, is a major one. Functional results of repair have left much to be desired. A degree of fatalism, with passive resignation to inadequate functional results, has sprung from the traditional view of tendon repair. We have tried to show that the traditional view is not entirely correct.

Conclusions to be drawn from experiments on tendon repair are not as bleak as some have made them. Careful attention to surgical technique, and deliberate manipulation of the reparative process (as we now see it) with drugs and with physical therapy, improves results. We have not yet reached the stage where full preinjury function can be restored on every occasion—far from it. But, in the hands of those who have mastered these concepts and techniques, results are approaching this goal.

BIBLIOGRAPHY

Bergljung L: Vascular reactions after tendon suture and tendon transplantation; a stereo-microangiographic study on the calcaneal tendon of the rabbit. Scand J Plast Reconstr Surg (Suppl) 4:7–63, 1968

Birdsell DC, Tustanoff ER, Lindsay WK: Collagen production in regenerating tendon. Plast Reconstr Surg 37 (6): 504–11, 1966

Duran RJ: Controlled passive motion following flexor tendon repair in zones two and three. In AAOS Symposium on Tendon Surgery in the Hand, St. Louis, Mosby, 1975, p 105

Eiken O, Lundborg G, Rank F: The role of the digital synovial sheath in tendon grafting. Scand J Plast Reconstr Surg 9: 182–89, 1975

Ellis H: The etiology of post-operative abdominal adhesions Br J Plast Surg 50: 10, 1962

Kappel D, Ketchum LD, Zilber S: In vivo electrophysiology of tendons and applied current during tendon healing. In Llaurado A, Sances A Jr, Battocletti JH (eds): Biologic and Clinical Effects of Low-Frequency Magnetic and Electric Fields.Springfield, Ill, Thomas, 1974

Ketchum LD: Effects of triamcinolone on tendon healing and function. Plast Reconstr Surg 47:47 1, 197 1

Ketchum LD, Martin N, Kappel D: Factors affecting tendon gap and tendon strength at the site of tendon repair. Plast Reconstr Surg 59: 1977

Kleinert HE, Kutz JE, Atasoy E, Storm A: Primary repair of flexor tendons. Orthop Clin North Amer 4:865, 1973

Lindsay WK, Birch JR: The fibroblast in flexor tendon healing. Plast Reconstr Surg 34 (3): 223–232, 1964

Lundborg G, Myrhage R, Rydevik B: The vascularization of human flexor tendons within the digital synovial sheath region—structural and functional aspects. In press.

Lundborg G, Rank F: Experimental Intrinsic Healing of Flexor Tendons Based upon Synovial Fluid Nutrition. In press.

Mason ML, Allen HS: The rate of healing of tendons: An experimental study of tensile strength. Ann Surg 1 13:424–59, 194 1

Matthews P, Richards H: The repair potential of digital flexor tendons. J Bone Joint Surg 56-B (4): 6 18–625, 1974

Peacock EE Jr: A study of circulation in normal tendons and healing grafts. Ann Surg 149:4 15–28, 1959

Potenza AD: Tendon healing within the flexor digital sheath in the dog. J Bone Joint Surg 44-A (1): 49–64, 1962

Verdan CE: Half a century of flexor-tendon surgery. J Bone Joint Surg 54-A (3):472–490, 1972

Fracture and Cartilage Repair
R. Bruce Heppenstall

524

Bone is a unique structure with several specific characteristics. It is the major reservoir of calcium in the body and serves to support the human frame. It also serves as an anchor for the origin and insertion of the surrounding musculature and protects vital soft tissue structures. The skeleton plays an important role in locomotion. In spite of its vital role in providing body support and strength, it is light, constituting only one-tenth of body weight. Bone is extremely strong with a breaking strength comparable to medium steel, and yet it is a flexible and elastic structure. Bone may be bent or twisted and will still return to its former shape following removal of the deforming force provided the force has not exceeded the limits of elasticity. Although it is able to resist axial stresses, bone is limited in its ability to resist rotational forces. One important point to remember is that bone, like liver, is one of the few organs that is able to undergo spontaneous regeneration with restoration of lost structure.

STRUCTURE

Bones are divided into two major structural types: tubular and flat. Tubular bone functions to provide normal weight bearing and locomotion. Flat bone, such as the skull, serves to protect vital soft tissue structures. Anatomically, tubular bones consist of the diaphysis (the central portion), and the epiphysis (ends of the bone) or the secondary ossification center. Diaphyseal bone has a lamellar structure. This is mature bone with collagen fibril bundles that are arranged in layers, strata or lamellae. Fibrous bone, on the other hand, is primitive nonlamellar bone that is seen in embryonic life, at fracture sites and at the metaphysis during new bone formation. At the junction of the diaphysis and epiphysis is a major growth area called the epiphyseal plate. This is the area where normal longitudinal growth occurs. Flat bone has no epiphyseal plate.

Bone is surrounded by a fibrous sheet called the periosteum. This is subdivided into an outer fibrous layer and an inner layer called the cambium. New bone cells arise from the cambium. The periosteum appears to have its greatest osteogenic potential in children. This potential may be important to fracture healing, since nonunion is rare in children.

The inner portion of bone (marrow cavity) is lined with a

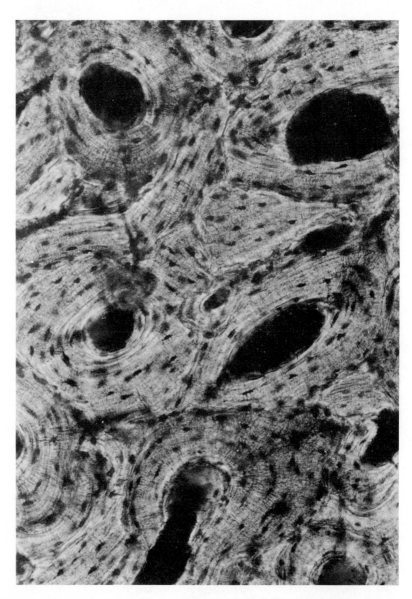

Figure 7.21 Cross section of bone under polarizing light microscopy illustrating the osteon unit, central canal surrounded by lamellae of bone containing osteoblasts (x200).

fibrous sheet called the endosteum. The Haversian system, or osteon, is the functioning unit in mature bone. It is composed of a central Haversian canal surrounded by concentric layers of bone as depicted in Figure 7.21. The surrounding lamellae have lacunae each containing an osteocyte with a cytoplasmic process extending through canaliculi to communicate with the Haversian vessels. The size of the osteon is limited by the fact that the Haversian canal supplies nutrition, and bone cells in general cannot survive further than 0.1 mm away from a capillary.

BONE FORMATION

Bone is generated by two separate mechanisms: endochondral and membranous bone formation. Endochondral bone formation occurs at the epiphyseal plate in long bones and accounts for growth in length. It requires laying down of a preformed cartilage model. The cartilage is gradually resorbed and replaced by bone. This sequence of events has also been described in fracture healing and will be dealt with later. Growth in width occurs by subperiosteal appositional bone formation.

Membranous bone formation does not involve a cartilage model. Mesenchymal cells differentiate into osteoblasts that lay down osteoid, which is then mineralized to form bone. This type of bone formation occurs in the calvarium, most facial bones, the clavicle, the mandible, and subperiosteal bone. The type of bone formation has a direct bearing on repair of a particular bone. For example, skull heals, in general, with fibrous union and not with new bone formation.

BONE COMPOSITION

A typical lamellar bone has a composition of approximately 8 percent water and 92 percent solid material. The solid is divided into 21 percent organic phase and 71 percent inorganic phase.

Organic Constituents

The organic material, known as the matrix, supplies form to bone and supporting structure for the deposition and crystallization of inorganic salts. The matrix is more than 90 percent collagen, with the remainder being proteoglycans. Bone collagen, as discussed in the first chapter, is Type I and consists of two α-1 (1) chains and one α-2 chain. This type of collagen is similar to skin and tendon collagen. However, during normal fracture healing a persistence of Type II collagen (which is characteristic of cartilage) has been demonstrated, well into the period when the bone is clinically united. This adds evidence that normal fracture healing takes place by endochondral bone formation within the callus. If compression plating is employed in the fixation of fractures very little callus forms and the collagen formed is then a Type I collagen. The principal carbohydrate component of the protein-polysaccharide (proteoglycans) is chondroitin sulfate A, with a small amount of keratosulfate.

Inorganic Constituents

The principal inorganic salt is crystalline hydroxyapatite $Ca_{10}(PO_4)_6(OH)_2$. The mineral crystals are extremely small being 25 to 75 A in diameter and approximately 200 A long. This provides a very large surface to volume ratio. There is a shell of water surrounding the surface crystals (hydration shell) and ions may move freely between the hydration shell and the crystalline surface. Glimcher has demonstrated that bone crystals align in a specific pattern within collagen. The long axis of the crystal is parallel to the longitudinal axis of the fiber, in a band pattern within the collagen fibril. In other words, they appear in the "hole" zone of the collagen fibril, increasing the surface area of the fiber. For example, a skeleton of a 150 lb man contains enough hydroxyapatite to cover about 100 acres.

Cellular Components of Bone

There are three principal cells identified during bone formation and remodeling. These bone cells consist of the osteoblast, osteocyte, and osteoclast. A similar series of cells has been demonstrated during cartilage formation and are known as chondroblasts, chondrocytes, and chondroclasts.

In bone, the osteoblast forms the matrix. The osteocyte has a dual function, both as a bone-forming cell and also as a bone-destroying cell. The osteoclast is charged with bone destruction

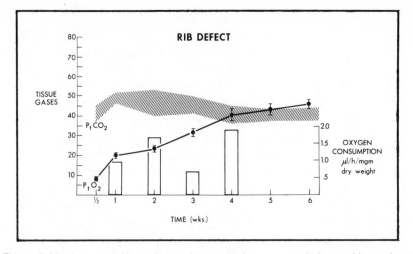

Figure 7.22 Low oxygen tension and consumption present during rapid new bone formation at two to four weeks. *(From Heppenstall, RB, et al. Clin Orthop 106:357–65, 1975.)*

and resorption, and also plays a role in remodeling. It is felt that the normal day-to-day resorption occuring during bone remodeling is mediated in the osteocyte, whereas pathologic resorption would be mediated by the osteoclast. The osteocyte produces collagen, and it is felt that it elaborates the glycoproteins and protein-polysaccharides. The osteocyte is found within the Haversian system in lamellar bones and is seen in lacunae communicating with Haversian canals where bone obtains its nourishment and oxygen supply.

During fracture repair osteoblasts appear to originate from cells of the cambium layer of the periosteum and also from the endosteum. Several names have been attached to these cells in the past, including fibroblast, osteoprogenitor, and undifferentiated mesenchymal cells. It is still felt by many investigators that the periosteum contains osteogenic cells and participates in the formation of external callus; and it should therefore be preserved, if at all possible, during the surgical treatment of fractures. However, as will be discussed, the endosteum makes the most important contribution to fracture healing. Bone cells predominantly rely on anaerobic metabolism. Bone formation, both at the epiphyseal plate in the zone of the metaphysis and at a fracture site, normally occurs under conditions of "relative hypoxia" as depicted in Figure 7.22.

BIOPHYSICAL PROPERTIES OF BONE

Live nonstressed bone exhibits a low magnitude steady-state electrical potential that is negative in the metaphyseal region and approaches isopolarity in the midshaft of bone. However, following a fracture, the entire shaft of bone reverts to an electronegative charge, with the metaphyseal electronegativity becoming even higher, and a secondary increase of electronegativity appearing over the fracture site. During subsequent healing the pattern of electropolarity returns to normal. The steady-state potential that exists in resting bone appears to depend on a summation of electromotive forces in actively metabolizing cells. It is not dependent upon nerve or vascular supply. The exact source of the potentials, whether it be metabolic products, membrane ionic gradients, or ion flux in the bone, has not been determined. However, it has been proved that the source of potential in unstressed bone is dependent on cell viability.

Several laboratories, including our own, have been able to demonstrate that fracture healing may be stimulated by the application of an electrical current through the fracture site. Initially, fractures in animals healed under electrical stimulation of 10 to 20 μamp direct current. This study was then advanced into the clinical investigation of fracture healing in humans. This is a multicenter study and results to date seem to indicate that delayed healing may be hastened and nonunions may be stimulated to heal under applied electrical current.

Osseous tissue follows Wolff's law. Simply stated, this law is "form follows function." If bone is gradually stressed under its breaking limit, the response of the osseous tissue will be to produce more bone to combat the compressing force. *Bone forms in compression and bone fails in tension* (Fig. 7.23). This is an important observation and has a direct clinical application to the management of fractures. If a patient with a fracture is treated with internal fixation, the bone must be placed in compression and not in tension. In other words, if a compression plate is employed in the treatment of an irregular fracture, compression may be achieved directly under the plate, but on the opposite cortex the bone may be in tension and this will alter fracture healing. It is for this reason that bending com-

530

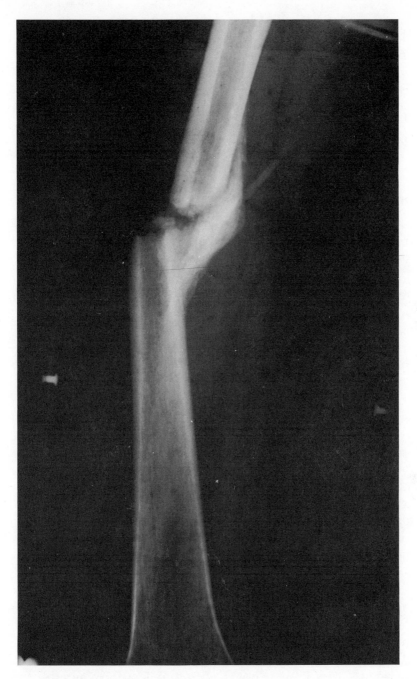

Figure 7.23 Note callus laid down on the compression side of a fractured femur and absence of callus on the tension side of the fracture.

pression plates has been suggested to obtain uniform compression across the fracture site, and to avoid compression of one cortex with tension on the opposite cortex. Initially, several years ago it was felt that compression plates produced their excellent results by applying pressure at the fracture site. At present, the function of compression plates is thought to provide excellent apposition and rigid immobilization. This will be dealt with later.

PRIMARY BONE HEALING

Primary bone healing is only possible with rigid internal fixation and excellent anatomic apposition. These two goals are only obtained by primary internal fixation. It has been adequately shown that fractures treated in this manner demonstrate evidence of primary bone healing with no signs of fibrous tissue or cartilage during healing. There is no evidence of external callus formation with this type of treatment.

The local destruction of osteons close to the fracture site, initiated by the destruction of the local blood supply, stimulates an intensive regeneration of new Haversian systems in the local area. Osteoclasts form spearheads at the ends of the Haversian canals close to the fracture site and these become enlarged in preparation for the formation of a new system. The osteoclast spearhead, or "cutting cone," can advance through bone at a rate of 50 to 80 μ per 24 hours up to and through the fracture surface, with the production of enlarged Haversian canals that cross from one fragment to the other. It is followed immediately by osteoblasts and new vessels to form new osteons that traverse the fracture site. This is the concept of the wound module (see Chap. 1 on normal repair) expressed in terms of bone.

If rigid internal fixation is employed, it will take approximately five to six weeks for new osteons to be constructed. The repair is produced by new osteons developing and crossing the fracture site, replacing the old osteons that had been deprived of their local blood supply. If a gap exists between the fracture fragments, or if there is not rigid immobilization, then this type of healing does not occur.

532

Stages of Repair

Stage of Impact   Bone will absorb energy until mechanical failure occurs. Bone can absorb more energy if it is applied rapidly. The amount of energy that can be absorbed by the bone is inversely proportional to the modules of rigidity, but it is directly proportional to the volume of bone.

Fracture lines will follow the path of least resistance. If drill holes have been placed in bone prior to impact, a fracture line will pass through the drill holes because they produce areas of stress concentration. This is extremely important to remember when large plates are removed following internal fixation. The limb must be protected (usually three to four weeks) until the osseous tissue around the drill holes has a chance to react to the new stress and abolish the stress concentrations. If compression plates have been left on for a prolonged period, osteoporosis can develop under them and this, of course, will further weaken the resistance to impact.

Stage of Induction   The duration of the stage of induction is unknown. It may occur any time from impact to the completion

Figure 7.24   Pictorial representation of fracture hematoma with disruption of periosteum and endosteum.

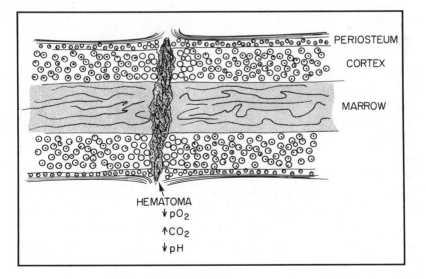

PERIOSTEUM

CORTEX

MARROW

HEMATOMA
$\downarrow pO_2$
$\uparrow CO_2$
$\downarrow pH$

of the stage of inflammation. Cells in the area of the fracture are induced to form new bone.

There are two separate mechanisms of induction. In the first mechanism, the periosteal cell, endosteal cell, and osteocyte modulate to produce new osteoblasts. The second mechanism involves differentiation of fibroblasts, endothelial cells, and muscle cells from other, undifferentiated, mesenchymal cells.

The actual stimulus to modulation and differentiation is also unknown. It is possible that the initial disruption of the blood supply and the consequent hypoxia with a large oxygen gradient may aid the stimulation of osteoblasts from their precursors (Fig. 7.24). An acidic pH rapidly develops in the local area and this, too, may be a stimulus. Lysosomal enzymes are released following cell disruption. As stated, each is a possible initial stimulant, but it is probable that the stimulation is multifactorial.

Stage of Inflammation   This stage begins immediately following the production of the fracture and persists until cartilage or bone formation is initiated, usually for three or four days. Clinically, the end of this stage is usually associated with a decrease in pain and swelling.

In this stage, there is a gross disruption of the vascular supply with attendant hemorrhage and hematoma formation. Hypoxia and acidosis dominate the environment. The bone at the edge of the fracture site, both the periosteal and endosteal surfaces dies. Osteons and lacunae are disrupted, and lysosomal enzymes escape. Mast cells invade during this period bringing vasoactive substances as well as heparin. (They are thought to play an active role in repair at this stage.) As in other areas of inflammation, the macrophage plays an active role in removing metabolic byproducts and dead tissue. Recent work suggests that the macrophage may be the activator of fibroblasts in soft tissue repair and it is conceivable that the same mechanism operates in the case of fracture repair. Osteoclasts begin to mobilize and osteolytic activity can be seen along the ruffled border of the cell.

Stage of Soft Callus   This is a very active phase in which both an external and internal soft callus are formed. (Fig. 7.25). The external callus plays an important initial role by helping to im-

534

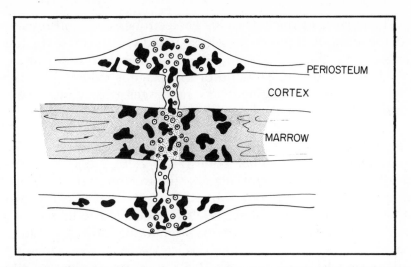

Figure 7.25 Pictorial representation of soft callus stage. Note reaction in periosteum away from the fracture site.

mobilize the fracture fragment. This is achieved by an active proliferation of the osteoblasts in the cambium layer of the periosteum. This is evident not only at the fracture site, but also along the under surface of the periosteum away from the fracture site. In effect, this produces two collars of soft tissue callus approaching each other from each fragment. The fibrous layer of the periosteum is elevated for a distance proximal to the fracture site by the proliferation of the underlying osteoblasts. In the proximal portion of the periosteum the osteoblasts form new bone directly. However, as the fracture site is approached, cartilage cells, as well as active osteoblasts, may be seen. There is also an associated gradual ingrowth of new vascularity. New cells are also collecting, and they advance beyond the vascular supply, producing a state of relative hypoxia.

The endosteal circulation, and not the periosteal circulation, plays the major role in fracture nutrition. Normally blood flows centrifugally from the endosteal area outward into the cortex and periosteal areas. The endosteal vessels are thought to supply at least the inner two-thirds to three-quarters of the cortex. The periosteal blood supply is not felt to be as important and is effective only in local areas of fascia and muscle attachments. Eventually the endosteal blood supply is reconstituted and the blood once more flows in a centrifugal direction.

The surface of the soft callus is electronegative and remains so throughout this stage, which usually lasts three to four weeks until the bony fragments are united by fibrous and/or cartilaginous tissue. The end of this stage is evident clinically when the osseous fragments are no longer grossly mobile and have reached a "sticky" phase.

Stage of Hard Callus.   In this stage, external and internal callus gradually convert to fiber bone (Figs. 7.26, 7.27). If internal fixation has not been employed in the treatment of these fractures, endochondral bone formation predominates. However, if the fragments have been well immobilized with use of a compression plate, membranous bone formation will predominate.

During this stage there is a definite increase in vascularity, but there is also an abundant increase in cellularity. Therefore, much of the cellular structure is still operating under conditions of relative hypoxia. The pH of the matrix now reverts to neutral, but the external and internal surfaces of the callus remain electronegative. The endosteal blood supply continues to develop, and osteoclasts are still actively removing dead bone.

This stage begins at three to four weeks and continues until the fragments are firmly united with new bone. The fracture site is now clinically and radiologically healed. The average

Figure 7.26 Pictorial representation of hard callus. New fiber bone occurs in both the periosteal and endosteal collars.

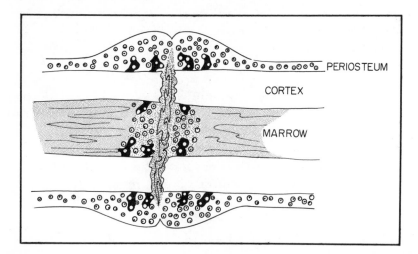

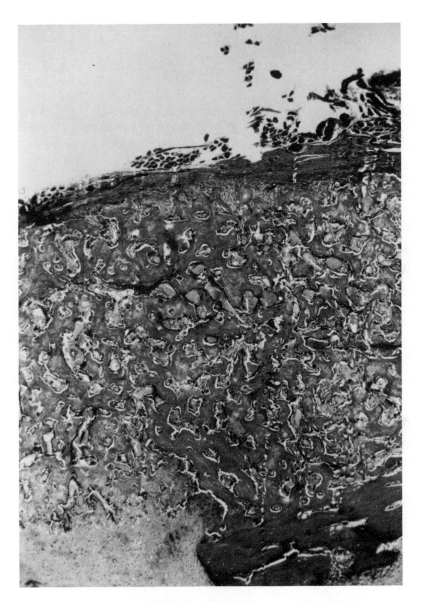

Figure 7.27 Photomicrograph demonstrating the external callus.

elapsed time from fracture is three to four months for major long bones.

Stage of Remodeling   In this stage, the newly formed fiber bone is gradually converted to lamellar bone. Osteoclasts remodel the bone to decrease the size of the callus or "bump," and reconstitute the medullary canal. During this phase the local tissue oxygen reverts to normal. The surface charge of the fracture site is no longer electronegative. The duration of this stage is variable. It may last for a few months, but there is evidence in human biopsy studies that it may continue for several years.

Special Types of Repair

Small Osseous Defects   This type of repair has been studied in animals with the use of a small drill hole in bone. The periosteum is destroyed at the penetration site. As in a fracture, the surrounding bone and marrow for at least a few millimeters around the hole becomes necrotic. A small hematoma develops in the osseous defect. Polymorphonuclear leukocytes are evident in the hematoma almost immediately, and by 24 hours plasma cells, lymphocytes, and macrophages are evident. Granulation tissue gradually replaces the hematoma. The periosteum reacts as it does to a normal fracture. The cambium layer becomes thickened by the preparation of new osteoblasts, elevating the fibrous layer. This reaction extends for some distance from the drill site. The osteoblastic cells from the periosteum eventually bridge the defect in a peculiar sort of manner that resembles the external callus of normal fracture healing, but the transformation of undifferentiated mesenchymal cells is more rapid with this type of defect. The endosteum responds similarly. Intramembranous bone formation occurs within the central portion of the defect. In general the major portion of the trabeculae are orientated at right angles to the osseous shaft. Lamellar bone gradually replaces fiber bone within the osseous defect and large intertrabecular spaces are gradually abolished. By three weeks, a mixture of fibrous and lamellar bone bridges the gap. There is no definite evidence of endochondral bone formation in this type of defect. Cutting cones gradually replace the reactive bone with new bone oriented in the same

538

direction as the remainder of the shaft. The excess periosteal and endosteal callus remodels as described.

Intramedullary Fixation   This type of fixation was introduced by Küntscher in 1940 when he reported the results of intramedullary rod fixation of femoral fractures. The femoral region is still the area of its most useful application. New devices have appeared over the past two decades. The Schneider, Hanson-Street, and the fluted Sampson devices are available, just to mention a few.

The femoral cavity must be reamed extensively to insert any of these devices. The effect of reaming has been thoroughly studied by Rhinelander using excellent microangiographic techniques. He demonstrated that the majority of the cortical diaphyseal bone is supplied by the endosteal nutrient vessel system. The main intramedullary vascular supply is destroyed during the reaming prior to insertion of the devices. The periosteal vessels, which usually supply only the outer one-quarter to one-third of the cortex, then increase their function to compensate for the destroyed endosteal circulation. The deficit is compounded if the periosteum is "stripped" during the insertion of the intramedullary device. Rhineland demonstrated that the best intramedullary device is one with a "fluted" design which permits control of rotation but at the same time allows regeneration of the endosteal vascular blood supply between the flutes.

If there is solid fixation of the intramedullary device, the small amount of external callus that develops will have a decreased amount of endochondral bone formation. If there is motion between the fragments due to a loose-fitting rod, the major portion of the bone deposited between the bone fragments will be by endochondral bone formation.

Clinically, it is difficult to decide when the fracture site is completely healed, since a portion of it is obscured by the intramedullary device. Most authors feel that at least one and a half years should pass before the device is removed. An important point to remember is that if there is evidence of comminution at the fracture site, a bone graft from the iliac crest should be used along with the internal fixation. We have seen cases presenting with initial comminution that are bone grafted in this manner and the rod removed at a later date. Following

539

removal of the rod, one sometimes sees a fracture line in the intramedullary area that was once occupied by the rod. However, there is usually extensive bone around this area bridging the two main fragments. We interpret this to mean that if the fracture had not been bone grafted initially it would not have healed as well, even with the internal fixation device. Therefore, it is a good "rule-of-thumb" to use a bone graft as well as internal fixation for open reduction of a comminuted femoral fracture.

Compression Plating   The role of a compression plate is to provide rigid internal fixation, reducing motion at the fracture site and allowing excellent apposition of the osseous fragments. Several outstanding studies have been performed by Perrin et al. of the AO Group in evaluating the beneficial effect of compression plates. (The AO Group was formed for the study of internal fixation and is based in Switzerland.)

Following the use of compression devices one often observes "primary" bone healing. In other words, the osseous fragments unite with osteonal bone of normal orientation. The bone fragments directly underneath the plate are usually approximated almost anatomically, but the cortices opposite it are often poorly approximated due to the differing configurations of the bone and the plate. *To achieve primary repair, it is important to ensure good apposition by bending the plate to prevent this. Remember, bone heals under compression and fails under tension.* Therefore, it is theoretically sound to obtain good apposition of both cortices. It is also very practical.

In this type of healing a hematoma does not form between the bone fragments as apposition is greatly improved and there is, in fact, no room for a hematoma. there is a mild inflammatory reaction in the soft tissues adjacent to the periosteum and in the marrow. New cutting cones (see section on primary bone healing) originate at the junction of live and dead bone. Osteoclasts lead the cutting cones and migrate directly across the fracture site along an empty Haversian canal resorbing the matrix. They cross the fracture site and enter another opposing empty Haversian canal, or begin to cut into the necrotic bone on the other fragment. This means that a new living osteon is produced immediately behind the cutting cone.

The obvious question that arises is what is the significance of the finding of an external callus? By inference it means that there has been motion at the fracture site. This implies that if motion at the fracture site can be eliminated, an external callus does not form but is replaced by primary bone healing. It also implies that with an external callus, endochondral bone formation is present; whereas, with compression plating, and the consequent absence of an external callus, primary bone healing, without intervening cartilage, occurs.

It is also important to remember that a compression plate, if left in place, will continue to absorb a major portion of the stress normally placed on this bone. Osteoporosis underneath the plate is the ultimate result. To avoid, this, the compression plates should be removed as soon as bone is healed. Protective weight bearing should be prescribed following removal of the plates if a fracture through the osteoporotic bone is to be avoided. When flexible compression plates are employed instead of rigid fixation plates, the severe osteoporosis underneath the plate does not develop. The design of improved plates, and the timing of their removal, are subjects of extensive investigation.

BLOOD SUPPLY, OXYGEN TENSION, AND ANEMIA IN BONE HEALING

Excellent independent studies by both Kelly and Rhinelander have revealed that blood supply plays an important role in fracture healing. As previously stated, endosteal blood supply appears to be the most important source of new blood for healing fractures. The author has also demonstrated that fractures, like soft tissue wounds, normally heal in a state of "relative hypoxia." Systemic hypoxia definitely delays fracture healing, as depicted in Figure 7.28; and in normal bone, hyperbaric oxygen increases osseous resorption relative to new bone formation. We feel that the large oxygen gradient that exists at a wound margin may well play an active role in initiating repair. A working scheme is depicted in Figure 7.29. There are clinical counterparts to these studies. For example, conditions marked by increased blood flow produce bone resorption. Conversely, calcification is frequently seen in association with areas of hypovascularity such as seen in the region of the rotator cuff in the shoulder. The unanswered question is: What is the effect of

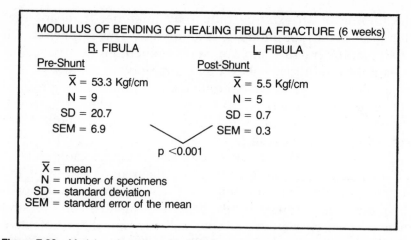

Figure 7.28 Modulus of bending of healing fibula fracture at six weeks. The strength of fractures made in chronically hypoxic dogs (after construction of a central arteriovenous shunt) is less than their counterparts made prior to shunting. *(From Heppenstall RB, et al.: J. Bone Joint Surg 58-A (8):1153–56, 1976).*

Figure 7.29 Theoretical scheme of events leading to fracture healing.

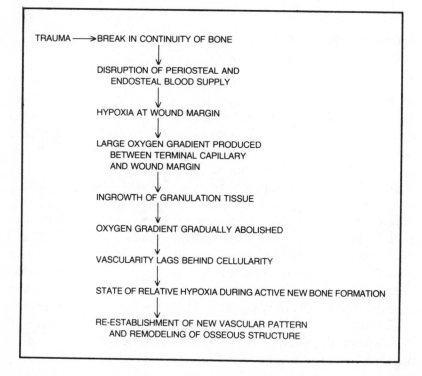

mild elevation of oxygen supply in vivo on both bone turnover and fracture repair? Investigations are presently in progress.

The question of the effect of anemia on bone repair frequently arises. Iron deficiency anemia delays repair in young animals as iron is required for the hydroxylation of proline and lysine in the formation of collagen and is also vital for function of the electron transport mechanism within the cell. However, an uncomplicated normovolemic anemia (the usual clinical situation) does not delay repair. If hypovolemia is associated with the anemia then repair is delayed. Therefore, in the usual case of moderate normovolemic anemia, blood transfusion does not stimulate fracture repair.

REMODELING

Fractures in the pediatric age group have an almost unbelievable ability to remodel. In children it is not necessary to obtain end-to-end apposition inasmuch as remodeling will produce a straight bone even if there is overlap initially. Healing adult bone makes an attempt at remodeling an overlap, but it is minimal compared to that seen in children. This implies a governing role of the epiphyseal plate, as this is the only significant anatomic variation between bones of the two age groups. It is also common knowledge that if a child's bone is fractured and end-to-end apposition is achieved, there is frequently an overgrowth of that particular bone in later life. It is for this reason that fractures of some long bones in children, particularly the femur, can be reduced with a slight overlap to compensate for the anticipated overgrowth.

EARLY FUNCTIONAL TREATMENT

In the past two decades there has been a definite trend toward returning the injured part to early functional use. When this is done several events occur. First of all, there is active contraction of the surrounding musculature that will help to stimulate increased blood flow around the fracture. This, in effect, will deliver more nutrients and will also aid in the production of a negative charge by means of the negatively charged red blood cells. Secondly, the intermittent contraction of the surrounding musculature will produce intermittent compression across the fracture site. Intermittent compression is definitely advantageous to fracture healing. Thirdly, if active motion of the proximal and distal joints is encouraged, contractures and stiffness will be avoided. Finally, early functional weight bearing on the fracture of the lower extremity will tend to produce a "hydraulic" effect if the applied cast is snug. That is, weight bearing produces a constant pressure across the entire fracture surface, and there is no area of localized stress directly at the fracture site. The pressure is evenly distributed along the bone rather than concentrated at the fracture site itself. Active compression at the fracture site tends to increase the generation of negative potential across it. Several clinical studies in the past decade have proved that this principle is valid. It used to be said that a fractured part should be put to rest and immobilized in plaster in order to promote healing. This type of thinking has gradually given way to early return of the injured part to functional activity.

EFFECT OF VITAMINS ON BONE HEALING

Vitamin A has been reported to decrease the time required for fracture healing by promoting cell proliferation and matrix formation. The specific mechanism of action is not evident. Vitamin A deficiency produces a thickening of osseous tissue, particularly in the calvaria. On the other hand, severe vitamin A deficiency can also result in a gross thinning of the cortical bone increasing the susceptibility to fracture.

Vitamin C deficiency produces scurvy. This vitamin plays a vital role in the hydroxylation of proline and lysine. Since this plays such an important role in the production of collagen, a deficiency of vitamin C will produce a decrease in matrix synthesis. This will delay bone repair as well as bone growth.

Vitamin D metabolism has been extensively investigated in recent times. DeLuca has made some very important observations on the role of vitamin D and calcium metabolism. In brief, vitamin D is converted to 25-hydroxycholecalciferol (25-HCC) in the liver. In the kidney this is then converted to 1,25-dihydroxycholecalciferol (1,25-HCC). This is the active form of vitamin D that is involved in initiating synthesis of a calcium binding protein within intestinal epithelial cells. Therefore, one of the major functions of vitamin D is involved in the intestinal absorption of calcium. Evidence has been presented that vitamin D increases the solubility of bone minerals and increases lactate production, thereby affecting bone cell metabolism directly. Vitamin D is also involved in the conversion of pyruvate to oxaloacetate, which is eventually converted to citrate. If this vitamin is given in excess concentration, osteoblasts will hypertrophy, and the size of the endoplasmic reticulum and golgi apparatus is increased.

Finally vitamin D appears to affect calcium metabolism by three distinct mechanisms. First, it is directly involved in the active transport of calcium and phosphorus from the intestine to the blood stream. Second, it plays a direct role in regulating movement of both calcium and phosphorus ions across renal tubular epithelium. Finally, it increases citrate production in bone cells. The increased citrate chelates calcium thereby removing ionized calcium and secondarily promoting mobilization of calcium from bone.

Deficiency of this vitamin plays a direct role in rickets and bone repair. Patients with rickets heal fractures poorly. If large doses of vitamin D are provided, fracture healing may progress normally. Recently, vitamin D has also been reported of value in healing fractures in patients taking high doses of anticonvulsants, particularly Dilantin. These patients develop osteomalacia with concomitant fractures. If large doses of vitamin D and calcium supplementation are given along with the anticonvulsant therapy this complication may be avoided.

COMPLICATIONS OF FRACTURE REPAIR
Nonunion

Simply stated, this occurs when the repair process has come to a halt and healing will not occur without some external stimulus. This is seen at varying time intervals, depending on the particular bone involved. For example, it has been stated that the average time for healing of an adult fracture is three to six months. Therefore, if healing has not occurred by six to nine months, a state of nonunion should be assumed. The accepted manner of treating this complication is to perform an open reduction and internal fixation, along with a bone grafting procedure. It is very important to provide "rigid" internal fixation for the treatment of a nonunion. Several centers around the country are attempting to heal these difficult cases with the application of a steady-state current of 10 to 20 μamps. This is exciting new research, but the final results will not be available for two to three years. Therefore, this procedure is now considered completely experimental. It has the potential advantages of requiring only limited surgical exposure for insertion of electrodes and eliminating the necessity of a bone graft.

Pseudarthrosis

This complication occurs when all repair has ceased and a false joint, with a synovial lining, has developed between the fracture fragments. Treatment of this problem is difficult at best. It occurs on a congenital basis in the clavicle and the tibia where it is particularly difficult to treat. The standard form of treatment is open reduction and internal fixation, with destruction of the false joint between the bone ends and application of a bone graft.

Avascular Necrosis

This complication is seen following fractures in three specific areas:

1) Fractures of the femoral neck in the hip that may cause avascular necrosis of the femoral head. These may require insertion of artificial prostheses.
2) Fractures of the navicular in the wrist, particularly ones through its waist, resulting in avascular necrosis of the proximal pole. Frequently, these are managed by bone grafting procedures.
3) Fractures of the neck of the talus with avascular necrosis of the proximal body. These may require bone grafting, excision of the talus, or ankle fusion.

Osteomyelitis following Open Injury

The only way osteomyelitis can be prevented is through aggressive early treatment of open ("compound") fractures. It is extremely important to debride and irrigate all open fractures thoroughly if this complication is to be avoided. It is not sufficient to attempt a minimal cleansing in the emergency room. Affected patients should be taken to the operating room for a formal cleansing procedure with antibiotic administration intraoperatively and postoperatively.

CARTILAGE REPAIR

Cartilage repair differs from osseous repair in that cartilage is unable to reconstitute its basic structure perfectly following injury. Repair is not always complete, and this problem is partially related to its blood supply.

There are four basic types of cartilage:

Elastic cartilage. This contains elastin fibers and is found in such areas as the ears and nose. It has a wide elastic range.

Fibrocartilage. This is poorly organized and is found in uncalcified bodies associated with joints, such as the intervertebral disc, or in slightly movable joints such as the symphysis pubis, and pseudarthroses. Its function is to provide stability and act as a shock absorber.

Articular cartilage In contrast to the above, this type is well organized and layered, covering most articular surfaces. In common with other types of cartilage, it contains collagen. Its function is to provide a smooth surface for the gliding motion of opposing osseous structures, and also to act as a shock absorber to decrease the cyclic loading of the underlying cancellous bone.

Hyaline cartilage. This type is similar to articular cartilage but is found in nonarticular locations, such as the epiphyseal plate and the tracheal rings. In the epiphyseal plate it is a precursor for normal bone formation.

Fibrocartilage Repair

Commonly encountered fibrocartilagenous structures are the menisci located within the knee joint. This cartilage spreads a film of nutrient synovial fluid over the articular surfaces; it protects the opposing articular surfaces as a shock absorber; it increases the stability of the knee joint by deepening the articular surfaces; and it facilitates complex movements. However, it is also susceptible to injury. The meniscus obtains its blood supply through its extreme peripheral edge. The vessels extend inward from the periphery for short distances and arise both from the capsule and from folds of synovial membrane. The innermost portion of the cartilage is devoid of blood supply. Therefore, it depends on the synovial fluid for its nutrition.

Due to this vascular anatomic relationship this cartilage is unable to repair itself once it is torn within its substance. If a tear occurs along the peripheral portion that does have a blood supply, then repair can take place. However, in the usual clinical setting the tear of the meniscus occurs within its substance and repair is not possible. If a meniscus is surgically excised in the treatment of an internal derangement, a new fibrocartilage is regenerated. It is not as thick as the original but it does provide for function. A similar situation exists within an intervertebral disc. It is also supplied with vessels only in its periphery, and nutrition enters its center through diffusion. Therefore, like a meniscus, an intervertebral disc is unable to repair itself following injury within its substance. A typical example of this is a disc in which the nucleus pulposus ruptures out through the annulus fibrosus.

Articular Cartilage Repair

The repair of articular cartilage takes place with the formation of fibrocartilage. The normal sequential layering of the articular surface is disrupted following repair with fibrocartilage. The only blood supply available to normal articular cartilage is at its base at the bone-cartilage junction. An injury to the superficial zones of the articular cartilage must depend upon diffusion for its nutrition. If the injury is complete and extends down to the subchondral bone then vascular invasion from below may hinder repair. A typical attempt at repair is noted in Figure 7.30.

Hyaline Cartilage Repair

The best example of hyaline cartilage is that found in the epiphyseal plate. In this location the cartilage is a precursor for normal bone formation. The blood supply to this cartilage, similar to that noted above, arises from a fine network of vessels at the base of the cartilage, at the bone-cartilage junction. An injury to this type of cartilage usually occurs in the zone of

548

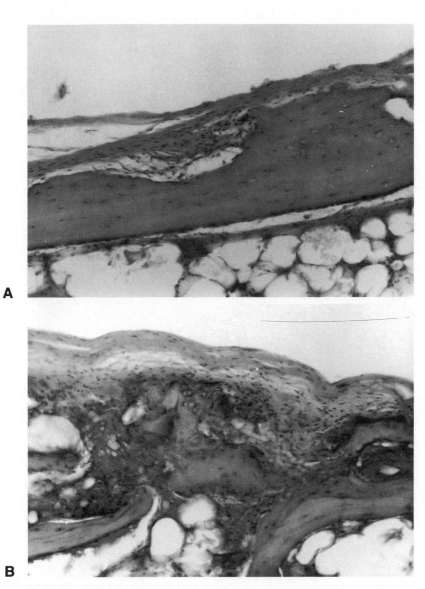

Figure 7.30 **A.** Attempt at fibrous repair in articular cartilage following superficial injury. **B.** Fibrocartilage repair of deep injury to articular cartilage involving the bone-cartilage junction. *(From Heppenstall, RB, et al.: Clin Orthop 103:136–42, 1974.)*

549

hypertrophic cells and may extend upward in a cleavage pattern to the zone of cell columns. It is extremely important to obtain as accurate an anatomic reduction as possible in order to aid the repair of hyaline cartilage. If the sequential zones of the epiphyseal plate are destroyed then the blood supply extends upward through the bone-cartilage junction in an attempt to repair the substance, producing a typical fibrocartilage. This can interfere with normal growth at the epiphyseal plate, producing gross distortions of subsequent growth.

In summary, it can be seen that the repair of cartilage is less than satisfactory. The type of cartilage generated in normal repair is a form of fibrocartilage that has neither the resilience and shock absorbing capacity, nor the structural organization, of normal cartilage.

REFERENCES

Collagen and Mineralization

Glimcher MJ: A Basic Architectural Principle in the Organization of Mineralized Tissues. Clin Orthop, 61:16–36, 1968

Cell Function

Belanger LF; Robichon J, Migicovsky BB, Copp DH, Vincent J: Resorption without osteoclasts (osteolysis) in mechanism of hard tissue destruction. In Sognnaes RF (ed): Washington, D.C. American Assn. for Advancement of Science, 1963, pp. 531–56

Bioelectric Properties

Brighton CT, Friedenberg ZB, Mitchell EI, Booth RE: Treatment of nonunion with constant direct current. Clin Orthop 124:106, 1977

Friedenberg ZB, Harlow M, Heppenstall RB, Brighton CT: The cellular origin of bioelectric potentials in bone/calcified tissue research. 13:52–63, 1973

Friedenberg ZB, Roberts PG, Didizian NH, Brighton CT: Stimulation of fracture healing by direct current in the rabbit fibula. J Bone Joint Surg 53-A: 1400–08, 1971

Blood Flow, Oxygen Tension, and Anemia

Heppenstall RB, Brighton CT: Fracture healing in the presence of anemia. Clin Orthop 123:253–58, 1977

Heppenstall RB, Goodwin C, Brighton CT: Fracture healing in the presence of chronic hypoxia. J Bone Joint Surg 58-A: 1153–56, 1976.

550

Heppenstall RB, Grislis G, Hunt TK: Tissue gas tensions and oxygen consumption in healing bone defects. Clin Orthop 106:357–65, 1975

Rhinelander FW: The normal microcirculation of diaphyseal cortex and its response to fracture. J Bone Joint Surg 50-A: 784–800, 1968

Rhinelander FW: Effects of Medullary Nailing on the Normal Blood Supply of Diaphyseal Cortex. Instruction Course Lectures, A.A.O.S., St. Louis, Mosby, 1973, p 161

Sim FH, Kelly PJ: Relationship of bone remodeling, oxygen consumption and blood flow in bone. J Bone Joint Surg 52-A: 1377–89, 1970

Compression Plating

Perrin S: Cortical bone healing. Act Orthop Scand (Suppl.) 125, 1969

Morphology of Repair

Ham AW: A histological study of the early phases of bone repair. J Bone Joint Surg (Am) 12:827, 1930

Ham AW, Harris WR: Repair and transplantation of bone. In Bourne G (ed): Biochemistry and Physiology of Bone, 2nd ed. Vol 3. New York, Academic Press, 1972, pp 337–97

Cartilage References

King D: The healing of semilunar cartilages. J Bone Joint Surg 18:333, 1936

Meachin G: The effect of scarification on articular cartilage in the rabbit. J Bone Joint Surg 45-B: 150–61, 1963

Burns
Thomas K. Hunt

Spontaneous healing can be both a curse and a blessing to burn victims. Superficial, or first degree, burns in which little or no cell death occurs and damage is confined to the epidermis, will heal spontaneously with no apparent scarring. Second degree burns, in which cell death is confined to the epidermis and upper dermis, will usually heal spontaneously by epithelization resulting in excellent function and good cosmetic appearance. In contrast, spontaneous healing of deep second degree burns (in which a few viable epithelial sources remain in the burn) or in third degree or deeper burns in which no epithelial elements remain alive, ends frequently in contracture and hypertrophic scars that become the causes of subsequent disability.

THE THERMAL INJURY

It seems common sense to regard the burn wound as an inalterable necrosis determined within a few seconds of the thermal injury. Investigation has shown, however, that this is not true. The extent of injury is determined by the temperature of the burning object, the length of the exposure, the thickness of

552

skin exposed to the injury, and the ability of the skin to conduct the heat away (usually proportional to blood flow). Deep, severe thermal trauma injures different components of tissue in various ways. The thermal injury may kill surface tissue outright. However, deeper into the skin, blood vessels may be only "partly injured." Soon after the injury, large quantities of plasma begin to exude from the injured vessels into the surrounding tissue, blood flow becomes sluggish, the cell volume of the blood in the small vessels rises, and soon the vessels thrombose. Whether endothelial injury contributes or not is not known. This vascular thrombosis slowly progresses during the first three days after deep second and third degree burns. As the blood supply stops, the area of necrosis deepens due to advancing ischemia. In other words, the depth of many burns is not determined immediately by the thermal exchange. The burn, instead, deepens due to ischemic necrosis and reaches its maximum depth between 48 to 72 hours after injury.

The hard leathery eschar that results immediately from searing burns does not participate in this edema, but tissue deep to it does. The loss of fluid within the burn due to increased vascular permeability may be extensive, but even so it does not account for the total loss of fluid from the intravascular spaces in burn patients. For reasons not thoroughly understood, the burn edema is also seen in tissues remote from the burn. The increase in vascular permeability is, to some extent, generalized. Some investigators have postulated that the release of toxic substances from burns increases vascular permeability elsewhere; and others have pointed to a loss of serum protein and the infusion of large amounts of protein-free fluids as the cause. Obviously, these hypotheses are not mutually exclusive.

Since the depth of tissue necrosis is frequently determined by vascular factors, a "transition zone" must exist where necrotic and live tissue come together. This "transition zone" is unstable and its fate remains precarious until the patient's circulatory hemodynamics stabilize. Even when the situation becomes stable, the viable deep tissue has barely enough circulation to remain alive, and no reserve with which to heal or resist infection. It is easily infected. Infection tends to compromise the local vessels further, and a second deepening of the burn may result. Other factors may be acting on the vasculature, but the progressive vascular thrombosis certainly seems to be the major event in the evolution of the burn. The major evidence for this point of view is the fact that in laboratory conditions, burned skin, which is destined to become necrotic if left in situ can be transplanted early after burning to an unburned area and can be made to survive. This simple but elegant observation has opened the hope that medical measures that might limit the advancing vascular occlusion may also limit the depth of the burn.

As we have noted before in Chapter 1, a vascular supply sufficient for mere tissue survival is not adequate for repair. Healing requires greater vascularity. Therefore, healing of a burn must often be delayed until a neovasculature appears or until the burn is debrided to a level where adequate vascularity already exists upon which skin grafts can be nourished. Scalpel wounds begin neovascularization within a few days. Burn injuries, however, do not show much neovascularization until well over a week has passed. In contrast, if the burn is excised soon after it is made, neovascularization seems to proceed normally in the bed of the wound. For this reason, a number of investigators have postulated that a burn "toxin" prevents normal neovascularization, but the idea remains controversial. The inflammatory reaction and neovascularization are both delayed even in tiny deep burns.

SEPARATION OF DEAD TISSUE

After the vascular injury (if any) has reached its maximum, a slow process of demarcation of the living from the dead begins. In first degree burns, very little tissue is devitalized and little must be removed. In superficial second degree burns, only epithelial elements become necrotic and only separation of superficial epithelium need occur. In deep burns, subcutaneous tissue or even bone or fascia must be separated and removed. The first sign of this process is seen when the still functional small vessels regain their normal permeability and start to remove the local edema. Inflammatory cells migrate to the burn from the working vasculature and accumulate in the plane between viable and nonviable tissue. Small vessels proliferate into the viable tissue and migrate toward the inflamed and necrotic areas.

The eschar, or dead burned tissue, is separated by the inflammatory reaction. It has been assumed that the presence of necrotic tissue is the factor that incites inflammation. Though this is certainly true, it may not be the whole cause. We know that each of us has an immunity to his own collagen. Normally, this immunity is masked by the proteoglycans molecules that cover the collagen fiber and the fact that the vast majority of the antigenic sites in collagen are unreachable in the central portions of large collagen fibers. When collagen is injured, antigenic sites undoubtedly become more accessible. The level of circulating anticollagen antibody rises very quickly after burning, and thus it seems possible that immune factors may play a role in the inflammatory reaction to burned tissue. The exact cause of the inflammation may not be important to the separation of the eschar. However, it could become extremely important to the manner in which the burn heals.

Regardless of cause, a dense inflammatory exudate collects. The polymorphonuclear leukocytes and macrophages secrete collagenase and other proteases that can hydrolyze denatured connective tissues. Bacteria also secrete such enzymes. Therefore, an infected eschar will separate more quickly than one which is not infected. In fact, when modern topical antibacterial agents were first used, many surgeons objected to them because they "delayed" the separation of eschar. We now recognize that the early separation to which we were accustomed came about largely by infection, and was very much a mixed blessing.

Separation of tissue can also occur in second degree burns since epithelial cells also secrete collagenase. The thin eschar over superficial second degree burns usually separates from unburned tissue as epithelium grows beneath it. When the eschar falls off, a healed wound usually appears beneath.

Natural lysis is usually too slow a process on which to depend for separation of deep burns. If the burn is not infected the eschar may take many weeks to separate, and surgical separation is usually preferable. Unfortunately, the surgeon cannot see easily the exact depth of the burn wound. Therefore, there is a fine art to debriding burned tissue. The problem is not difficult if the burn is obviously third degree to begin with, or has only a few small areas of superficial injury that can be sacrificed. The fine judgment comes into play when the surgeon is faced with debriding a burn that may have a significantly large second degree component. In this case, he may want parts of the eschar to separate spontaneously, or will debride the burn in such a way that epithelial remnants remain and some spontaneous epithelization is possible. It is not usually valuable to preserve small islands of epithelium, but large areas deserve saving.

Recent experiments with bacterial enzymes, particularly bacterial subtilains, show them an effective means of debriding burned tissue. Viable tissue seems unaffected by them. On the negative side, it is extremely difficult to maintain surface asepsis and still keep the effectiveness of the enzyme. Although the problems seem on their way to solution, infection remains a major risk in burns debrided by topical enzyme therapy; and the technique has limited value now.

REGENERATION OF VASCULATURE AND CONNECTIVE TISSUE

After inflammation is established, a rich plexus of new vessels develops in the inflamed area. This circumstance is already described in Chapter 1. Large numbers of fibroblasts also appear. When the eschar separates from a third degree burn, "granulation" tissue is disclosed. The granulation tissue blends subtly into the deeper normal tissue.

The surface of granulation tissue advances slowly by the same means as described in Chapter 1. The vessels of the "inflammatory" plexus coalesce and new small vessels advance into the volume previously filled by necrotic tissue to support its replacement with fibroblasts and inflammatory cells.

While granulation tissue is theoretically capable of filling even large defects, the process has limitations. As epithelium covers the granulation tissue, the inflammatory vessels disappear and the connective tissue contracts. Therefore, large defects remain misshapen because epithelization usually progresses before the normal contours can be restored.

If the surgeon, for any of a number of reasons, chooses to allow spontaneous healing to occur, the granulation tissue remains uncovered for prolonged periods. It becomes contaminated. It is exposed to foreign body as well as to physical and thermal injury. Therefore, a number of possible stimuli to inflammation and subsequent fibrous proliferation may persist in the tissue. If small islands of injured (or foreign) collagen persist as well, an immune stimulus may remain. Under these stimuli, fibroblasts synthesize a dense layer of collagen fibers under the surface granulation. Unfortunately, scar collagen shrinks as it ages and remodels. The mechanism for the shrinkage is discussed under contraction and contracture in Chapter 2. The older and thicker the layer becomes, the stronger is the force of contracture. The only real defenses against scar contracture are to excise the eschar and cover the deep tissue early with skin graft.

Skin grafts reduce contracture not only because of their epithelium, but especially because they contain flexible and tough dermis. The rejoining of the vasculature from wound to skin graft is quick, and the healing process thus circumvents the stimulus to continued connective tissue proliferation which is normally present in open wounds. The flexible dermis protects the tissue from reinjury. Therefore, the scar between normal tissue and skin graft tends to remain thin and supple. Antigenic or foreign body or mechanical stimuli to continued repair could still remain and skin grafts do not always obviate hypertrophic repair, but they usually minimize it.

In the long-term healing of burns, when epithelization is complete, a contest between remodeling and contracture ensues. In flat, relatively immobile protected skin of trunk, thighs, and scalp, remodeling usually wins the battle. Though the scar may temporarily become hypertrophic, thick, and brittle, the stimulus to continue collagen synthesis eventually subsides. Between a few months after epithelial coverage to a year or a year-and-a-half thereafter, the scar may "resolve" remarkably. However, a contracture is much more likely to be the winner when tissue is frequently moved or injured; for example, around joints, in the neck, and on the face. The brittle new tissue in these sites is easily reinjured by motion, trauma, and exposure. With each new injury, the healing sequence is reactivated with deposition of more collagen and consequent shortening of scar. Furthermore, scar collagen tends to orient along lines of tension and subsequently shortens along these lines.

Fortunately, as noted in Chapters 1 and 2, there are ways of conquering this tendency to thicker and shorter scar. New collagen is a plastic substance, and its deposition and resorption can be influenced. The rapidly "turning-over" collagenous scar can be "stretched" if put under mild constant traction. Furthermore, if pressure is applied to the area, (usually about 25 mm Hg, approximately the critical closing pressure of capillaries), the blood flow to the rapidly metabolizing collagenous tissue presumably decreases. The collagenolytic process is not affected since it is mediated mainly by enzymes deposited into the extracellular space. Therefore, the balance of collagen dynamics turns to lysis, and the scar under direct pressure tends to resorb. The modern treatment of the burn wound often relies on traction and direct dressing pressure, especially for burns in the vicinity of joints.

EPITHELIZATION

Epithelium regenerates by mitosis beginning near the injury, and by subsequent migration of new epithelial cells over the defect. New epithelium can become thick or multilayered only a limited distance from each natural source—usually about 10 mm. Beyond this, spontaneous epithelization produces thin, friable epidermis. Once again, if one procrastinates and waits for spontaneous epithelization, the result tends to be unsatisfactory.

In second degree burns, many sources of epithelium persist in the depths of hair follicles, sweat glands, and eccrine glands. When proper local conditions permit, epithelial cells migrate onto the granulation tissue forming mounds of epithelial cells at the vestiges of skin appendages, and these cells then rapidly migrate centrifugally. If the burn is superficial, there is little distance between these "volcanoes" of epithelium, and the burn heals quickly with little scarring. In deeper burns, fewer sources of epithelium survive, and spontaneous epithelization is proportionately slower. Unfortunately, the sophisticated collagenous architecture of dermis can never regenerate, and the tendency to scarring of third degree and deep second degree burns is therefore greater. Epithelium depends on the mechanical properties of dermis for its durability. Healing after thick skin grafts (with more dermis) is generally preferable to healing after thin ones.

Undoubtedly, epithelization and connective tissue regeneration interact. Epithelial coverage normally halts connective tissue proliferation and eventually causes regression of neovascularization. It may not exert its normal effects over keloids and hypertrophic scars.

Surprisingly, allografts placed on second degree burns may become vascularized much like the "take" of a split-thickness isograft on granulation tissue. Biopsies have confirmed that a blood supply crosses the burned epithelium and joins with that of the foreign split-thickness graft. The vascularized allografts may not "reject" until the second or third week. When they do "reject," they develop a cyanotic hue, become desiccated, and spontaneously separate. Beneath them is a well-healed wound surface. Graft separation occurs earlier in areas of superficial second degree burn and later in deeper ones. Biopsy suggests that the grafts do not actually "reject" in the immunologic sense. Histologic studies suggest instead that vascular supply to the graft is progressively occluded by the growth of the epithelium resurfacing the second degree burn beneath the allograft. No microscopic evidence of immune rejection is seen. No intermingling of host and allograft collagen is seen.

INFLUENCE OF DEHYDRATION

Dehydration suppresses the rate of epithelization. Most manuals on emergency management of burn wounds advises blister debridement on the theory that the blister fluid aids bacterial growth. In clinical practice, however, except for rare streptococcal infections usually seen in children, wound sepsis arising in superficial second degree burns is rare. Epithelization is more rapid under an intact blister. The burn will heal to functional integrity 10 percent to 20 percent faster if the blister is left undamaged and dehydration is prevented.

If the blister is removed, microporous tape or a cadaver allograft can be placed to protect the wound. Once again, epithelization is more rapid than when the tender deep epithelium is exposed to air and allowed to dry.

The quality of coverage is also much better when epithelization occurs in a protected environment. Biopsies of adjacent areas, covered and uncovered, reveal mature, flexible epithelium in the protected situation and thinner dyskeratotic and acanthotic epithelium in the exposed dehydrated burn (Fig. 7.31).

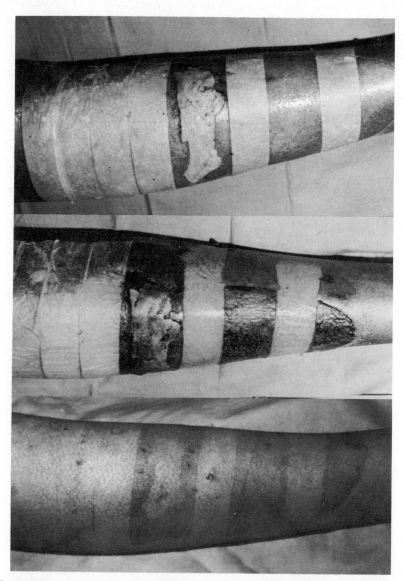

Figure 7.31   Top. The anterior aspect of the left lower leg six hours after a moderate depth second degree burn. The blister has been debrided and the wound covered with strips of microporous tape and fresh cadaver allograft. Note fluid on burn surface which is exposed. **Center.** Seven days postburn. Note thick crust overlying exposed wounds. The allograft is adherent and vascularized. The two lower tape strips have been removed. The underlying epithelial surface is well healed. **Bottom.** Six weeks postburn. The areas that were previously covered can be easily distinguished from those that had been exposed. *(From Miller TA, White WL: Plast Reconstr Surg 49:522, 1972. The Williams & Wilkins Co., Baltimore.)*

Areas covered with microporous paper adhesive tape (Micropore brand surgical tape) heal about 25 percent faster than exposed second degree burn (when the tape can be made to adhere). This is an argument against any humoral stimulatory effect that allograft might have on epithelization, and an argument for the superior epithelization being due to environmental factors.

All of these situations have one thing in common. Evaporative water loss from the wound is known to be diminished by skin grafts and microporous tape. After a second degree burn, or any deep burn as well, water loss through the destroyed epithelium increases to as much as 100 times normal. Intact blisters, allograft, and microporous tape all diminish water loss. If major areas of increased water loss can be so treated, the metabolic heat loss can also be significantly diminished.

BURN WOUND MANAGEMENT

The subject of burn management in general cannot be summarized here. Recently, major advances have been made. The basic principles are (1) rapid and complete restoration of fluid balance and blood volume, (2) exclusion of bacteria, (3) early debridement and closure, and (4) maintenance of nutrition and resistance to infection. Unless the patient is well supported, his wound cannot be healed.

Exclusion of bacteria may be attempted in several ways. The most common is the use of a topical antibacterial agent. Currently, silver sulfadiazine, silver nitrate, and providone iodine are the most commonly used. Each has its own advantages and drawbacks. The first two are the most thoroughly tested and give about the same results in terms of mortality rates. Many burn units use allografts and xenografts liberally usually on the debrided and healing burn surface. However, as noted above, allograft can be a most effective dressing over second degree burns. A newer method, reserved currently for massive burns, is massive debridement done as soon as fluid and hemodynamic stability is reached followed by allografting with immune suppression to allow early and prolonged "take" of the allografts. Obviously, this course has many pitfalls, but results are encouraging.

Debridement is still done surgically in most cases. Debriding enzymes are effective, but it is difficult to use them and at the same time exclude bacteria. Surgical debridement can be done by taking successive thicknesses of burn with the dermatome until viable tissue is reached, the so-called tangential excision technique. However, the scalpel is still used as well. Laser excisions are used in a few units so equipped.

In general, the earlier the excision and homografting, the better are the cosmetic and functional results. Xenografts and allografts can preserve soft wound for a while until autograft can be obtained. After a long debate, most experts now agree that allografts are preferable to xenografts. Procurement is expensive, but freeze banking techniques are good, and skin banks can be maintained. A useful rule is to autograft sensitive functional areas such as hands, face, and elbows first to make use of the thicker dermal sections one can get. Second cropping of autograft donor sites can be done, but quality of graft slowly deteriorates with successive crops.

DONOR SITE HEALING

The partial thickness donor site is usually thought of as an iatrogenic second degree burn. A moment's reflection on the mechanism of injury will reveal that this is an oversimplification. There is no vascular injury. There is no dead tissue on the surface.

Many means of treating donor sites have been devised, and are often the subject of passionate advocacy. However, donor sites almost always heal without complication when covered by a single layer of fine mesh gauze or left exposed without any coverage. No one has yet improved significantly on this method of treatment. Unfortunately, it is difficult to cover donor sites with microporous tape because the immediate exudation and bleeding prevents contact of tissue with the adherent.

It would seem that coverage of donor sites with allograft would prevent metabolic losses and accelerate repair. However, the allografts usually "take," and at about two to three weeks, graft deterioration appears and a classic imune rejection reaction occurs. The added inflammation and tissue damage can produce a third degree injury and complicated repair. Hypertrophic scar (with microscopically visible allograft collagen) often results, an interesting observation which may reflect on the cause of hypertrophic scar.

It remains a mystery why second degree burn separates an allograft by epithelizing under it and can be protected from this immune reaction whereas a donor site is not so protected. However, these are the facts as they are seen in the clinic and laboratory. The only unifying theory that has been set forth that explains this difference is that in order for epithelial migration to occur, a nonviable plane (the burn) must exist (see Miller in Bibliography).

Epithelization in donor sites is more rapid under water-impermeable/oxygen-impermeable dressings, such as Teflon, as opposed to other plastics—such as polypropylene—which are less permeable to oxygen. Regrettably, both plastics tend to promote infection. If infection does occur, the acceleratory effects of oxygen are lost. The principle has been established, however, that epithelization occurs more rapidly in moderately hyperoxic conditions.

HYPERTROPHIC SCAR

No injury is so frequently followed by hypertrophic scars as burn injuries (Fig. 7.32). Microscopic examination of hypertrophic scars (Figs. 7.33–7.35) shows small islands of cellular activity surrounded by "whorls" of connective tissue. The scar is vascular and remains so for many months, or even years. Traction and pressure are useful in countering hypertrophic healing, but often they must be used for many months before the tendency to hypertrophy is gone.

Unfortunately, no animal models exist that can be used to explain hypertrophic scar. This author tends to believe that the burn is contaminated by many bacteria, not all pathogenic. It is probably contaminated with viruses, and certainly with foreign substances. This author suspects that the tendency to hypertrophy remains as long as irritative and antigenic substances (some of which may be autologous tissue) persist in the wound. There is a tendency for hypertrophy to diminish with time, and this would seem to correlate with the removal of macrophage-stimulating substances. It has been suggested that the antigenic sites in collagen exposed by the burning process tend to remain in tissue causing a continued macrophagic in-

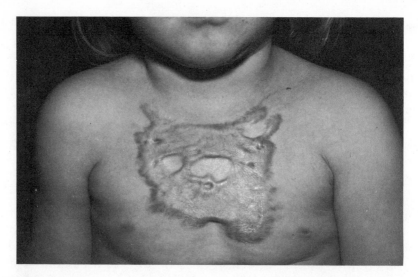

Figure 7.32 This burn scar has characteristics of both keloid and hypertrophic scar. The "invasive" appearance at its edges suggests keloid.

Figure 7.33 Scanning electron microscopic view of hypertrophic scar. Note the nodular arrangement of the fibers (approximately × 250). *(Courtesy of Paul S. Baur, M.D., Division of Cell Biology, University of Texas, Medical Branch, Galveston, Texas.)*

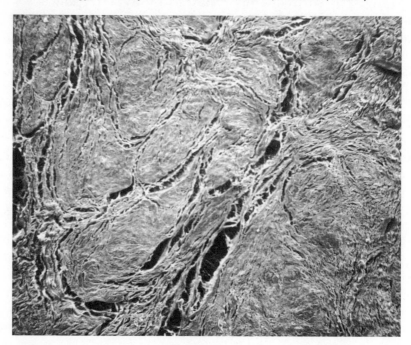

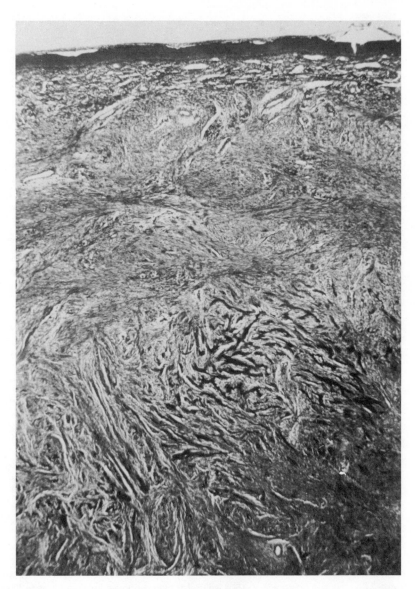

Figure 7.34 Light microscopic view of hypertrophic scar. Note whorls and nodules (×
25). *(Courtesy of Hugo A. Linares, M.D., Chief Pathologist, Shriners Burns Institute,
Galveston, Texas.)*

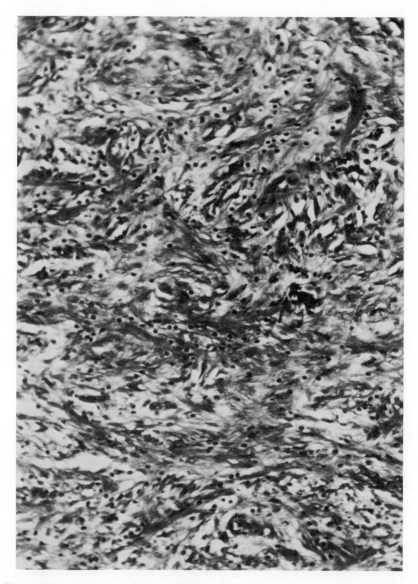

Figure 7.35 Higher powered (× 150) view of a hypertrophic scar nodule. Note fibro-blasts and macrophages. *(Courtesy of Hugo A. Linares, M.D., Chief Pathologist, Shriners Burns Institute, Galveston, Texas.)*

flammatory response that in turn stimulates collagen deposition. This theory is supported by the occurrence of hypertrophic scars in donor sites treated with allografts.

CONTRACTION

Burn wounds usually become thick and brittle; and contraction, as defined above and in Chapter 1, plays a relatively minor role in the healing of major burns. However, as the wrinkles in healed skin grafts often demonstrate, contraction, or contracture, may persist even after skin graft coverage.

SUMMARY

Burn injuries heal rather differently than mechanical injuries. The differences tend to express themselves in prolonged healing, susceptibility to infection, and excessive scarring. It seems likely that we fail to appreciate many aspects of burn injury and repair. It is fair to say that there are few places in surgery where well directed research is as likely to make "revolutionary" changes in therapy as it is in repair of burn injuries.

BIBLIOGRAPHY

Baur P, Barr G, Linares HA, et al.: Wound contractions, scar contractures, and myofibroblasts: A classic case study. J. Trauma 18(1): 8–22, 1978
Burke J, Quinby WC, Bondoc CC, et al.: Immunosupression and temporary skin transplantation in the treatment of massive third degree burns. Ann Surg 182(3): 183, 1975
Burke JF, Quinby WC Jr, Bondoc CC: Primary excision and prompt grafting as routine therapy for the treatment of thermal burns in children. Surg Clin North Am 56:477, 1976
Hinshaw J, Payne F: The restoration and remodeling of the skin after a second degree burn. Surg Gynecol Obstet 117:738, 1963
Ketchum LD, Cohen IK, Masters FW: Hypertrophic scars and keloids: A collective review. Plast Reconstr Surg 53:140, 1974
Larson DL, Baur P, Linares HA, et al.: Mechanisms of Hypertrophic Scar and Contracture Formation in Burns. Burns 1:119, 1975
Miller TA: The deleterious effect of split-skin homograft coverage on split-skin donor sites. Plast Reconstr Surg 53:316, 1974
Miller TA, White WL: Healing of second degree burns. Plast Reconstr Surg 49:522, 1972

Order SE, Moncrief JA: The Burn Wound. Springfield, Ill, Thomas, 1965

Peacock EE Jr, Van Winkle W, Jr: Surgery and Biology of Wound Repair. Philadelphia, Saunders, 1976

Pruitt BA, Jr: Burns. In Manual of Surgical Nutrition by Committee on Pre- and Postoperative Care, American College of Surgeons, Philadelphia, Saunders, 1975, p 396

Surgical Clinics of North America, Synposium on Burns. vol. 58 #6, Dec., 1978. This is the most recent symposium on burns with many of the current experts represented.

Wheeler ES, Miller TA: The blister and the second degree burn in guinea pigs: The effect of exposure. Plast Reconstr Surg 57:74, 1976

Wilson JS, Moncrief JA: Vapor pressure of normal and burned skin. Ann Surg 162:30, 1965

Winter GD: Movement of epidermal cells over the wound surface. In Montagna W, Billingham RE (eds): Advances in Biology of Skin, vol V. Oxford, Pergamon Press, 1964, pp 113–27.

Zaroff LI, Mills W Jr, Duckett JW Jr, Switzer WE, Moncrief JA: Multiple uses of visible cutaneous homografts in the burned patient. Surgery 59:368, 1966

Zawacki BE: Reversal of capillary stasis and prevention of necrosis in burns. Ann Surg 180:98, 1974

Wound Healing in the Gastrointestinal Tract

Clifford W. Deveney
J. Englebert Dunphy

MECHANISMS OF WOUND HEALING

The response to injury in the gastrointestinal tract is similar to those that occur elsewhere in the body, but the details of healing to functional integrity are often unique.

569

Immediately following an injury to the bowel there is *hemorrhage* followed by *hemostasis,* which is accomplished by retraction and contraction of vessels, platelet clumping within the vessels, fibrin formation, and clotting of blood. Fibrin initially seals the wound and forms a lattice upon which cells may later migrate. The adequacy of hemostasis, the amount of tissue trauma, and the quantity of spillage or contamination occurring at this time all have a major effect on the healing of the anastomosis. Attention to hemostasis is most desirable because extravascular clot provides a culture medium for bacteria and creates unnecessary wound dead space. The degree of bacterial contamination at the time of anastomosis may affect the character of the healed anastomosis. Although the peritoneal cavity is capable of controlling or removing a large number of bacteria, gross contamination in combination with foreign bodies can overcome the resistance of the host. Bacterial growth can lead to a myriad of complications such as abscess, anastomotic leakage, bacteremia, and late anastomotic stricture secondary to excess collagen production.

Once fibroblasts have appeared and collagen synthesis has begun, the wound gains strength. The normal wound in the gastrointestinal tract is at its weakest until the third day after the anastomosis, after which time the wound rapidly gains strength and at the seventh to tenth day, it resists bursting as well as it did prior to injury. This rapid gain in strength corresponds to total collagen content (Fig. 7.36). (Within 7 to 14 days new circulation from budding capillary endothelium will bridge the anastomosis.)

The collagen that is laid down is in constant flux; collagen turnover is especially rapid in the GI tract. The new collagen tends to adapt itself to the stresses that are placed on the wound. This remodeling process produces an alignment of the new collagen and proteoglycans in a manner which produces greater strength per milligram of collagen and tends to allow the small anastomosis to dilate. As the anastomosis continues to heal, the total amount of collagen decreases but the tensile strength of the wound becomes greater.

Although one would hope that gastrointestinal anastomoses would heal by first intention, most actually heal by a process more like second intention. Some mucosa sloughs at the wound edge leaving an open wound; the amount of slough is inversely proportional to the excellence of the surgical tech-

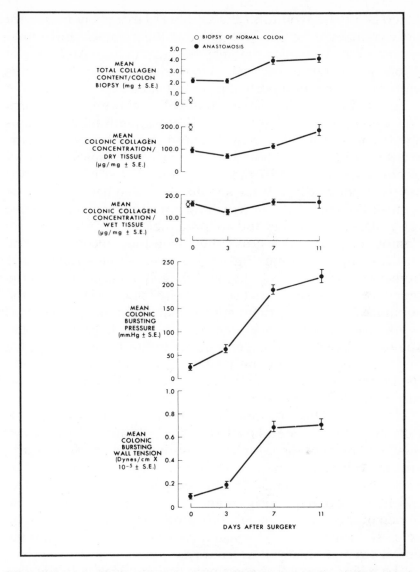

Figure 7.36 Anastomotic strength increases from Day 3 through Day 11. Note also the concomitant increase in total colonic collagen content and in the mean collagen concentration in dry colon tissue. *(From Irvin TT, Hunt TK: Surg Gynecol Obstet 138:741–746, 1974 by permission of Surgery, Gvneocology, and Obstetrics.)*

nique. Reepithelization of these open areas is similar to the process seen in the skin. The mucus-secreting columnar epithelial cell reverts to a more primitive cuboidal cell at the edge of the anastomosis and then divides rapidly, migrating over the granulation tissue to reepithelize the anastomosis. Mucosal coverage of any wound in the GI tract is extremely important since completion of this layer inhibits the excessive inflammation and fiber formation that may lead to stricture. Additionally it forms a barrier to bacteria. When coverage is complete this mucosa matures into normal gastrointestinal epithelium.

To construct an anastomosis that will heal primarily requires delicate apposition of mucosa and serosa, with minimal damage to the edges of the bowel. These should be cleanly transected, and bleeding should be controlled by judicious use of electrocoagulation and ligation of vessels. If crushing clamps are used, the crushed tissue should be excised before the anastomosis is completed. Noncrushing bowel clamps are available (i.e., Glassman clamps) and are preferable to Allen and Kocher clamps, both of which crush the tissue they encompass. The sutures approximating the anastomosis should not be too numerous or tied too tightly, and they should not include too much tissue. The authors use small bites of tissue securing the submucosa and place them approximately 4 mm apart.

The use of diathermy to transect bowel devitalizes more tissue than a scalpel and experimental studies have shown a lag period of two days in the healing of bowel transected with diathermy compared to cold knife. For this reason a scalpel is recommended to transect bowel.

The GI tract has several characteristics that might theoretically lead to poor wound healing: 1) Bacteria are always numerous in all parts of the GI tract except the stomach, duodenum, and the biliary system; and in certain instances may even be present in these areas. 2) The stomach secretes both hydrochloric acid and pepsin, both of which injure tissue. 3) The lumen of the duodenum contains proteolytic enzymes. In spite of these factors most GI anastomoses heal and regain normal bowel strength in seven to ten days.

The major factors that contribute to good healing in the gastrointestinal tract are the same as for tissues elsewhere in the body:

A good blood supply
Absence of tension
The absence of gross contamination
The absence of foreign material (i.e., sutures, feces) in the area
    (Figs. 7.37–7.39).

572

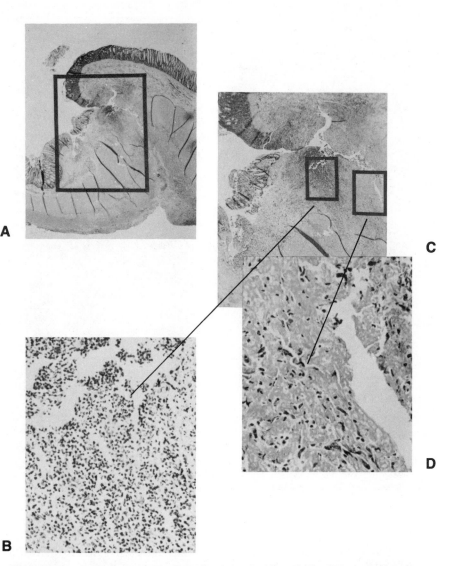

Figure 7.37 A bowel anastomosis at two days. **A.** Although the tissue edges are opposed, there is no tissue connecting the edges. At this point the anastomosis is dependent on suture for strength. **B.** A small mucosal slough is apparent at the anastomosis. **C.** Inflammatory cells mainly polymorphonuclear cells and lymphocytes are present. **D.** An area of necrotic tissue next to an area of fibroplasia.

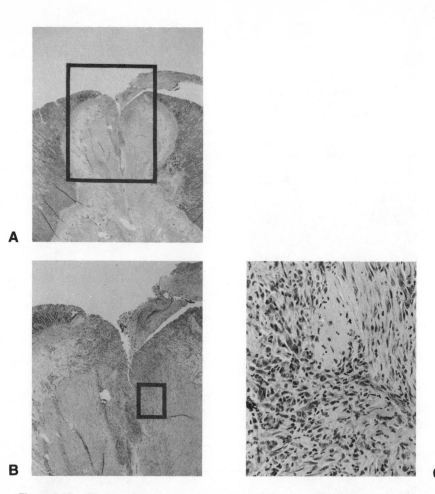

Figure 7.38 A bowel anastomosis at seven days. **A.** The wound edges are now bridged by tissue. **B.** The mucosa is still absent over a small area of the anastomosis. **C.** The predominant cells now are fiberblasts and granulocytes.

A watertight anastomosis may be provided by a continuous layer of fine rapidly absorbable suture material to the mucosa with an interrupted inverting serosal layer of fine nonabsorbable sutures. The excellent results reported for the use of selected types of single layer anastomosis indicate that when properly used, these also provide a nonleaking anastomosis. Figures 7.37–7.39 show a typical sequence of intestinal repair from two to fourteen days after anastomosis.

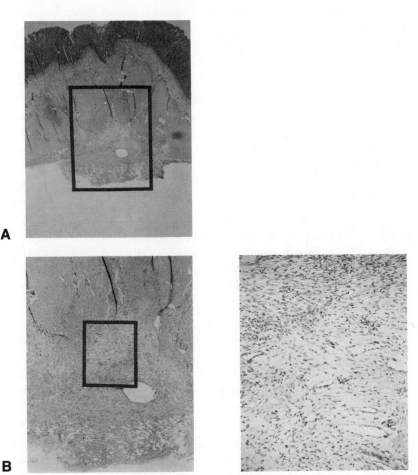

Figure 7.39 A bowel anastomosis at fourteen days. **A.** The mucosa has now covered the anastomosis. The anastomosis has been bridged by fibrous tissue, and it is difficult to determine where bowel was transected. **B.** An area of granulation tissue with budding capillaries on either side of the anastomosis. **C.** Granulation tissue consisting of thin walled capillaries and fibrocytes. Vessels have bridged the anastomosis.

ANASTOMOTIC TECHNIQUES

Description

Segments of the gastrointestinal tract can be joined together in different ways (i.e., end-to-end, end-to-side, or side-to-side), and the anastomosis can be performed over clamps in a "closed" technique or with the lumen of both ends of bowel open. The anastomosis can be performed with an inner layer of sutures passing through the full thickness of the bowel wall and an outer layer penetrating to the submucosa only; or it can be performed with a single layer of sutures either going through the entire bowel wall or going down to submucosa. The anastomosis may be *inverted* so that the opposing edges of serosa are approximated, or the anastomosis may be *everted* with the mucosae being approximated.

The majority of surgeons agree that inversion of the anastomosis with approximation of serosa is preferable to the eversion technique. A more normal sequence of wound healing occurs in the inverted anastomosis with revascularization between the segments occurring at a much earlier date than with eversion. Clinical trials comparing eversion to inversion have shown a significantly greater incidence of anastomotic leakage and peritoneal adhesions occuring with eversion. It appears that when everting anastomoses are accomplished with staplers, the incidence of complications is less than when they are performed with everting sutures.

The single layer inverting anastomosis is performed with one layer of interrupted sutures that either encompass all layers except mucosa, or that are placed by the method of Gambee (Fig. 7.40). This anastomosis heals in a fashion similar to the two layer inverting anastomosis. However, the absence of a continuous inner suture causes the single layer anastomosis to leak bacteria for about one hour after construction. The rates of clinical complications following single or double layer anastomoses are about the same in most reports.

The use of staplers to perform GI anastomoses is becoming increasingly popular. The stapler has several appealing aspects. It performs a more uniform anastomosis because the staples are equally spaced and each exerts the same pressure on the tissues. In addition, the staples are constructed so that they do not occlude all the blood supply of the tissue through which they pass. Finally, an anastomosis can often be performed more rapidly with the stapler. Although these are all desirable characteristics, a potential drawback is that the anterior row of the anastomosis must often be performed in an everting manner, thus predisposing to adhesions. Nevertheless, few complications of stapled anastomoses have been reported to date.

Some anastomoses are more easily performed end-to-side.

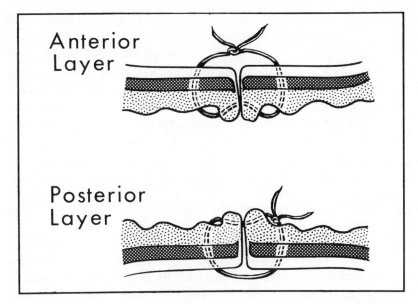

Figure 7.40 The single layer inverting suture of Gambee.

Esophagojejunostomy after total gastrectomy is often performed most easily and accurately with the end of the esophagus anastomosed to the side of the jejunum. Similarly, in a low anterior resection the side of the left colon may be anastomosed to the end of the rectal stump. The primary indication for end-to-side anastomosis is a difference in luminal diameter between the two portions of bowel to be joined.

Complications

The three principle complications associated with gastrointestinal anastomoses are *obstruction, bleeding,* and *leakage.* The occurrence of these complications can be minimized by proper surgical technique and judgment.

Obstruction can occur early if too much tissue is inverted. This problem can be avoided by proper surgical technique. Obstruction also occurs late in the form of an anastomotic stricture. The cause of late obstruction is excess fibrous tissue that accumulates secondary to paraanastomotic infection, excessive devitalized tissue, or hematoma in the anastomosis. Aseptic technique, a water-tight anastomosis, meticulous hemostasis, and minimal tissue trauma are essential factors in the prevention of late anastomotic stricture as well as facilitating the immediate healing of an anastomosis.

Bleeding can be minimized by careful hemostasis before construction of the anastomosis and/or by use of a continuous hemostatic inner suture. The need for a continuous hemostatic suture is greatest in the stomach and duodenum, and is minimal in colon and esophageal anastomoses.

METHODS EMPLOYED TO PROTECT ANASTOMOSES OR TO MINIMIZE THE CONSEQUENCES OF LEAKAGE

Leakage rarely occurs in anastomoses of the stomach and small bowel, but is more frequent in colonic and esophagus. Most authors report leakage rates in these latter two structures of 5 to 25 percent. When constructing an anastomosis, it is well to keep in mind that the major requirements for healing are (1) excellent blood supply, (2) absence of tension, (3) water-tight apposition of the edges, and (4) gentle handling of the tissues (Figs. 7.41, 7.42). Impaired blood supply may result from too many sutures, sutures tied too tightly, pressure from an intramural hematoma or ligation of critical mesenteric vessels. The strongest layer in bowel is the submucosa, and it must be included in the principle layer of sutures.

Drains

Drains are used to provide a route of egress for serum, shed blood, or pus that might collect around an anastomosis, and to provide a route for external drainage if the anastomosis should leak. In deciding whether to use drains one must weigh the possible morbidity of the drains against benefit from their use. Drains are foreign bodies and they often serve as a nidus for infection. In addition, drains may provide a route for the ingress of bacteria and can lead to an infection along the drain tract. Drains placed against an anastomosis can cause erosion and leakage at the point of contact.

It is not necessary to drain most intestinal anastomoses within the peritoneal cavity since drains will become walled off within a few hours or days. Hence, it is not prudent to drain

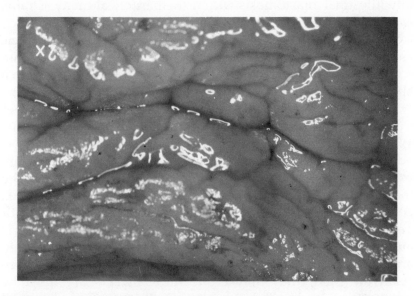

Figure 7.41 An anastomosis after seven days performed with minimal tissue trauma. Note minimal inflammation and good apposition of mucosa.

Figure 7.42 An anastomosis after seven days in which the mucosa was damaged. There is no apposition of mucosa and healing must occur by second intention.

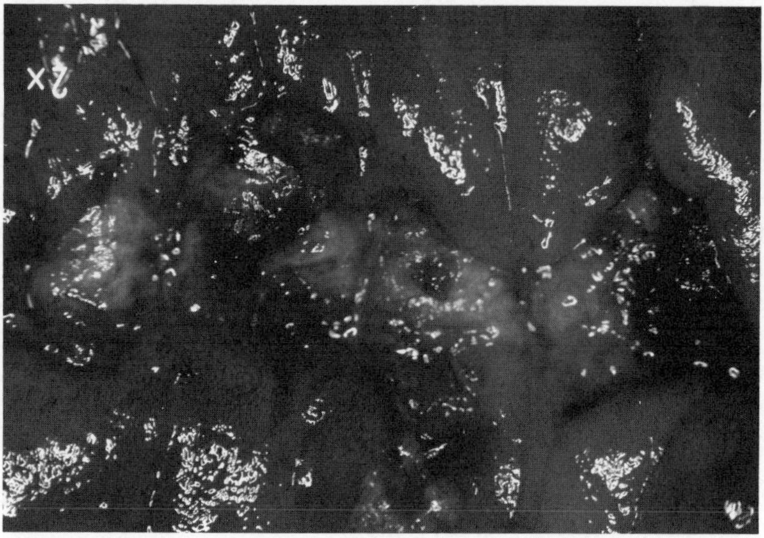

any intestinal anastomosis within the peritoneal cavity. Drains *may* be indicated in the following: operations of the biliary tract, extraperitoneal low colonic anastomoses, and intrathoracic esophageal anastomoses. Each of these anastomoses is associated with a high incidence of leakage, and is performed in a space that is amenable to drainage.

There are essentially two types of drains: the soft, rubber Penrose drains and the more rigid tube and sump drains. When simple drainage is indicated, the Penrose drain is adequate in most instances. Because both suction and irrigation may be accomplished through rigid tube drains, they may be indicated for (1) drainage of a cavity or abscess where copious continuing drainage is expected (i.e., a cavity connecting with an enteric fistula), and (2) irrigating a cavity to flush out debris and viscous material. Sump drains are preferable because they are not likely to become occluded. Because all tube drains are relatively rigid, they may erode into bowel. Care must be taken not to leave rigid drains in contact with the bowel, and all drains should be removed as soon as possible.

Diverting Enterostomy

Although a diverting enterostomy (colostomy in most cases) does not prevent anastomotic dehiscence or leak, it does lessen the morbidity and mortality of a leak since the anastomosis can be placed out of the fecal stream. However, if the surgeon is unduly concerned over the integrity of an anastomosis, he is often wiser to refashion his anastomosis or avoid anastomosis altogether rather than attempt to protect a tenuous anastomosis with a proximal colostomy.

The primary use of the diverting colostomy is for the decompression of obstructed colon (i.e., carcinoma of the colon) or for bypass of inflamed or infarcted colon. These colostomies are performed weeks before anastomosis and may often be left in place for a time after the anastomosis is done.

LOCAL FACTORS DETRIMENTAL
TO HEALING OF THE ANASTOMOSIS

Even though an anastomosis is done with the best surgical technique, there are sometimes local and/or systemic factors that may mitigate against adequate healing. Local factors that significantly hinder proper healing are:

Infection
Local and distant trauma
Fecal spillage
Extraperitoneal location
Blood in the peritoneal cavity
Abnormal bowel

Infection and trauma increase the collagenase activity within the colon, which leads to increased collagen destruction and hence weakening of a healing anastomosis. Infection can also cause thrombosis of small vessels adjacent to the wound with subsequent ischemic necrosis of bowel. In many instances a leak in the presence of infection does not occur at the anastomosis but instead occurs adjacent to the suture line secondary to ischemic necrosis.

Feces, in addition to containing large numbers of bacteria, also contain foreign material that enhances infection. In elective large bowel surgery, preparation of the bowel eliminates much of the risk of fecal contamination since stool bulk and the number of bacteria are markedly reduced.

Extraperitoneal anastomoses performed in the presacral space have a notably higher incidence of leakage than intraperitoneal anastomoses. The peritoneal cavity has an immense capacity to disperse bacterial contamination and remove most of the bacteria from the area of anastomosis. The presacral space is an ideal area for para-anastomotic infection to occur because it has no peritoneum and often contains a hematoma. In addition, the low rectal anastomosis is technically more difficult than most intraperitoneal anastomoses. Some surgeons place a drain near (but not *on*) extraperitoneal anastomoses, either transsacrally or through the abdominal cavity, since these anastomoses suffer a moderately high incidence of leakage.

Blood in the peritoneal cavity enhances bacterial growth and predisposes to infection and abscess formation. Any infection close to an anastomosis promotes collagenase activity, decreases anastomotic strength, and increases the potential for anastomotic leakage.

581

Abnormal bowel is also associated with an increased incidence of anastomotic leakage. *Edematous, obstructed, inflamed,* and *ischemic bowel heal poorly. Irradiated bowel* also heals poorly because of the progressive obliteration of its blood supply.

SYSTEMIC FACTORS DETRIMENTAL TO ANASTOMOTIC HEALING

In addition to local factors there are several systemic factors that lead to poor healing:

Malnutrition (to about 20 to 25 percent of body weight loss)
Impaired oxygen delivery
Drugs (E.g., some cancer chemotherapeutics, antiinflammatory corticosteroids
Advanced age, obesity, diabetes, cardiopulmonary disease, chronic renal failure, and advanced liver disease
Distant or local trauma
Any diseases that depress the immune system (e.g., leukemia)

Because of recent advances in oral and intravenous nutrition, any malnourished patient should undergo nutritional repletion, if possible, before a critical anastomosis is attempted. Drugs that impair the immune system, such as antiinflammatory corticosteroids, should be tapered off and discontinued prior to operation, if possible. Anastomoses in the traumatized patient heal poorly because of the shock associated with the trauma, the metabolic demands that the traumatic episode make on all parts of the body, and because trauma impairs the flow properties of blood.

GENERAL CONSIDERATIONS IN PERFORMING AN ANASTOMOSIS

When considering whether or not to perform an anastomosis, the surgeon must consider all of the adverse factors affecting anastomotic healing. Anastomoses in the stomach and small bowel are usually performed even in the presence of suboptimal systemic conditions because there is no satisfactory alternative to doing the anastomosis; and also because the anastomoses usually heal in spite of adverse factors. Consequently, a perforated gastric ulcer may be treated by a subtotal gastrectomy performed in the face of early peritonitis. However, anastomoses in the colon and in the esophagus do not heal nearly as reliably.

When adverse factors are present and the surgeon is faced with a decision of whether to do a colonic anastomosis, he may elect simply to do a colostomy, resect the involved segment of bowel and leave the anastomosis for a later date. These factors are often considered when operating on acute diverticulitis or obstructing carcinoma of the colon.

In a study of 1,700 large bowel anastomoses performed at the University of California, San Francisco, anastomotic leakage occurred in only 1.7 percent of patients who had no adverse factors present, whereas leakage occurred in 6.7 percent of those patients in whom one or more adverse factors were present. Other investigators have presented higher incidence of leakage, but the same relationships hold.

Elective primary resection and anastomosis is practiced by many surgeons for acute diverticulitis. The results are excellent provided there is no significant contamination of the peritoneal cavity prior to or during the operation. At the University of California, in a series of selected cases in which primary anastomosis was performed for acute diverticulitis, leakage occurred in 0.6 percent of the patients. It must be noted, however, that a leakage rate of 6.7 percent occurred when there were adverse factors such as free pus in the peritoneal cavity.

CHOICE OF SUTURE MATERIAL

There are at present many types of sutures available. They may be divided into absorbable and nonabsorbable materials. The absorbable sutures are plain and chromic catgut, polyglycolic acid, and polyglactin 910. The nonabsorbable, or very slowly absorbed, sutures are silk, cotton, wire, and such synthetic sutures as nylon, polypropylene, and braided polyester.

Almost all surgeons performing single layer anastomoses use a nonabsorbable suture, whereas those performing a two layer anastomosis use an inner layer of absorbable and an outer layer of nonabsorbable suture.

Of the absorbable sutures, polyglycolic acid and polyglactin 910 may offer some advantages over catgut. They have longer life in the GI tract than catgut (Table 7.1), and they produce less

Table 7.1 Time of Dissolution of Intraluminal Sutures in Various Parts of the Gut, in Median Number of Days to Dissolution

Suture	Stomach	Duodenum	Jejunum	Colon
Plain catgut	1	1	3	4
Chromic catgut	2	1	3	7
Polyglycolic acid	28	22	21	21
Polyglactin	28	22	22	21

(From Deveney, K. University of California Medical Center, Department of Surgery, San Francisco, California.)

inflammation than catgut. However, to date, clinical studies have failed to demonstrate a conclusive advantage of these sutures over catgut as the inner suture layer.

Cotton and silk are the most commonly used nonabsorbable sutures. Ease of handling probably accounts for this choice. Stainless steel wire, nylon, and polypropylene all produce less tissue inflammation, but are more difficult to tie.

SPECIAL PROBLEMS

Esophagus

The major problem with a primary wound of the esophagus is a high rate of anastomotic leakage. This can be explained by several factors: (1) poor tissue strength, (2) lack of a serosal (collagenous) outer layer, (3) a marginal segmental blood supply, (4) constant motion of adjacent organs, and (5) the absence of omentum or serosa that could wrap around the anastomosis and seal it.

When a segment of esophagus is electively resected the ends are rarely reanastomosed since the tenuous segmental blood supply prohibits extensive mobilization. The segment of esophagus may be replaced with a segment of colon, stomach, or small bowel that is transposed to the chest on its vascular pedicle. To preserve the tenuous blood supply, only interrupted sutures should be used; and, if possible, a segment of omentum should be rotated up to cover the anastomosis. Esophageal resection is best performed through the right chest, and following surgery ample drainage of the chest and mediastinum is always indicated.

Esophageal perforation may occur secondary to a foreign

584

body or instrumentation, or "spontaneously" following vomiting. When esophageal perforation is recognized, prompt repair of the perforation by reapproximation of the esophagus should be performed when feasible. Although such closures frequently disrupt, early closure with drainage will substantially reduce the morbidity from mediastinal abscess, empyema, and late esophageal stricture.

Stomach and Small Bowel

The excellent healing properties of stomach and small bowel are attributed to an abundant blood supply, ample tissue strength in the submucosal layer, minimal intraluminal bacterial counts, and rapid mucosal turnover and regeneration.

In general, traumatic injuries to the stomach and small bowel are treated by minimal resection of the injured tissue and reanastomosis of normal tissue. Any laceration or perforation of the stomach should be closed in two layers including a hemostatic inner layer. If a large segment of small bowel is injured, it may usually be resected and a primary anastomosis performed.

Biliary Tract

The most common circumstance in which the biliary tract requires surgical repair is stricture or injury of the extrahepatic bile ducts. The stricture may be secondary to gallstones but occurs most often following surgical operations.

In general, one can say that healing of the extrahepatic biliary tree will occur, unless there is inflammation or distal obstruction. Because the bile duct is relatively small, magnification is often helpful in biliary reconstruction. The surgical procedure for treating bile duct injuries will differ if the problem is acute or chronic.

If the bile duct is accidentally completely transected and the injury is immediately recognized, the proximal duct should be anastomosed to the distal duct in an end-to-end fashion, providing the anastomosis can be made without tension. Most surgeons employ a T-tube to drain the common bile duct with one limb of the T-tube used to stent the anastomosis. The T-tube should remain in place for two weeks or longer. In repair of a common duct which is not scarred, it is debatable whether a T-tube stent is necessary to maintain patency, and some would argue that it is detrimental to healing because it acts as a foreign body and also creates pressure on the mucosa. However, the T-tube does serve to decompress the common bile duct, and it allows radiographic visualization of the bile ducts postoperatively. It provides drainage for a bile leak and it allows sampling of bile for culture.

If the common bile duct is only partially transected, or if a portion of the anterior wall of the duct is accidentally removed during cholecystectomy, these injuries can be treated by anastomosing the duct to itself. If an anterior defect is large enough to obviate anastomosis but the posterior wall is intact, it can be successfully treated by using a vein patch graft. Alternatively, a piece of gallbladder or cystic duct can be used as a graft. The patch graft functions temporarily as a seal while the bile duct regenerates to fill the defect. The common duct should be drained according to individual surgeon preference. Prolonged stenting is not necessary.

The repair of an injury to the common duct recognized during operation may be by end-to-end anastomosis provided there is no tension. Under these ideal circumstances, the results are very satisfactory. Whenever there are any unfavorable factors such as scarring or inflammation, reconstruction by means of a Roux-en-Y loop is preferred.

The principles underlying the repair of chronic stricture are (1) resection of scarred bile duct back to normal pliable bile duct, (2) performing the anastomosis without tension on the suture line, and (3) approximating the mucosa of bile duct to the mucosa of the bowel. In the relatively normal duct a stent need not be employed but proximal drainage of the anastomosis should be provided, if necessary, by a Smith catheter passed through the liver. However, if the bile duct is scarred and the mucosal lining is compromised, the stent should remain in for as long as it functions well. The anastomosis should be performed in one or two layers, depending on the size of the duct, using a 5-0 or smaller suture. Under favorable circumstances, the success rate is about 85 percent. However, even under the best of circumstances late stricture formation may occur. We have encountered stenosis as long as 10 to 20 years after what appeared to be very satisfactory function. The most reliable indicator of an anastomotic stricture is the appearance of frequently recurring episodes of cholangitis.

In addition to external drainage of the bile duct, drainage of the subhepatic space should be performed because bile leaks are common after operation.

Colon

Factors responsible for leakage in colon anastomoses are (1) poor blood supply, (2) increased collagenase activity, (3) high intraluminal bacterial counts, (4) particulate intraluminal foreign material (i.e., feces), and (5) extraperitoneal location.

The surgeon can drastically reduce the bacterial count and eliminate the bulk of stool with use of proper bowel preparation. The bowel preparation should consist of a clear liquid diet and a combination of oral cathartics and cleansing enemas. Oral antibiotics acting intraluminally have lowered the morbidity associated with colonic resection and anastomoses. The desirable characteristics of antibiotics used to prepare the colon are: broad spectrum activity against aerobic and anaerobic colonic organisms and minimal or no absorption from the GI tract. These antibiotics do substantially alter the gastrointestinal flora and have been associated with staphylococcal enterocolitis. When oral antibiotics are used, they should not be given for more than two days since maximal reduction of colonic bacterial counts occurs at 24 to 48 hours and subsequently resistant strains emerge. Our practice is to give oral antibiotics only on the afternoon and evening before surgery.

One of many satisfactory regimens for colonic preparation has been outlined by Nichols. A clear liquid or elemental diet is given for three days before operation. Cathartics are begun in the evening three days before operation. Oral antibiotics are begun the day before operation and consist of neomycin, 1 g., and erythromycin base, 1 g., by mouth at 1:00, 2:00, and 11:00 P.M. Enemas are discontinued two days before operation. In the experience of one of the authors (J.E.D.), catharsis and enemas may be kept to a minimum provided a low residue diet is started five to six days before operation.

Colonic anastomosis is contraindicated in the presence of peritonitis or paracolic abscess, as may occur in acute diverticulitis. Also when colonic obstruction is present anastomosis should be avoided. The obstructed colon is edematous and dilated with decreased tensile strength, and its vascular supply has been compromised by the pressure of dilation. The obstructed colon should be treated initially by a colostomy proximal to the obstruction, or cecostomy. Resection of the obstructing lesion can be performed with safety after the colon is decompressed and the bulk of feces has been removed. Avoidance of primary colonic anastomosis in the presence of inflammation and obstruction has greatly reduced the incidence of anastomotic leakage.

Acute rectal perforation presents special problems for the surgeon. The rectum is mostly an immobile retroperitoneal structure and thus the perforation cannot be mobilized and brought out as a colostomy. Treatment consists of (1) proximal diverting colostomy, (2) removal of intraperitoneal foreign bodies, (3) drainage of the presacral space, (4) closure of the perforation, and (5) evacuation of stool from the rectum at the time of operation. This last measure is extremely important.

Peritoneal Adhesions

Peritoneal adhesions may occur after any intraabdominal operation. Nevertheless, it should be the goal of the surgeon to minimize these adhesions since they can cause bowel obstruction.

While diffuse fibrinous adhesions occur after all abdominal surgery, most of them are absorbed within two weeks. Adhesions become organized with fibroblasts and capillaries to produce fibrous changes only in certain instances. These organized adhesions occur primarily around (1) ischemic tissue and (2) foreign material. Small amounts of ischemic tissue are created wherever surgical dissection is performed. The more meticulous the technique the less the ischemic tissue. Closure of peritoneal defects by suturing the edges together often stretches the peritoneum, compromises its blood supply, and consequently leads to the formation of adhesions in that area. Indeed, if nothing is done to repair a peritoneal defect, reperitonealization with minimal adhesions will occur rapidly whatever the size of the defect. The implication is that peritoneal defects should not be repaired since reperitonealization occurs rapidly and with fewer adhesions. Foreign material such as blood, bacteria, sutures, ties, fragments of material from sponges and laparotomy tapes, and powder from gloves all can initiate adhesion formation.

Since adhesions are almost certain to form in response to local ischemia and foreign material in the abdominal incision and in the anastomotic line, the surgeon should insure that adhesions form to innocuous moveable structures such as omentum or falciform ligament rather than to bowel. The placement of omentum around the anastomosis or the placement of omentum between the incision and bowel will lessen the adhesions of bowel to the wound or to the anastomosis. These simple techniques may not lead to diminished adhesions but tend to reduce their morbidity.

The initial step in the formation of adhesions is the deposition of fibrin. This occurs diffusely within the peritoneal cavity following surgery. Where ischemia and foreign body are present, macrophages collect, new vessels and fibroblasts "organize" the fibrous adhesion, and vascularized collagenous adhesions form.

Efforts to reduce adhesion formation have been aimed at (1) prevention of fibrin deposition, (2) enzymatic digestion of fibrin (fibrinolysis), and (3) inhibition of fibroblast proliferation. Most, if not all, of these attempts have met with failure. Intraperitoneal administration of agents such as anticoagulants and antiinflammatory drugs has been used in an effort to reduce intraperitoneal fibrin deposition. The use of anticoagulants was associated with a significant morbidity and has been abandoned. Mechanical removal of fibrin, by irrigation or by the use of digestive enzymes such as pepsin or trypsin, has been shown to be ineffective, probably because the irrigation substance is rapidly absorbed and the enzymes are quickly inactivated. The fibrinolytic enzyme streptokinase has been used experimentally with inconclusive results. Antiinflammatory corticosteroids are known to inhibit fibroplasia. In high enough doses they will inhibit adhesion formation, but their deleterious effect on wound healing and resistance to infection in the rest of the organism prevents their use.

Thus, the prevention of adhesions remains the responsibility of the surgeon at operation. Measures that will help limit adhesion formation are (1) minimal tissue trauma, (2) mechanical removal of foreign bodies, (3) the placement of the omentum near areas where adhesions are likely to form, (4) avoidance of peritoneal closure under tension, and (5) removal of all ischemic tissue or preservation of normal blood supply.

BIBLIOGRAPHY

General

Agrama HM, Blackwood JM, Brown CS, Machiedo GW, Rush BF: Functional longevity of intraperitoneal drains on experimental evolution. Am J Surg 132:418, 1976

Daly JM, Steiger E, Vors HM, Dudrick SJ: Postoperative oral and intravenous nutrition. Ann Surg 180:709, 1974

Dunphy JE: The cut gut. Am J Surg 119:1, 1970. Note: An Historical Review.

Kott I, Lurie M: The effects of electrosurgery and the surgical knife on the healing of intestinal anastomoses. Dis Colon Rectum 16:33, 1973

Rosin RD, Exarchakos G, Ellis H, et al.: An experimental study of gastric healing following scalpel and diathermy incisions. Surgery 79:555, 1976

Shilling JA: Wound healing. Symposium on response to infection and injury I. Surg Clin North Am 56: 859, 1976. Note: A good review of the physiology of wound healing.

Temple WJ, Voitk AJ, Snelling CFT, Crispin JS: Effect of nutrition, diet and suture material on long term wound healing. Ann Surg 182:93, 1975

Tera H, Aberg C: Tissue holding power to a single suture in different parts of the alimentary tract. Acta Chir Scand 142:343, 1976

Esophagus

Akiyama H, Hiyama M, Hashimoto C: Resection and reconstruction for carcinoma of the esophagus. Br J Surg 63:206, 1976

Hardy JD, et al.: Esophageal perforations and fistulas. Ann Surg 177:788, 1973

Hix WR, Mills M: The management of esophageal wounds. Ann Surg 172:1002, 1970

Rosoff L, White EJ: Perforation of the esophagus. Am J Surg 128:107, 1974. Note: A retrospective study of 68 patients with esophageal perforation. This paper deals with the etiology as well as treatment of this condition.

Thal AP, Hatafuku T: Improved operation for esophageal rupture. JAMA 188:826, 1964

Small Bowel

Abromowitz HB, McAlister WH: A comparative study of small bowel anastomoses by angiography and microangiography. Surgery 66:564, 1969

Seidel BJ, Maddison FE, Evans WE: Pedicle grafts of ileum for the repair of large duodenal defects. Am J Surg 121:206, 1971

590

Wise L, McAlister W, Stein T, Schuck P: Studies on the healing of anastomoses of small and large intestines. Surg Gynecol Obstet 141:190, 1975. Note: A valuable experimental study with clinical applications.

Biliary Tract

Belzer FO, Watts J McK, Ross HB, Dunphy JE: Auto-reconstruction of the common bile duct after venous patch graft. Ann Surg 162:346, 1965

Dunphy JE: Some observations, practical and impractical, on the function of the common bile duct. J R Coll Surg Edinb 11:115, 1966

Dunphy JE, Stephens FO: Experimental study of the effect of grafts in the common duct on biliary and hepatic function. Ann Surg 155:906, 1962

Michie W, Gunn A: Bile-duct injuries. A new suggestion for their repair. Br J Surg 51:96, 1964

Rand RW, Cannon JA, Rodriguez RS: Microsurgery of the common bile duct. An experimental and clinical study. Am J Surg 120:215, 1970

Warren KW, Jefferson MF: Prevention and repair of strictures of the extrahepatic bile ducts. Surg Clin North Am 53:1169, 1973

Way LW, Dunphy, JE: Biliary stricture. Am J Surg 124:287, 1972. Note: A comprehensive retrospective study of the treatment of biliary stricture. The study spans three decades and examines the changes in treatment of this lesion.

Colon

Chilimindris C, Boyd DR, Carlson LE, et al.: A critical review of management of right colon injuries. J Trauma 2:651, 1971

Cronin K, Jackson DS, Dunphy JE: Changing bursting strength and collagen content of the healing colon. Surg Gynecol Obstet 126:747, 1968

Cronin K, Jackson DS, Dunphy JE: Specific activity of hydroxyprolinetritium in the healing colon. Surg Gynecol Obstet 126:1061, 1968

Golligher JC, Smiddy FG: The treatment of acute perforation and obstruction in carcinoma of the colon and rectum. Br J Surg 45:270, 1957

Hawley PR, Hunt TK, Dunphy JE: Etiology of colonic anastomotic leaks. Proc R Soc Med 63:28, 1970

Haygood FD, Polk HC: Gunshot wounds of the colon. A review of 100 consecutive patients, with emphasis on complications and their causes. Am J Surg 131:213, 1976

Herrmann JB, Woodward SC, Pulaski EJ: Healing of colonic anastomoses in the rat. Surg Gynecol Obstet 119:269, 1964

Hunt TK, Hawley PR: Surgical judgment and colonic anastomoses. Dis Colon Rectum 12:167, 1969. Note: A practical appraisal based on clinical and experimental study

Irvin TT: Collagen metabolism in infected colonic anastomoses. Surg Gynecol Obstet 143:220, 1976

Irvin TT, Bostock T: The effects of mechanical preparation and acidification of the colon on the healing of colonic anastomoses. Surg Gynecol Obstet 143:443, 1976

Irvin TT, Hunt TK: Reappraisal of the healing process of anastomosis of the colon. Surg Gynecol Obstet 138:741, 1974

Lung JA, Turk RP, Miller RE, Eiseman B: Wounds of the rectum, Ann Surg 172:985, 1970

Morgenstern L, Yamakawa T, Ben-Shoshan M, Lippman H: Anastomotic leakage after low colonic anastomosis. Am J Surg 123:104, 1972

Schrock TR, Deveney CW, Dunphy JE: Factors Contributing to Leakage of Colonic Anastomoses. Ann Surg 177:513, 1973. Note: A large retrospective study analyzing the factors which increase the morbidity of colonic anastomoses.

Schrock TR, Christensen N: Management of Perforating Injuries of the Colon. Surg Gynecol Obstet 185:65, 1972

Welch JP, Donaldson GA: Perforated carcinoma of colon and rectum. Ann Surg 180:734, 1974. Note: The treatment of colonic perforation is delineated from a retrospective analysis.

Peritoneal Adhesions

Belzer FO: The role of venous obstruction in the formation of intra-abdominal adhesions: An experimental study. Br J Surg 54:189, 1967

Buchman RF, et al.: A unifying pathogenetic mechanism in the etiology of intraperitoneal adhesions. J Surg Res 20:1, 1976

Ellis H: The cause and prevention of postoperative intraperitoneal adhesions. Surg Gynecol Obstet 133:497, 1971. Note: An excellent, well-referenced review article.

Anastomotic Techniques

Akiyama H: Esophageal anastomosis. Arch Surg 107:512, 1973

Goligher JC, Morris C, McAdam WAF, DeDombal FT, Johnston D: A controlled trial of inverting versus everting suture in clinical large bowel surgery. Br J Surg 57:817–22, 1970

Ravitch MM: Observations on the healing of wounds of the intestines. Surgery 77:665, 1975

Limpi HD, Khubchandovic IT, Sheets JA, Stasik JJ; Advances in intestinal anastomoses. Dis Colon Rectum 20:107, 1977

Trueblood HW, Nelsen TS, Kohatsu S, Oberhelmon HA Jr: Wound healing in the colon: comparison of inverted and everted closure. Surgery 65:919, 1969

Goligher JC: Visceral and parietal suture in abdominal surgery. Am J Surg 131:130, 1976

Radiation Injury to Bowel

DeCosse JJ, Rhodes RS, Wentz WB, et al.: The natural history and management of radiation induced injury of the gastrointestinal tract. Ann Surg 170:369, 1969

Deveney CW, Lewis FR, Schrock TR: Surgical management of radiation injury of the small and large intestine. Dis Colon Rectum 19:25, 1976

Suture Material

Deveney KE, Way LW: Effect of different absorbable sutures on healing of gastrointestinal anastomoses. Am J Surg 133:86, 1977. Note: An excellent experimental study that examines the anastomotic strength and tissue reaction with different absorbable sutures.

Howes EL: Strength studies of polyglycolic acid versus catgut sutures of the same size. Surg Gynecol Obstet 137:15, 1973

Miln DC, O'Connor J, Dalling R: The use of polyglycolic acid suture in gastrointestinal anastomosis. Scott Med J 17:108, 1972

Hastings JC, Van Winkle H Jr, Barker E, Hines D, Nichols W: Effect of suture materials on healing wounds of the stomach and colon. Surg Gynecol Obstet 140:701, 1975

Colon Preparation and Prophylactic Antibiotics

Clarke JE, Condon RE, Bartlett JG, et al.: Preoperative antibiotics reduce septic complications of colonic operations. Ann Surg 186:251, 1977. Note: A prospective study comparing the use of neomycin-erythromycin base colon preparation with placebo; but the incidence of infection in controls was unusually high

Condon RE, Nichols RL: The present position of the neomycin-erythromycin bowel prep. Surg Clin North Am 55:1331, 1975. Note: A good description of a popular bowel preparation.

Farmer RG: Preoperative preparation of the patient with carcinoma of the colon. Surg Clin North Am 55:1335, 1975

Judd ES: Preoperative neomycin-tetracycline preparation of the colon for elective operations. Surg Clin North Am 55:1325, 1975

Karl RC, Mertz JJ, Veith FJ, Dineen P: Prophylactic antimicrobial drugs in surgery. New Engl J Med 275:305, 1966

LeVeen HH, Wapnick S, Falk G, et al.: Effects of prophylactic antibiotics on colonic healing. Am J Surg 131:47, 1976

Washington JA, Dearing WH, Judd E, Elveback L: Effect of preoperative antibiotic regimen on development of infection after intestinal surgery: prospective, randomized, double-blind study. Ann Surg 180:567, 1974

Index

Burns (cont.)
  blisters and, 559
  collagen and, 555, 557
  contraction and, 567
  contractures and, 160–61, 557
  debridement of, 561–62
  dehydration and, 559–61
  donor site healing, 562–63
  dressing for, 561, 563
  epithelization of, 44, 45, 558–59
  excision and prompt closure of, 216–17
  granulation tissue and, 296, 556
  host defense defects and, 259, 268–69
  hypertrophic scars and, 563–67
  incision healing and, 303
  infection and, 216–17, 251, 268–69,
    561–63
  inflammation and, 555
  keloid scars and, 112
  neovascularization and, 554
  nitrogen balance and, 290–91
  nutritional problems and, 295–97
  protein metabolism and, 307
  regeneration of vasculature and
    connective tissue, 556–58
  scars from, 112, 557–58, 563–67
  separation of dead tissue and, 554–56
  skin grafts and, 297, 557, 559, 562–63
  sloughing of, 296, 297
  temperature and, environmental,
    352–54
  thermal injury in, 552–54
  transition zone of, 553
  vitamin C and, 318–19
  wound management, 561–62
Burst abdomen, 135. See also Dehiscence.

Calcification, arterial healing and, 480
Calcium, vitamin D and, 326, 545
Callus
  hard, 536–38
  soft, 534–36
Caloric expenditure, 346–47
Cambrium, 525
Camper, chiasma of, 508
Cancer
  chemotherapy for, 275
  immune response effects of, 273–74
  nutritional problems and, 298
  as wound complication, 141–42
Carbohydrates, 309–10
  dietary, 347–48
Carcinoid syndrome, 121–23
Cardiac valvular disease, prophylaxis for,
    231
Carotene, 323

Cartilage, 547–50
  articular, 547, 548
  bone formation and, 527
  elastic, 547
  fibrocartilage, 547–48
  hyaline, 547, 548–50
    proteoglycans and, 40
  repair, 547–50
Case reports of repair disorders, 152–62
Catabolic reaction to injury, 299, 306–8
Catecholamines, 311–12
Catgut sutures, 583, 584
Cavity, temporary, 376–77
Cecostomy, 588
Cell-mediated immunity, 256–58
Cellular interactions in wound, 53–61
Cellular response to infection, 254
Cellulitis, 219, 220
Cephaloridine, 201
  prophylactic, 232, 234
Cephalosporins, time sequences and
    concentrations of, 198, 201
Chemotaxis, 81
  neutrophil, 263–64, 266
  trauma and, 266–68
Chemotherapy, 274–75
  cancer, 275
  protein synthesis inhibition by, 103
Chest wounds, dehiscence of, 137
Chiasma of Camper, 508
Chloramphenicol, prophylactic, 232
Chlorhexidine, 404
Cholecalciferol, 544
Chondroitin sulphate, arterial healing
    and, 480, 481
Chromium, 336
Circulation, infection prevention and,
    184–86
Clamping of vessels, 382, 383
Classification, wound, 210–11, 236
Clay, 394
Cleansers, skin wound, 400–401
Cleansing
  of hands, 404–5
  mechanical, 408–13
  of skin of patient, 401–4
Clindamycin, 416
Clips, closure with, 427
Clostridial infections, 223–26
  interaction schema for, 249
  myositis (gas gangrene), 225–26, 249
  tetanus, 223–25
Closure, wound, 423–40
  clip and staple, 427
  dead space, 417–23
  debridement and, 408

597

600

Fibrin
    adhesions and, 143, 589
    endarterectomy and, 479
    prosthetic vascular grafts and, 487, 488,
        489
    tendon repair and, 502
Fibrinolysis, adhesions and, 589
Fibrinous coagulum, 413, 414
Fibroblasts, 7, 16−21
    arteriosclerosis and, 124−25
    arteriovenous anastomosis and, 483
    cellular interactions and, 54−58
    characteristics of, 17
    drugs inhibiting, 92
    macrophage stimulation of, 12
    micrographs of, 18−20
    module of repair and, 9
    proliferation of, 92−94
    prosthetic vascular grafts and, 488
    scurvy and, 315
    signals to, 7−8, 16, 54−55
    tendon repair and, 502−3
Fibrocartilage, 547−48
Fibrocontracture, 117
Fibrosis, 62
    carcinoid syndrome and, 121−23
    endocardial and endothelial, 124−25
    retroperitoneal, 122, 123
Fibrovascular tissue, tendon, 503
Fistula, intestinal, collagen balance and,
    120
Fixation, intramedullary, 539−40
Flexor tendons of hand, 507−9, 511, 521
5-Fluorouracil, protein synthesis
        inhibition by, 103
Folic acid, 320, 321
Foot, ischemic tissue in, 60
Foreign bodies
    contamination from, 393−95
    peritoneal adhesions and, 589
    phagocytes and, 89−91
    puncture wounds and, 217
Fractures, 530−33. See also Bone.
    calcium and phosphorus and, 326
    incision healing and, 303−4
    mobility and, 543−44
    nonunion of, 545−46
Fragmentation injury, 376−77

Gambee suture method, 576, 577
Gas gangrene, 225−26, 249
Gastrointestinal tract, 569−90
    anastomoses. See Anastomoses,
        gastrointestinal.
    epithelium, 46−48
    granulation tissue, 575

Gastrointestinal tract (cont.)
    healing, 569−90
        factors affecting, 572, 580−82
        mechanisms of, 570−74
    hemorrhage and hemostasis, 570, 572
    microflora of, 389−91
    mucosa, 47, 388−89, 571−72, 575, 579
    serosa, 572, 576
    sutures for, 436−37, 576, 583−84
Globulin, immune human, for tetanus,
        225, 239
Gloves, surgical, 404
Glucocorticoids, 311
Glucose, 309−10
    healing and, 108−9
    infection and, 339
    intake of, 350
Glutaraldehyde, activated, 179
Glycine, 21
Glycoprotein, collagen, 21−22
Glycosaminoglycans, 39−41
Gortex, 495
Grafts
    arteriovenous, 482−84
    bovine, 495
    mandril, 493, 495
    nerve, 470
    prosthetic arterial, 486−96
    skin. See Skin grafts.
    umbilical, 495
Gram-negative organisms, 223, 263
Gram-positive organisms, 263
Gram stain, 218
Granulation tissue
    burns and, 296, 556
    cellular interactions and, 57, 59
    delayed closure and, 216
    gastrointestinal, 575
    open wound repair and, 9n, 10, 29
Granules, cytoplasmic, 83
Granulocytes, 91
    ingestion by, 82
Granulomas, talc and, 143
Granulomatous disease, chronic, 85−86
Gravel, 393−94
Ground substance, glycosaminoglycans
        and, 39
Growth hormone, 312

Hair removal, preoperative, 397−98
Hand
    bacteria on, 387, 404−5
    flexor tendons of, 507−9, 511, 521
    zones of, 501
Handwashing, 404−5
Haversian system, 527

Healing of wounds. *See* Repair of wounds.

Heart
 scar tissue, 71, 72
 valvular disease, prophylaxis for, 231

Heat exposure indicators, 178

Hematoma, 133–34
 fracture, 533, 538

Hemorrhage, 133–34
 gastrointestinal, 570
  anastomosis and, 578
 host defense effects of, 270
 vitamin K and, 327–28

Hemostasis
 coagulation and, 75
 electrosurgical, 381–83
 gastrointestinal, 570, 572

Hernia
 Ehlers–Danlos syndrome and, 127, 161–62
 incisional, 139–41, 158
 recurrent, 130–31, 159
 ventral, 159–60

Hexachlorophene, 400, 404

Histidine, urinary excretion of, 307

Homeostasis, 244–45

Homocystinuria, 128–29
 endothelial injury and, 125

Homotropism, 465

Hormones, 311–12
 steroid. *See* Steroids.

Host resistance, 247–83. *See also* Defense mechanisms, host.
 understanding of, 189–200

Humoral response to infection, 253–54

Hyaline cartilage, 40, 547, 548–50

Hyaluronic acid, 40
 arterial healing and, 480, 481

Hydraulic force, 409

Hydrogen peroxide, 84

Hydroxyapatite, 528

Hydroxylation
 collagen, 23, 26, 96–98, 103–4
 proline and lysine, 21, 22, 23, 103–4
  vitamin C and, 315, 317

Hyperglycemia, healing and, 108–10

Hypertrophic scar, 114–16
 burns and, 563–67

Hypesthesia, 133

Hypoalbuminemia, 307

Hypoprothrombinemia, 328

Hypotension, infection and, 185

Hypovolemia, repair of wound and, 98–102

Hypoxia, repair of wounds and, 8, 61
 bone healing and, 529, 541

Hypoxia, repair of wounds and (cont.)
 collagen synthesis and, 8, 96–99
 host defense effects of, 270
 infection and, 86, 87–88

Ileum, microbes of, 390

Immobilization
 of injury site, 446
 nonhealing and, 146
 tendon repair and, 518–19

Immune globulin for tetanus, 225, 239

Immunity. *See also* Defense mechanisms, host.
 components of, 247
 congenital and acquired disease and, 187–88
 nonspecific (natural), 190
 phagocytes and, 80
 specific (acquired), 189

Immunization, tetanus, 224, 238–39

Immunodeficiency, 258–59

Immunodilating agents, 282–83

Immunoglobulins, 253–54

Immunosuppression
 infection and, 250, 274
 steroids for, 274–75

Impact injuries, 371–75
 antibiotics for, 416
 debridement and, 408

Incision
 burn injury effect on healing of, 303
 fracture effect on healing of, 303–4
 histologic appearance of, 300–301
 infection and, 182, 183
 scalpel design and, 370–71
 techniques for, 370–71, 373

Incisional hernia, 139–41, 158

India-Rubber-Man disease, 129

Infection, 171–283
 "acceptable" rates of, 173
 anticomplement and, 194–95
 aseptic technique and, 178–81
 burns and, 216–17, 251, 268–69, 561–63
 cancer and, 273–74
  chemotherapy and, 275
 causative organisms, 222–26, 237, 244–46
 cell-mediated immunity and, 256–58
 cellular response to, 254
 chemotherapy and, 274–75
 clinical manifestations of, 219–22
  abscess, 220–21
  blood and lymphatic, 221–22
  cellulitis, 220
  surgery-requiring, 222

Infection (cont.)
clostridial, 223–26, 249
collagen synthesis and, 110
contamination and, 174–81. See also
Contamination.
sources of, 174–77
dead space, 416–23
debridement and, 213–14, 405
decisive (early) period for, 192–96
delayed closure and, 214–16, 424
determinants of, 366–95
contaminants, 384–95
interactions of, 248–52
mechanisms of injury, 366–84
diabetes and, 276
drainage and, 220–21, 278, 442–43
dressings and, 443–45
electrosurgery and, 380
environment and, 176–77, 246–52
epinephrine and, 194, 195
established, 218–22
foreign bodies and, 89–91, 393–95
gastrointestinal anastomosis and, 581
gram-negative, 223, 263
gram-positive, 263
hernia recurrence and, 159–60
host resistance to, 181–212, 247–48,
252–76
abnormalities of, 258–59
identification of patient with defects
in, 259–66
supplementing weakened, 189–211,
276–83
understanding of, 189–200
humoral response to, 253–54
hypotension and, 185
hypoxia and, 86, 87–88
immunologic support and, 276–83
immunomodulating agents and,
282–83
immunosuppression and, 250, 274
incidence of, by wound classification,
236
intensive care unit and, 251–52
interactions of determinants of,
248–52
iron and, 342
laser surgery and, 384
monocytes and, 255–56
number of organisms required for,
182–83, 190–91
nutrition and, 187, 271–73, 279–82,
336–42
patient as source of, 175–76
perfusion and, 88–89
phagocytes and, 80

Infection (cont.)
physiologic maintenance and, 183–88,
276–78
circulation and, 184–86
congenital and acquired disease and,
187–88
nutrition and, 187, 271–73, 279–82
polymorphonuclear (PMN) activity
and, 254–55
preventive antibiotics and, 196–211,
232–35
prophylaxis protocols, 231–35, 238–41
puncture wounds and, 217–18
risk assessment, 211–12
scalpel usage and, 371, 374
sepsis and, 269–70
serum collections and, 134–35
shock and, 185, 270
skin test predictability of, 261–66
staphylococcal, 176, 190–91. See also
Staphylococcal infections.
sterilization and, 177–78
steroids and, 274–75
streptococcal, 220, 222–23
surgical team and, 174–75, 177
surgical technique and, 182–83, 371,
374
susceptibility to, 206
sutures and, 89–91, 183, 429–34
tape and, 91
tetanus, 223–25, 238–41
transplantation and, 250, 274
trauma and, 266–68
treatment of, 212–41
uremia and, 276
in vascular prosthesis, 493
vascular response to, 253
vitamin A and, 187, 340–41
vitamin B and, 187
vitamin C and, 187, 340
Infection-potentiating fractions, 395
Inflammation, 75–80, 252–58
aspirin and, 79–80
bone, 534, 546–47
burns and, 555
cell-mediated immunity and, 256–58
cellular response and, 254
early, as decisive period, 192–96
exaggerated, in exposed wounds, 413
humoral response and, 253–54
hypertrophic scars and, 115
macrophage's role in, 12
monocyte and, 255–56
polymorphonuclear cell and, 254–55
prolongation of repair and, 75–80
steroids and, 76–77, 79

Inflammation (cont.)
tendon, 502—4, 516
vascular response and, 253
vitamin A and, 77—79
Ingestion, phagocytic, 83
Injury. *See also* Trauma.
antibiotic indications for, 414—16
bullet, 375—77, 408
catabolic reaction to, 299, 306
character of, 73—74
collision, 375
impact, 371—75, 408, 416
massive, repair process and, 74
mechanisms of, 366—84
electrical energy, 377—83
mechanical energy, 367—77
radiant energy, 383—84
scalpel and, 367—71
traumatic compression and, 371—77
nerve, 463—64
response to, 6—8
Insulin, healing and, 108—10, 310—11, 339
Intensive care unit, infection and, 251—52
Intestines. *See also* Colon.
anastomosis of, 585
epithelium of, 46—47
fistula of, collagen balance and, 120
microbes of, 390—91
Intima, 477
prosthetic grafts and, 488, 489
stripping of, 478—82
venous, 483
Intramedullary fixation, 539—40
Iodine, antimicrobial activity of, 401—3
Iodophors, 400—405
Iron, 333
infection and, 342
vitamin C and, 317
Irrigation, 409—11
gastrointestinal anastomosis and, 580
Ischemia
adhesions and, 509, 588, 589
burns and, 553
in foot, 60
infection and, 86
tendon, 509, 511

Jaundice, healing and, 111
Joint, contracture of, 118. *See also* Contracture.

Kanamycin, 416
Keloids, 112—13
melanocyte-stimulating hormone and, 113

Keratin, 41
Kidney transplant, infections and, 250
Knitting, vascular grafts with, 487, 490
Kupffer cells, 256

Lacerations, tape closure of, 439
Lactate as collagen stimulator, 8
Langer's lines, 116
Laparotomy, repair of, in burned animals, 303
LaPlace's law, 492
Laser surgery, 383—84
Lateral trap, 512
Lathyrism, 29
Lathyrus ororatus, 105
Leakage, gastrointestinal anastomosis, 578—80
Leg ulcers, 146—48
Leukocytes, 11—13
arterial wall infiltration of, 479, 480
diabetes and, 109
nutrition and, 338—39
phagocytic. *See* Phagocytes.
polymorphonuclear, 11, 82, 253, 254—55
repair of wound and, 11—13
Lidocaine hydrochloride, 395—97
Linoleic acid, 310
Linolenic acid, 310
Lipoic acid, 320
Liver, protein metabolism and, 305—6
Lung, scar tissue of, 71
Lymphangitis, 219, 221—22
Lymphatics, regeneration of, 16
Lymphocytes
B, 255
T, 255, 256—57
testing of, 263
Lymphokines, 257
Lysine, 21, 26
hydroxylation, inhibitors of, 103—4
vitamin C and, 315, 317
Lysosomes, 83, 255
Lysozyme, 83
Lysyl hydroxylase, 105, 317—18
Lysyl oxidase, 29, 105

Macrophages, 254, 255—56
activation factor, 257
alveolar, 256
arterial healing and, 480
cellular interactions and, 55—57
collagen and, 31
as director cells, 11—12
hypertrophic scars and, 563, 567
repair of wounds and, 8—9, 11—13

Macrophages (cont.)
  vitamin A and, 12
  wandering (resident), 255−56
Magnesium, 330−31
Malnutrition, 279−82
  immunologic abnormalities and,
    271−73, 279−82
  infection and, 187
  protein-calorie, 280, 309, 338
  therapy for, 344−54
Mandril grafts, 493, 495
Manganese, 335
Marfan's syndrome, 128
Marjolin's ulcer, 141
Mason suture technique, 512
Mast cells, nerve injury and, 463
Matrix, 527−28
Mechanical cleansing, 408−13
Mechanisms of injury, 366−84
  electrical energy, 377−83
  mechanical energy, 367−77
  radiant energy, 383−84
  scalpel and, 367−71
  traumatic compression and, 371−77
Media, vascular, 477
Median nerve, 473
Melanocyte-stimulating hormone,
    keloids and, 113
Mesh, plastic, for incisional hernia
    closure, 141
Metabolic rate, 346−47
Metabolism
  anaerobic, 8, 61
  infection and, 337
  starvation and, 306
  temperature and, 351−52
  traumatic derangements of, 288−99
Methicillin, prophylactic, 232
3-Methyl-histidine, protein breakdown
    and, 307
Methysergide, 122, 123
Microflora, 387−93
  digestive, 389−91
  mucosal, 388−93
  respiratory, 388−89
  skin, 387−88
  urogenital, 391−92
Migration inhibition factor, 257
Minerals, 330−36
  macrominerals, 330−31
  parenteral preparations for, 351
  in soil, 393−94
  trace, 331−36
Missile injury, 375−77, 408
Mobilization
  fracture healing and, 543−44

Mobilization (cont.)
  tendon repair and, 515−16, 518−19
Module, wound repair, 8−21, 53−61
Molybdenum, 335
Mouth, bacteria of, 389−90
Mucopolysaccharides, 39−41
Mucopolysaccharidoses, 130
Mucosa
  gastrointestinal, 47, 388−89, 571−72,
    575, 579
  microflora of, 388−93
  respiratory tract, 388−89
  urogenital, 48, 391−92
Muscle, debridement of, 405−6
Myelin sheath, 460, 461, 464
  regeneration of, 465
Myeloperoxidase, 83, 84
Myofibroblasts, 17
  contraction of, 50, 51, 117
Myointima, 480, 481
  arteriovenous anastomosis and, 483
Myositis, clostridial, 225−26

Nafcillin, prophylactic, 234
Neck, contracture from burn of,
    160−61
Necrosis, burn, 546, 552−56
Neoendothelization, vascular, 477, 480,
    481, 485
Neomycin, 587
Neovascularization, 7, 13−16
  burns and, 554
  cellular interactions and, 59−60
  inhibitors of, 91
Nerves, peripheral, 459−74
  anatomy of, 459−61
  blood supply of, 462, 463
  conduction testing of, 471
  function of, 461−62
  grafts of, 470
  healing of, 459−63
  injury of, 463−64
  median, 473
  monitoring of recovery of, 470
  pattern of recovery of, 473−74
  regeneration of, 465−66
  repair techniques for, 466−74
  suturing of, 437, 467−68
  tendon repair and, 519
  tension on, 469−70
Neurolysis, 471
Neuroma, 471
  pain from, 133
Neuropathy, diabetic, 108
Neutropenia, 255
  cancer chemotherapy and, 275

606

Sebaceous follicles, 388
Secondary intention, healing by, 9n, 29
Selenium, 336
Separation of wound, 135. *See also*
    Dehiscence.
Sepsis
    acquired defensive defects and, 259–60
    definition of, 244n, 261
    gram-negative, 223
    host defense defects and, 269–70
    skin testing for prediction of, 261–66,
        269
Septicemia, 219
Serosa, gastrointestinal, 572, 576
Serotonin, carcinoid syndrome and, 122
Serum collections in wounds, 134–35
Sex hormones, 52, 91, 124
Shaving, preoperative, 397–98
Shear, 367
Shock
    infection and, 185, 270
    repair delay and, 74
Shrapnel wounds, 292–95
Silicone-coated sutures, 433, 434
Silk sutures, 434
    for vascular anastomoses, 492
Silver nitrate, 561
Silver sulfadiazine, 561
Sinus, suture, 139
Skin
    disinfecting property of, 388
    grafts, 146–47
        burns and, 297, 557, 559, 562–63
        contraction and, 51
        for hypertrophic scars, 116
        neovascularization and, 13–16
        nonhealing wounds and, 146–47
    microflora of, 387–88
    preparation of, preoperative, 175,
        401–4
    testing
        hemorrhage and, 271
        sepsis prediction and, 261–66, 269
        trauma and, 266–68
Small bowel. *See also* Intestines.
    anastomosis, 585
    microbes of, 390–91
Soil, contamination from, 393–95
Solutions
    irrigating, 410
    parenteral, 350
    scrub, 400, 404
Specific gravity, projectile injury and, 377
Sponges, scrubbing with, 411–13
Staphylococcal infections
    abscesses, 221

Staphylococcal infections (cont.)
    antibiotics for, 203–5
    dead space, 417
    delayed closure and, 424
    enhancement of, 195, 196
    epidermidis, 263, 442
    interaction schema for, 248
    number of organisms for, 190–91
    penicillin-resistant, 415
    sources of, 176
Staples, closure with, 427
    gastrointestinal anastomosis and, 576
Starch powder, adhesions and, 142–43
Starvation
    collagen synthesis-lysis balance and,
        120–21
    infection and, 187
    metabolic rate and, 306
Steam sterilization, 177–78
Steel sutures, 434
Stem cells, radiation effects on, 93
Stents, respiratory scarring and, 46
Sterile technique, 178–81
Sterilization of equipment, 177–79
Steroids
    anabolic, 77, 79
    diabetes and, 110
    esophageal dilatation and, 162
    infection and, 274–75
    for nonhealing wounds, 147
    repair of wounds and, 52, 76–77, 79
    tendon healing stopped by, 517
    vitamin A and, 77–79
Stomach, 585
    epithelium of, 47
    microbes of, 390
Stones, soil, 393–94
Strength of wound, 34–35. *See also*
        Dehiscence.
Streptococcal infections, hemolytic
    cellulitis, 220
    treatment of, 222–23
Streptokinase, 589
Stress, mechanical, repair and, 37–38
    dehiscence and, 135
Stricture, 118
Subcutaneous tissue, defensive weakness
        of, 88
Suction, drainage and, 442
Sump drains, 580
Superoxide, phagocytes and, 84, 86
Surfactants, 400–401, 403
Surgical intensive care unit (SICU),
        infection and, 251–52
Surgical team, bacterial contamination
        by, 174–75, 177

609

Surgical technique, meticulous, 182—83
Sutures, 427—38
  absorbable, 429, 431, 583—84
  Allen technique for, 512
  biliary tract, 436
  biochemical properties of, 434—36
  catgut, 583, 584
  choice of material for, 90
  configuration of, 429, 431—32
  cotton, 434
  Dacron, 432—34
  dead space closure with, 417—23
  degradation of, 429, 431
  dehiscence and, 135—36
  epineurial, 468, 469
  fascial, 436
  Gambee method for, 576, 577
  gastrointestinal tract, 436—37, 576,
    583—84
  infection and, 89—91, 183, 429—34
  lateral trap, 512
  Mason technique for, 512
  monofilament, 429, 431, 432, 436, 437,
    438
  nerve repair, 437, 467—68
  nonabsorbable, 429, 431
  nylon, 431
  perineurial, 468—69
  PGA, 431
  phagocytes and, 89—91
  polyglactin, 583—84
  polyglycolic, 583—84
  polypropylene, 431, 492—93
  scarring and, 44
  silicone coating for, 433, 434
  silk, 434, 492
  sinus tracts from, 139
  stainless steel, 434
  staple, 427, 576
  tape closure vs., 439
  technique for, 429—30
  Teflon coating for, 433, 434
  tendon repair, 437—38, 511—12, 518
  urinary tract, 436
  vascular, 437
    anastomotic aneurysm and, 492—93
    artery-to-artery anastomosis, 485,
      486
  wire, 137
Synovial fluid, 507
Syringe, irrigating, 409—11

T cells, 255, 256—57
Talc, adhesions and, 142—43
Tape closure, 438—40
  burns and, 561

Tape closure (cont.)
  infection and, 91
Technical factors, 395—447
  anesthesia, local, 395—97
  antibiotics, 413—16
  antisepsis, 398—405
  closure, 423—40
  dead space, 416—23
  debridement, 405—8
  drainage, 440—43
  dressing, 443—45
  hair removal, 397—98
  immobilization, 446
  mechanical cleansing, 408—13
Teeth, microflora of, 389
Teflon
  donor site dressing with, 563
  sutures coated with, 433, 434
  vascular grafts with, 487, 494, 495
Temperature, metabolism and, 351—52
Tendolysis, 520
Tendons, 500—522
  adhesions of, 509—10, 516
  antiinflammatory agents and, 516, 519
  blood supply of, 507—14
  epitenon growth of, 505
  fibrovascular tissue surrounding, 503
  freeing of, 520
  gliding of, 515—16
  healing of, 500—518
    collagen organization and
      remodeling, 514—17
    intrinsic, 504—7
    sequence in, 502—4
  inflammation of, 502—4, 516
  ischemia of, 509, 511
  management of injuries of, 518—20
  mobilization and repair of, 515—16,
    518—19
  nerve damage and, 519
  sutures for, 437—38, 511—12, 518
  tension on, 513, 514—16
Tensile strength of wound, 34—35
Tensile stress, 371—77
Tension
  bone healing and, 530
  hypertrophic scars and, 114
  keloids and, 113
  on tendons, 513, 514—16
Testosterone, 312
Tetanus, 223—25
  equine antitoxin precautions, 241n
  immune globulin for, 225, 239
  immunization for, 224, 238—39
  prophylactic guide for, 238—41
  toxoid, 224, 238n, 239—41

612